Applying Continuous Quality Improvement in Clinical Practice

Second Edition

Billie Axley, MS, RN, CNN
Karen C. Robbins, MS, RN, CNN
Editors

ANNA

American Nephrology Nurses' Association
www.annanurse.org

Editors
Billie Axley, MS, RN, CNN
Director, Quality Initiatives
Fresenius Medical Center, Inc.
Brentwood, TN

Karen C. Robbins, MS, RN, CNN
Nurse Educator
Dialysis and Transplant Programs
Hartford Hospital
Hartford, CT

Associate Editor
Nephrology Nursing Journal
American Nephrology Nurses' Association
Pitman, NJ

Publication Management
Anthony J. Jannetti, Inc.
East Holly Avenue/Box 56
Pitman, NJ 08071-0056

Managing Editor: Carol M. Ford
Editorial Coordinator: Jamie Kalitz
Copy Editors: Linda Alexander and Katie Brownlow
Creative Design and Production: Jack M. Bryant, Melody Edwards, Bob Taylor and Darin Peters

American Nephrology Nurses' Association, East Holly Avenue/Box 56, Pitman, New Jersey 08071-0056
Web site: www.annanurse.org
Email: anna@ajj.com
Phone: 888-600-2662

Contents

Section 1: Overview of CQI Principles and Tools

Section 2: Clinical Applications

Contents

Section 3: Nephrology Community

This offering for 28.5 contact hours is being provided by the American Nephrology Nurses' Association (ANNA).

ANNA is accredited as a provider of continuing nursing education (CNE) by the American Nurses Credentialing Center's Commission on Accreditation.

ANNA is a provider approved by the California Board of Registered Nursing, provider number CEP 00910.

This CNE activity meets the Nephrology Nursing Certification Commission's (NNCC's) continuing nursing education requirements for certification and recertification.

Authors

Billie Axley, MS, RN, CNN
Director, Quality Initiatives
Fresenius Medical Center, Inc.
Brentwood, TN
Editor, and Chapters 4, 10, 12, 13, 14, and 21

Barbara Cortes, RN
Regional Quality Manager
Fresenius Medical Care North America
South Plainfield, NJ
Chapter 18

Helen Currier, BSN, RN, CNN
Assistant Director, Renal and Pharesis
Texas Children's Hospital
Houston, TX
Chapter 15

Linda Dickenson, BSN, RN, CNN, CQHP
Director of Education, Risk Management and Quality Assessment
Reliant Renal Care, Inc.
Altha, FL
Chapter 12

Lesley C. Dinwiddie, MSN, RN, FNP, CNN
Executive Director
Institute for Clinical Excellence, Education, and Research (ICEER)
Wheaton, IL
Chapter 8

Mary Fenderson, MSHSA, RN, CNN
Nephrology Nurse
FMQAI: The Florida ESRD Network
Tampa, FL
Chapter 20

Bonnie Greenspan, BSN, RN, MBA
Consultant, BBG Consulting, LLC
Member, CMS ESRD Transition Team
Alexandria, VA
Chapter 19

Debra Hain, DNS, ARNP, GNP-BC
Assistant Professor
Christine E. Lynn College of Nursing
Florida Atlantic University
Boca Raton, FL
Chapter 17

Raymond Hakim, MD, PhD
Senior Executive Vice President
Fresenius Medical Center, Inc.
Brentwood, TN
Chapter 21

Diana Hlebovy, BSN, RN, CHN, CNN
Director of Clinical Affairs
Hema Metrics
Kayseville, UT
Chapter 9

Judy Kauffman, BSN, RN, CNN
RN Administrative Coordinator
University of Virginia Health System
Charlottesville, VA
Chapter 13

Deuzimar Kulawik, MSN, RN
Quality Improvement Coordinator
FMQAI: The Florida ESRD Network
Tampa, FL
Chapter 20

Veronica Legg, MS, RN, FNP-BC
Director, Clinical Studies Department
Fresenius Medical Care North America
Battle Ground, WA
Chapter 22

Patricia McCarley, MSN, RN, ACPN, CNN
Nurse Practitioner
Diablo Nephrology Medical Group
Walnut Creek, CA
Chapter 16

Deborah H. Miller, MSN, RN, CNS, CNN
Clinical Nurse Specialist, Pediatric Nephrology
Inova Fairfax Hospital for Children
Falls Church, VA
Chapter 15

Jackie Miller, BS, RN, CNN, CPHQ
Six Sigma Black Belt
Vice President Quality, CBU
Fresenius Medical Care North America
Fort Wayne, IN
Chapter 4

Sylvia Moe, BSN, RN, CNN
Dialysis Home Training Coordinator
Mayo Clinic
Rochester, MN
Chapter 10

Linda Myers, BSN, RN, CNN, HP(ASCP)
Clinician III
Acute Care Renal/Apheresis Services
University of Virginia Health System
Charlottesville, VA
Chapter 13

Leonor P. Ponferrada, BSN, RN, CNN
Quality Management Coordinator
Dialysis Clinic, Inc.
Columbia, MO
Chapter 3

Regina M. Rohe, BS, RN, HP(ASCP)
Regional Vice President, Inpatient Services
Fresenius Medical Care North America
Mill Valley, CA
Chapter 13

Maggie Tatarek, RN, CNN
Clinical Quality Manager
Fresenius Medical Care North America
Latrobe, PA
Chapter 7

MaryKay Shepherd, RD
Dietitian
Fresenius Medical Care North America
Warsaw, IN
Chapter 6

Joan Camarro Simard, MS, RN, CNN
Information System Coordinator
Intermountain Healthcare Dialysis Centers
Salt Lake City, UT
Chapter 2

Tana Waack, BSN, RN
Area Manager
Fresenius Medical Center
Nashville, TN
Chapter 14

Pat Weiskittel, MSN, RN, CNN, ACNP,BC
Renal Hypertension Nurse Practitioner
Cincinnati VA Medical Center
Cincinnati, OH
Chapter 11

Gail Wick, MHSA, BSN, RN, CNN
Consultant
Atlanta, GA
Foreward, Chapters 1 and 5

Angeline F. Wieler, MSN, RN, CNN
Quality Improvement Coordinator
ESRD Network of Texas, Inc.
Dallas, TX
Chapter 20

Helen F. Williams, MSN, RN, CNN
Staff Nurse Acute Dialysis
Western Nephrology
Denver, CO
Chapter 14

Rebecca Wingard, MSN, RN, CNN
Vice President, Quality Initiatives
Fresenius Medical Care North America
Brentwood, TN
Chapter 6

Reviewers

Kim Alleman, MS, APRN, FNP-BC, CNN-NP
Nurse Practitioner
Hartford Hospital Transplant Program
Hartford, CT

Lynda K. Ball, MSN, BS, RN, CNN
Quality Improvement Director
Northwest Renal Network
Seattle, WA

Jeannette P. Berdowski, MSPH, RN, CNN
Regional Director of Education – New Jersey
Fresenius Medical Care North America
Kenvil, NJ

Jane K. Gardner, DNP, RN
Consultant
Jane K. Gardner, Inc.
Chicago, IL

Marriane Heffernan
Fresenius Medical Care
Corp. Director, Home Therapies
Waltham, MA

Maryann Lyon, BSN, RN, CNN
Speakers' Bureau, Amgen
Legal Nurse Consultant
Sidney, OH

Kathryn A. McDougall, MS, RN, CDE
Director, Quality Initiatives
Fresenius Medical Care North America
Greenbriar, TN

Glenda M. Payne, MS, RN, CNN
ESRD Technical Lead
Centers for Medicare and Medicaid Services
Dallas, TX

Regina M. Rohe, BS, RN, HP(ASCP)
Regional Vice President, Inpatient Services
Fresenius Medical Care North America
Mill Valley, CA

Suzann VanBuskirk, BSN, RN, CNN
Independent Consultant
VanBuskirk Consulting, LLC
Elkton, MD

Helen F. Williams, MSN, BSN, RN, CNN
Staff Nurse Acute Dialysis
Western Nephrology
Denver, CO

Statements of Disclosure

Lesley C. Dinwiddie, MSN, RN, FNP, CNN, disclosed that she is a Consultant and Advisor.

Debra Hain, DNS, ARNP, GNP-BC, disclosed that she is on the Consultant Presenter's Bureau for Amgen.

Diana Hlebovy, BSN, RN, CHN, CNN, disclosed that she is an educator for Hema Metrics.

Maryann Lyon, BSN, RN, CNN, disclosed that she is on the Consultant Presenter's Bureau for Amgen.

Patricia McCarley, MSN, RN, ACPN, CNN, disclosed that she is on the Consultant Presenter's Bureau for Amgen and Genzyme.

Karen C. Robbins, MS, RN, CNN, disclosed that she is on the Consultant Presenter's Bureau for Watson Pharma, Inc.

Suzann VanBuskirk, BSN, RN, CNN, disclosed that she is on the Consultant Presenter's Bureau for Watson Pharma, Inc.

Gail Wick, MHSA, BSN, RN, CNN, disclosed that she is on the Consultant Presenter's Bureau for Watson Pharma, inc., and Abbott Pharmaceuticals.

All other authors, reviewers, and editors reported no actual or potential conflict of interest in relation to this continuing nursing education publication.

Foreward

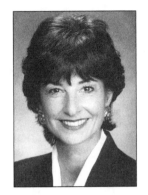

Improving performance and outcomes has always been a focus in the provision of health care, but they really came to the forefront in the 1990s as healthcare organizations developed new, formal approaches to quality assurance and improvement. The stimuli for this arose from increased expectations and standards of consumers and payers, and rising healthcare costs and deceasing resources, particularly manpower. Energy and resources were put into play in all arenas of health care as new structures and processes were designed to direct quality improvement and maintenance efforts. Recognizing the needs of our patients, nephrology-related organizations began a pursuit of improvement in all services provided to patients with renal impairment. The goal was to maximize the benefits of health care. Fortunately, there was a philosophy, structure, and process available that helped providers of services and products to become more quality-focused. This concept was continuous quality improvement (CQI).

As part of its mission to advance nephrology nursing practice and positively influence outcomes, and in response to the need for nephrology-specific CQI, ANNA published *Continuous Quality Improvement: From Concept to Reality* in 1995. In addition to ANNA's other resources, it paved the way to better practice as well as to the trending and documentation of the outcomes of quality efforts. With this 2nd edition, *Applying Continuous Quality Improvement in Clinical Practice*, ANNA continues its commitment to timely and relevant publications to help practitioners in their quest for excellence. A practical overview of CQI, case studies, and tools to use in the majority of practice areas within our specialty are contained within this book. In addition to being designed to guide practitioners in their quest for excellence, the contents of the 2nd edition are also geared toward satisfying mandates of oversight organizations, such as The Joint Commission and the Centers for Medicare and Medicaid Services (CMS). It is important to note that quality and formal programs ensuring quality outcomes are not optional in today's healthcare world; they are mandated. Therefore, implementing successful quality initiatives is not only the right thing to do, it is necessary to satisfy society's and government's mandate to provide the best services possible in the most economical manner.

While some case studies may not directly relate to one's area of practice, all will stimulate thinking and provide examples of structures and processes that can be used to address the various quality challenges nurses and healthcare professionals face. As you read each section, the questions to answer are, "How does this relate to my practice?" and "How can I adopt or adapt the content to suit the quality challenges my practice setting faces?" While this publication focuses on clinical quality initiatives, the concepts and principles can be applied to anything that needs improving, including technical, financial, and/or personnel issues.

Sound structures and processes aside, quality improvement and maintenance will not occur without commitment and perseverance on the parts of both the practitioner and organization. Nor will they occur overnight. Quality improvement is indeed continuous and ongoing. Fortunately, nurses are known for perseverance as well as for providing leadership within the interdisciplinary team. Your commitment to quality and passion for excellence when combined with the use of this manual's content can ensure that quality improvement can and will occur. Those we serve will benefit, but so will we, as we reap the satisfaction of continuously improving our professional practice as well as its outcomes.

Gail Wick, MHSA, BSN, RN, CNN
Co-Editor, **Continuous Quality Improvement: From Concept to Reality**
First Edition © 1995

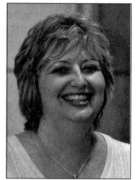

A prominent focus in health care has been the continuous challenge to provide quality care with limited resources. The first edition of ANNA's *Continuous Quality Improvement: From Concept to Reality* was published in 1995. This publication set the groundwork for nephrology nurses to develop a thorough understanding of the concepts and principles needed to implement a continuous quality improvement (CQI) plan in their work environment. The first edition gave us a solid foundation with useful tools to establish a plan to improve healthcare outcomes.

This second edition, *Applying Continuous Quality Improvement in Clinical Practice*, focuses on nephrology-specific clinical applications of continuous quality improvement. This edition addresses the application of CQI concepts in a wide range of clinical settings. It serves as a vital resource to all members of the nephrology community who seek quality outcomes in a challenging healthcare environment.

The ANNA Board of Directors join me as I commend Editors Billie Axley, MS, RN, CNN, and Karen C. Robbins, MS, RN, CNN, and all of the expert chapter authors and reviewers who contributed to the creation of this valuable publication. We appreciate their expertise and talent they have shared with all of us.

Enjoy this book and use it as a resource to promote and enhance quality outcomes as you care for patients with kidney disease. Both you and your patients will benefit from the knowledge you will gain from this valuable publication.

Sue Cary, MN, APRN, NP, CNN
ANNA President, 2008-2009

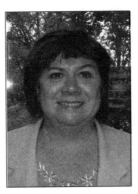

Research findings show what we, as nephrology nurses, have understood for many years: the contributions of nursing to patients' care have a significant effect on improving outcomes. Nurses' unique knowledge of what is involved in the care provided to patients places us in a position as being essential to the success of improving care processes. Nurses using continuous quality improvement (CQI) and participating in interdisciplinary improvement teams have the opportunity to share their knowledge to improve patient care. We ultimately have the ability to have an impact not only on the care processes, but also on the care delivery systems themselves. Our fundamental objective is for our patients' safety and improved outcomes.

My goal in serving as an editor for this manual has been to produce a resource in which all nephrology nurses will find information they can apply to patient care and realize the value of the application of CQI in their daily work. While many chapters contain an overview of their content, please listen to the authors' more extensive discussions as they share expertise from their experiences using CQI to improve their outcomes.

My sincere gratitude goes to those whose contributions resulted in the journey upon which the reader is about to embark in this manual of continuously looking for opportunities to improve, thereby benefiting all patients.

Billie Axley, MS, RN, CNN
Editor

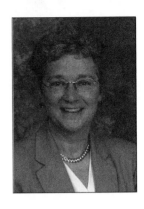

Fourteen years have passed since ANNA published *Continuous Quality Improvement: From Concept to Reality* under the talented nurses and editors, Gail Wick and Eileen Peacock. Much has changed in our world at large since then – health care in general and nephrology nursing in particular. Despite these changes, the aspiration to provide excellence in patient care with optimal outcomes remains an omnipresent objective.

The Centers for Medicare and Medicaid Services (CMS) published the *Conditions for Coverage* for transplantation in 2007 and for end stage renal disease facilities in 2008 (CMS, 2007, 2008). These regulations reflect people's expectations for quality care. There is an emphatic focus in these documents/regulations that quality is no longer optional, it is a mandate. Our patients deserve no less, and these regulations provide a structure by which we can approach and achieve this.

CQI initiatives provide a framework for objectively and critically examining outcomes and the processes involved. We believe this publication offers the background, information, and tools to get you started or to enhance your current practices. The contributors to this book are clinical experts and experts in the process of CQI. Please take advantage of all they have shared within these pages.

ANNA is the professional, organizational voice for nephrology nursing, and as such, is obligated to meet the needs of its membership. We, the editors, applaud the ANNA Board of Directors for their vision and decision to dedicate resources to this initiative at this time. I believe the publication of this robust resource will provide the needed resources for nephrology healthcare professionals to meet the challenge in providing quality care with the opportunity to continuously improve patient outcomes.

Karen C. Robbins, MS, RN, CNN
Editor

References

Centers for Medicare and Medicaid Services (CMS). (2007). *Conditions for coverage and conditions of participation for transplant.* Retrieved March 29, 2009, from http://www.cms.hhs.gov/Certificationand Complianc/20_Transplant.asp#TopOfPage

Centers for Medicare and Medicaid Services (CMS). (2008). *Conditions for coverage and conditions of participations for end stage renal disease facilities.* Retrieved March 29, 2009, from http://www.cms.hhs.gov/CFCsAndCoPs/13_ESRD.asp

This manual is dedicated to nephrology nurses everywhere.

Section 1:
Overview of CQI Principles and Tools

Concepts and Principles of Quality Management

Gail Wick, MHSA, BSN, RN, CNN

Objectives

Study of the information presented in this chapter will enable the learner to:
1. Define quality.
2. Discuss the basic principles and concepts of continuous quality improvement.
3. Describe a tested continuous quality improvement model for use in the nephrology setting.

Overview

The basics of quality management with a focus on continuous quality improvement (CQI) will be highlighted in this chapter. Quality, total quality management, and CQI will be defined, and an easy-to-implement CQI model will be presented.

Figure 1-1
Quality Management Diagram

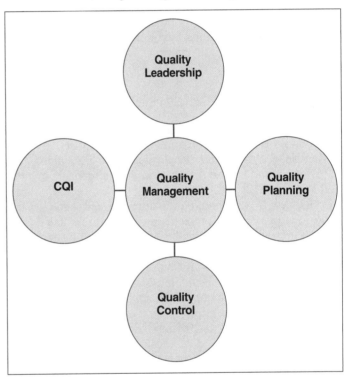

Source: Used with permission from Gail Wick.

Introduction

When faced with the need to do and document quality improvement activities on a formal basis in busy work settings, it is tempting for practitioners to say, "Why bother? We are far too busy taking care of patients to do more 'busy work!'"

Continuous quality improvement (CQI), if done correctly and with input from an interdisciplinary team, is not busy work. Nor is it optional when it comes to people's health and welfare. Striving to continually improve patient outcomes is mandatory, and ultimately, when CQI is practiced daily by the entire team, it saves time, since problems and suboptimal outcomes are reduced or eliminated.

Formal CQI does not need to be overwhelming, time consuming, or focused on paperwork. A simple process that can be implemented in any setting will be outlined in this chapter. Furthermore, while the principles of CQI apply to most structures and processes in any given setting, the application of CQI in this chapter will focus primarily on patient care and clinical outcomes.

What Is Continuous Quality Improvement?

CQI is a component of a broader concept called quality management (see Figure 1-1). Quality management encompasses all activities related to improving the quality of products or services as well as customer satisfaction with those products or services. The four components of quality management are *quality leadership, quality planning, quality control* and *quality improvement* (Hradesky, 1995).

Quality leadership provides the opportunity and guides the effort. Simply stated, quality leadership makes sure that quality improvement is pursued and provides the resources needed.

Quality planning involves 1) developing a plan for incorporating quality improvement efforts into everyday practice or activities, 2) identifying short-term and long-term quality needs, and 3) ensuring that resources, including knowledge, are available for CQI activities. An example of quality planning is establishing quality goals and projects for the year.

Quality control involves monitoring actual performance to see if expectations are being met. Data collection and analysis of the key indicators of quality are central to effective quality control. Monitoring and reporting water quality and clinical performance measures are two examples specific to the dialysis setting.

CQI, called quality assessment and performance improvement (QAPI) by some, is generally to describe, in the aggregate, the ongoing monitoring, evaluation and improvement of processes (Joint Commission on Accreditation of Healthcare Organization [JCAHO], 1992). Said another way, it is a formal process that 1) identifies improvement needs; 2) determines the causes of problems, needs, or gaps; 3) develops

> ## CQI monitors, evaluates, and improves the way we do things in order to optimize outcomes.

solutions; 4) implements those solutions; and 5) determines if the solutions work. There are many CQI methods or models to guide the process, but the one that is used in this chapter is an adaptation of the Shewhart Plan-Do-Check-Act (PDCA) Model promoted by W. Edwards Deming (Walton, 1986). The model will be discussed later in this chapter.

There are a number of formal definitions of quality improvement:

- A mind set, commitment, and process used in business in which teams continually improve all processes throughout the organization, with the intent of meeting and exceeding expectations, whether internal or external (Schroeder, 1994).
- A set of principles, policies, support structures, and practices designed to continually improve the efficiency and effectiveness of what is valued.
- Intelligent, focused teams making sound decisions about important issues in an organized, timely manner.
- Knowledgeable, caring people doing the right thing, the first time, and for the right reason in an organized manner (Hunt, 1992).

However it is defined, quality improvement identifies and solves real or potential problems. Problems are either 1) off-target (such as hemoglobins below an established target or parathyroid hormone [PTH] greater than an established upper limit target) or 2) unwanted (such as patients being hospitalized for preventable conditions). Another way of looking at problems is to say there is a gap between what is desired and what currently exists. For example, if the unit currently has 30% of its patients with a TSA < 20%, and the goal is 10%, that is a problem or a gap. When outcomes or situations are off-target or unwanted, or a gap exists, a quality improvement project to narrow the gap or resolve the problem is indicated.

What is Quality?

Quality means different things to different people, depending on their focus, values, and responsibilities. From a healthcare perspective, in the classic publication, *Medicare: A Strategy for Quality Assurance,* Lohr (1990) defines quality as "the degree to which health services for individuals and populations increase the likelihood of desired health outcomes and are consistent with current professional knowledge" (p. 4).

In *Quality in America*, Hunt (1992) discusses quality in two contexts: quality in perception and quality in fact. Examples of quality in perception include:

- Delivering the right service(s).
- Identifying and satisfying customers' needs.
- Meeting customers' expectations.
- Treating all customers with integrity, courtesy, and respect.

Hunt (1992) continues to define "quality in fact" as doing the right thing, doing it the right way, doing it right the first

Table 1-1
Improvements in the Nephrology Setting to Explore

Access function and type	Nutrition
Adequacy of dialysis	Patient adherence
Adverse occurrences	Patient knowledge and involvement
Anemia and iron management	Patient employment
Bone and mineral disorders	PD complications
Diabetes control and complications	Quality of life
Exercise	Re-use of dialyzers
Falls and patient safety	Rehabilitation
Family abuse	Regulatory compliance
Hospitalizations	Social functioning and support
Hyperlipidemia	Sodium/fluid/BP control
Machine maintenance	Staff attrition or job dissatisfaction
Missed treatments	Transplantation
Mortality	Water treatment

Source: Used with permission from Gail Wick.

time, and doing it on time. From the perspective of nephrology, examples of doing the right thing include:

- Using aseptic technique for catheter, fistula, and graft care.
- Providing adequate dialysis – correct dialyzer, full treatment time, full blood flow rate.
- Preventing or at least minimizing complications of dialysis, such as hypotension.
- Correcting the anemia of chronic kidney disease.
- Striving to improve patient compliance with the treatment regimen, whether it is transplantation, hemodialysis, or peritoneal dialysis.
- Collecting all billable charges.
- Being in regulatory compliance at all times.

Examples of doing it the right way include:

- Following accepted standards and practice guidelines.
- Using products, supplies, and devices correctly.
- Using aseptic technique consistently.
- Removing fluid without hypotension.
- Capture and collection of all billable charges in a timely fashion.

Doing it right the first time might include:

- Having practices and processes in place that prevent complications.
- Using needle insertion techniques that ensure consistent, adequate blood flow and no infection.
- Consistently administering the appropriate dose of erythropoietic stimulating agent (ESA) and iron.

Figure 1-2
Check – Plan – Do – Check – Act (CPDCA) Model

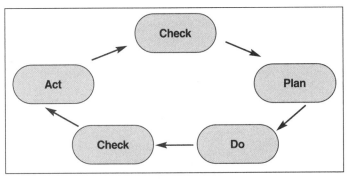

Source: Used with permission from Gail Wick.

- Preparing claims so that they are accepted and processed the first time.
- Using the structures, processes, and practices in place consistently so that survey is passed without deficiencies.

Doing it on time includes:
- Training patients for home therapy in an acceptable number of days.
- Monthly clinic visits for patients on home therapy.
- Safety and vital sign checks per policy.
- Obtaining target weight each dialysis.
- Billing cycle of 30 to 45 days.
- Comprehensive patient assessments by the interdisciplinary team within the first 30 days of treatment or the first 13 treatments.

What Is Needed for CQI to Be Effective?

For quality efforts to be successful, regardless of setting, a number of factors must be present (Hunt, 1992; Schroeder, 1994). They are:
- Leaders committed to quality and a formal CQI/QAPI process.
- Knowledgeable and dedicated employees committed to real time (daily) quality improvement.
- Accessible information, including data to help identify/prioritize projects and needs, upon which to base decisions and actions.
- Benchmarks.
- Easy-to-use tools for decision-making and documentation.
- Interdisciplinary team involvement in and accountability for quality outcomes.
- Ability to see the "big picture" of caring for a patient with kidney dysfunction, not just one specific treatment.
- Standards, guidelines, and evidence to guide practice and decisions.
- A formal CQI/QAPI structure and process used by all disciplines.

Potential Problems or Issues in the Nephrology Setting to Explore for Improvement

Processes and outcomes conducive to quality improvement fall into the broad categories of clinical, administrative, financial, technical, and regulatory. Improvements to explore are listed in Table 1-1.

Identifying Improvement Needs

If sound information and data collection and trending tools are in place, improvement needs can be easily identified and prioritized. Benchmarking or comparing one's self to others is frequently used in the nephrology setting for clinical issues. Examples of this include clinical performance measures, and the National Quality Forum (NQF) endorsed quality measures and internal corporate standards. Additionally, quality improvement teams often study the use of time as well as conduct surveys to identify customer needs and concerns. For example, do adverse occurrences, such as vascular access clotting, frequently occur? Is the facility being cited for regulatory issues? Do anemia and bone/mineral outcomes compare favorably to state and national benchmarks? Once identified, the top three or four problems or issues can be prioritized using the following criteria: 1) high risk, 2) high volume, 3) problem prone, and/or 4) high costs. While it is not practical to address all improvement needs at once, current projects and their status should be easily identifiable, and timelines should be set for future projects.

Basic Components of a CQI Program

Basic components of a CQI program include:
- Quality indicators based on internal and external expectations.
- Processes – clinical, managerial, or systems-oriented – to achieve outcomes.
- Data collection calendar.
- Trending tool, typically with 3 to 6 months of data.
- CQI model.
- Quality improvement meeting agenda.
- Meeting minutes that document analyses, discussions, actions, and results.
- Action plans focused on addressing the specific causes of problems or issues.

CQI Models

CQI methods or models simply provide a consistent set of steps to use in all improvement processes and projects. Documentation of quality projects and initiatives should follow the model or process used by the facility. While there are numerous CQI models available for use, such as the Shewhart PDCA cycle, FOCUS-PDCA, FADE, and IMPROVE models (JCAHO, 1992), the CPDCA model will be used in this chapter to explain the steps in CQI.

The CPDCA Model

The Check-Plan-Do-Check-Act (CPDCA) model (see Figure 1-2) is a modification of the Shewhart PDCA cycle developed by Walter Shewhart. Shewhart pioneered the application of statistical methods for controlling quality in manufacturing (Walton, 1986). His cycle has been modified to include the first check to emphasize the ongoing need to collect, trend, and analyze information. This cycle, as with any established CQI model, provides a structured and organized approach to evaluate how we are doing, what needs to be improved, how to improve, and if we succeeded.

Steps in the CPDCA Model

Check

1. Collect, trend, and analyze information on a consistent basis to monitor internally and externally established quality indicators. Information includes observations and patient symptoms/circumstances, as well as laboratory data.
2. Discuss the information at each monthly quality improvement meeting using a pre-established calendar. High-risk, problem-prone issues, such as those affecting patient health and safety, may need to be addressed on an accelerated basis.
3. Identify and prioritize projects using the "high-risk, high-volume, problem-prone, and/or has a negative effect on the mission of the facility and company" criteria. (JCAHO, 1994, p. 12).
4. Issues that cross all categories should receive top priority.

Plan

1. Select a quality improvement project team. Members should be knowledgeable of the process being studied as well as committed to a formal CQI process.
2. Analyze each process by using tools, such as cause and effect (fishbone) diagrams, flow charts, pareto charts, run charts, brainstorming, and the literature. Use observation, interviews, and audits to collect additional information on the possible causes or factors in the outcome. For efficiency, use automated reports as much as possible.
3. Based on the information, identify and document reasons for the problem or gap.
4. Develop a CQI action plan that:
   - Clearly states the improvement needed.
   - Identifies the specific goals of the project.
   - Includes what will be done, who will do it, the time frame involved, and how and when the outcome(s) will be measured or checked.

Brainstorming, flow charts, literature review, and communication with colleagues can be used to develop a "best practice" plan.

Do

1. Educate and train everyone who will be involved directly or indirectly in implementing the plan. Remember to include the patient and patient's family if the project is patient-centered.
2. Implement the plan on a small scale if it involves major policy or practice changes.

Check

1. Monitor the results of the action or improvement plan to see if the desired results have been achieved.

2. Share the information at the monthly quality improvement meeting, at staff meetings, and during patient rounds.

Act

1. Weigh the results against the desired outcome. If satisfied with the results, incorporate the changes into the facility's everyday policies, procedures, and/or practice, as well as the patient's plan of care.
2. If the outcome has not been achieved, make any necessary changes, modifications, or adaptations to the action or care plan and implement.
3. Communicate the outcomes and any procedure, practice, or policy changes to all appropriate parties.
4. Monitor outcomes on a regular basis to ensure that desired outcomes continue.

Application of this model is demonstrated in the Chapter 5, "Clinical Application: CQI in Anemia/Iron Management."

CQI Responsibilities

The commitment of work place leaders is essential to the success of a quality improvement program. The program should be comprehensive yet flexible enough to permit innovation and variation in assessment approaches. Regardless of its exact structure, it should contain all the necessary components discussed earlier in this chapter.

The Conditions for Coverage for End Stage Renal Disease Facilities, effective October 2008 (Centers for Medicare and Medicaid Services [CMS], 2008) are part of CMS' effort to "modernize regulations and improve the availability of quality-of-care information; to promote transparency; and to move toward a patient outcome-based system that focuses on quality assessment and performance improvement" (p. 20371). In keeping with this intent, the role of the medical director was expanded and clarified.

The medical director is responsible for the delivery of patient care and outcomes in the facility, which includes responsibility for the QAPI program, staff education, training, and performance, as well as policies and procedures of the end stage renal disease (ESRD) facility. To further strengthen the responsibilities of the medical director, the first paragraph of §494.150 (CMS, 2008) states, "the medical director is accountable to the governing body for the quality of medical care provided to patients" (p. 20483). While the medical director is ultimately responsible for the quality or QAPI program, physicians, nurses, dialysis technicians, social workers, dietitians, biomedical technicians, and secretaries are all potential members of CQI teams. These members and other staff serve on teams/committees to apply CQI techniques (such as CPDCA) to opportunities for improvement as they are identified via information review. In the case of outpatient dialysis clinics, quality improvement committees are accountable to the medical director of the facility, and ultimately, the governing board. Hospital-based programs will have their own reporting/accountability structure.

Although the frequency of quality improvement meetings is not mandated, they are routinely held monthly or more often as necessary to oversee quality initiatives. Based on issues identified, the quality improvement committee develops appropriate recommendations for changes to existing facility processes using a CQI model. These meetings are documented in minutes housed in the work setting. The quality improvement committee conducts assessments of action plan results and documents meaningful changes in service delivery as a result of the quality improvement activities.

Functions of the Quality Improvement Committee

The functions of a quality improvement committee generally fall into seven categories. These are:
- Coordinating the collection, review, and analysis of information to include outcome data.
- Identifying and prioritizing improvement opportunities.
- Selecting and preparing quality improvement teams.
- Overseeing the development of quality improvement projects and action plans; providing feedback.
- Assisting in the development and implementation of quality-related educational/training programs.
- Communicating quality initiatives and their outcomes to internal and external customers.
- Evaluating the overall quality improvement program at least annually.

What Should Happen if CQI/QAPI Is Being Practiced Consistently and Correctly?

If CQI/QAPI principles are being practiced consistently and correctly, both internal and external customers (patients, patients' families, doctors, staff, surveyors, payers) are more satisfied with the services and care provided. The ability to comply with federal and state regulations and to meet renal community standards is increased, and the likelihood of lawsuits is lessened. Patient complaints to the ESRD Network and State Department of Public Health are few to none. Most importantly, patient outcomes improve over time and are sustained.

From a practical perspective, less time is spent on dealing with problems and crises. Patient care is less fragmented, while at the same time, caregivers experience greater job satisfaction as they see their efforts improve care.

Summary

Quality and continuous quality improvement play a key role in health care. The specialty of nephrology is no exception. Quality and its ongoing improvement is the right thing to do because of the human lives at stake. It is also the business thing to do because of regulatory compliance and pay-for-performance expectations.

Quality improvement in health care is not a new concept. CQI, however, has at times been misunderstood, under used, and even misused. It is not simply paperwork to be completed for regulatory or corporate compliance. It is a time-tested, common-sense approach to quality that really works in helping to identify improvement needs, develop solutions, and assess results of actions taken, both in the short and long term. When all is said and done, CQI is a mindset – a way of thinking about and practicing for quality.

References

Centers for Medicare and Medicaid Services (CMS). (2008). *Medicare program; Conditions for coverage for end-stage renal disease facilities*. Washington, DC: Federal Register.

Hradesky, J.L. (1995). *Total quality management handbook*. New York: McGraw-Hill, Inc.

Hunt, V.D. (1992). *Quality in America*. Homewood, IL: Business One Irwin.

Joint Commission on Accreditation of Healthcare Organizations (JCAHO). (1992). *Using quality improvement tools in a health-care setting*. Oakbrook, IL: Author.

Joint Commission on Accreditation of Healthcare Organizations (JCAHO). (1994). *Forums, charts, and other tools for performance improvement*. Oakbrook, Il: Author.

Lohr, K.N. (Ed.). (1990). *Medicare: A strategy for quality assurance in Medicare*. Washington, DC: National Academy Press.

Schroeder, P.S. (1994). *Improving quality and performance: Concepts, programs, and techniques*. St Louis: Mosby.

Walton, M. (1986). *The Deming management method*. New York: Putnam Publishing Group.

| **Chapter 1** | **CONTINUING NURSING EDUCATION EVALUATION FORM** | **1.4 Contact Hours** |

Concepts and Principles of Quality Management   **ANNP0901**

Applying Continuous Quality Improvement in Clinical Practice contains 22 chapters of educational content. Individual learners may apply for continuing nursing education credit by reading a chapter and completing the Continuing Nursing Education Evaluation Form for that chapter. Learners may apply for continuing nursing education credit for any or all chapters.

Please photocopy this test page, complete, and return to ANNA.
You can also download this form from www.annanurse.org (choose Education - CNE Activities - Publications)
Receive continuing nursing education credit (CNE) immediately by completing the CNE evaluation process in ANNA's Online Library. Go to www.annanurse.org, and click on the Online Library icon for more information.

Name: _____
Address: _____
City: _____ State: _____ Zip: _____
E-mail: _____ Preferred telephone: ☐ Home ☐ Work _____
State where licensed and license number: _____

CNE application fees are based upon the number of contact hours provided by the individual section. CNE fees per contact hour for ANNA members are as follows: 1.0-1.9 – $15; 2.0-2.9 – $20; 3.0-3.9 – $25; 4.0 and higher – $30. Fees for nonmembers are $10 higher.

CNE application fee for Chapter 1: ANNA member $15   Nonmember $25
ANNA Member: ☐ Yes ☐ No   ☐ Member # (if available) _____
☐ Check or money order enclosed   ☐ American Express   ☐ Visa   ☐ MasterCard
Total amount submitted: _____
Credit card number _____ Exp. Date _____
Name as it appears on the card: _____
NOTE: Your evaluation form can be processed in 1 week for an additional rush charge of $5.00.
☐   **Yes, I would like this evaluation form rush processed. I have included an additional fee of $5.00 for rush processing.**

Instructions
1. To receive continuing nursing education credit for an individual study after reading the chapter, complete this evaluation form.
2. Detach, photocopy, or download (www.annanurse.org) the evaluation form and send along with a check or money order payable to **American Nephrology Nurses' Association** to: ANNA, East Holly Avenue Box 56, Pitman, NJ 08071-0056.
3. Test returns must be postmarked by **April 30, 2011**. Upon completion of the answer/evaluation form, a certificate will be sent to you.

This chapter was reviewed and formatted for contact hour credit by Sally S. Russell, MN, CMSRN, ANNA Director of Education Services.

> **CNE Application Fee for Chapter 1**
> **ANNA member = $15**
> **Nonmember = $25**

---

1. I verify that I have read this chapter and completed this education activity. _____ Date _____
                                                   Signature
2. What would be different in your practice if you applied what you have learned from this activity? (Please use additional paper if necessary.)
   _____
   _____
   _____
   _____

	Strongly disagree				Strongly agree
3. The activity met the stated objectives.					
a. Define quality.	1	2	3	4	5
b. Discuss the basic principles and concepts of continuous quality improvement.	1	2	3	4	5
c. Describe a tested continuous quality improvement model for use in the nephrology setting.	1	2	3	4	5
4. The content was current and relevant.	1	2	3	4	5
5. The content was presented clearly.	1	2	3	4	5
6. The content was covered adequately.	1	2	3	4	5

7. How would you rate your ability to apply your learning to practice?   ☐ diminished ability   ☐ no change   ☐ enhanced ability

Comments _____
_____

8. Time required to read the chapter and complete this form: _____ minutes

---

This educational activity is provided by the American Nephrology Nurses' Association (ANNA).
ANNA is accredited as a provider of continuing nursing education (CNE) by the American Nurses Credentialing Center's Commission on Accreditation (ANCC-COA).
ANNA is a provider approved of continuing nursing education by the California Board of Registered Nursing, provider number CEP 00910.
This CNE offering meets the Nephrology Nursing Certification Commission's (NNCC's) continuing nursing education requirements for certification and recertification.

Using Continuous Quality Improvement Tools

Joan Camarro Simard, MS, RN, CNN

Objectives

Study of the information presented in this chapter will enable the learner to:
1. Discuss strategies for using tools in a CQI/QAPI program.
2. Describe tools that can be used in a CQI/QAPI program.
3. Present examples of tools used for clinical performance measurements.
4. Describe tools that can be used in the evaluation process.

Overview

Continuous quality improvement (CQI) is a process where teams come together to review and identify areas of clinical practice and environment that require improvement or change in the processes, procedures, or policies (Donabedian, 2003). There is a wide variety of tools available for the collection, evaluation, measurement, and mapping of data to streamline the approach the CQI team uses to reach its goals. This chapter will highlight some easy-to-use tools to assist with the process of CQI and quality assessment and performance improvement (QAPI). For more in-depth explanations and instructions, refer to textbooks written for that purpose (several are listed in the References section of this chapter).

Introduction

Quality programs require tools to assist continuous quality improvement (CQI)/quality assessment and performance improvement (QAPI) interdisciplinary team members with the ability to identify, collect, and investigate data for assessment and evaluation. These assessments can direct the team to identify the appropriate improvement plans to obtain the desirable outcome for either clinical or facility programs (Kelly & Johnson, 2006). Knowledge of workable tools is essential to a successful CQI/QAPI program.

Tools that have been historically used in CQI include flow charts, cause and effect diagrams, tally sheets, run charts for trending, control charts, and statistical formats using histograms and Pareto charts (Fields & Glaser, 1997). Although they may sound intimidating, the use of these tools is quite simple and easy to adapt to any problem and/or situation where measurement and assessment can occur.

Quality improvement programs have sustained a long journey from the original ideas of Florence Nightingale to the present time (Nightingale, 1860). Whether investigating poorly ventilated healthcare wards in the 1800s or evaluating the effectiveness of an anemia management program, healthcare point-of-care providers continue to seek information that will identify the causes and effects of their processes and practices.

CQI: The Processes

Investigation is one of the processes performed by the professional nurse as part of the interdisciplinary team. This process could include observation, assessment, intervention, and evaluation not only of patients but also nursing practice itself. The methodology of these processes includes the use of the senses and knowledge plus the actual tools themselves. Nephrology nurses have standards of practice and guidelines for care that can be useful to identify their role in the the CQI process (see Figure 2-1) (Burrows-Hudson & Prowant, 2005).

Most healthcare programs have people, processes, procedures, policies, and products. Each component contributes to the "map" that can lead the investigator to the cause and effect of the problem. With this knowledge, a corrective action plan is possible. Implementation of this action plan on a trial sample can lead to an improved process outcome as defined in the flow chart of the process and or procedure (Brassard & Ritter, 1994; Cofer, Greeley, & Coburn, 1994; Fields & Glaser,

Figure 2-1
Nephrology Nursing Standards of Practice–Standards of Care

Assessment
"The nephrology registered nurse collects comprehensive data pertinent to the patient's health or the situation" (p. 7).

Outcomes Identification
"The nephrology registered nurse identifies expected outcomes for a plan individualized to the patient or the situation" (p. 7).

Planning
"The nephrology registered nurse develops a plan that prescribes strategies and alternatives to attain expected outcomes" (p. 8).

Implementation
"The nephrology registered nurse implements the identified plan" (p. 9).

Evaluation
"The nephrology registered nurse evaluates progress toward attainment of outcomes" (p. 10).

Source: Burrows-Hudson & Prowant, 2005.

1997; Hoggard-Green & Daines, 1990; Kelly & Johnson, 2006; Peacock, Sims, & Bednar, 1995).

Staff involvement is critical to an effective CQI program, and interdisciplinary teams broaden the non-bias knowledge of reviewers. Physicians, nurses, patient care technicians, dietitians, and social workers all bring practice-specific knowledge that will play a contributing role in the facility program (Donabedian, 2003). As a requirement of the Centers for Medicare and Medicaid Services (CMS) *Conditions for Coverage for End Stage Renal Disease Facilities*, Code § 494.110 Condition: QAPI, V625, each facility will look at aggregate data and perform assessment and improvement of care. §494.90 Condition: Plan of Care, V540 expects patient-based improvement of care (CMS, 2008b).

CQI/QAPI Team Members

The medical director/physician has medical knowledge and problem-solving techniques based on qualitative and quantitative data analysis (see Figure 2-2). The advanced nurse practitioner has clinical expertise with advanced practice knowledge and problem-solving techniques based on qualitative and quantitative information (University of California San Francisco School of Medicine, 2009). The registered nurse has clinical expertise at one of several levels of knowledge (novice nurse, proficient nurse, and expert nurse) and problem-solving techniques based on qualitative and quantitative information (Benner, 1982). Patient care technicians (PCTs) have expertise specific to their level of practice, whether they are novice, proficient, or expert. They develop problem-solving techniques based on qualitative data. The registered dietitian has clinical expertise with advanced practice knowledge and problem-solving techniques based on qualitative and quantitative information (Weber State University, n.d.). The social worker has clinical expertise with advanced practice knowledge and problem-solving techniques based on quantitative information (Education Portal, 2009).

CMS charges the QAPI team with oversight of the facility's CQI program. Members of the QAPI team will work as a group to function as a review body to:
- Define the areas of practice for review.
- Develop knowledge of clinical performance measures.
- Review established guidelines and regulations for clinical performance.
- Use creativity for a variety of ideas and viewpoints of clinical issues based on clinical practice areas and levels of expertise.
- Select tools to identify:
  - Program improvement opportunities.
  - Analysis of processes.
  - Change implementation.
  - Follow-up evaluation (CMS, 2008b).

Brainstorming as a CQI Tool

Brainstorming can be thought of as a "think tank" event where members come together to identify and share ideas about possible clinical and facility problems. They are obligated to work as a group and support any ideas or plans without criticism, praise, or endorsement.

Rules of brainstorming include (Brassard & Ritter, 1994; Fields & Glaser, 1997; Peacock et al., 1995; Schroeder, 1994):

**Figure 2-2
Qualitative vs. Quantitative**

Qualitative
Relating to quality; relating to or based on the quality or character of something, often as opposed to its size or quantity.

Quantitative
Relating to quantity; relating to, concerning, or based on the amount or number of something measurable; capable of being measured or expressed in numerical terms.

Source: MSN Encarta Online Dictionary, 2009a, 2009b.

- Create list(s) of problem(s). As a team, collectively submit processes and/or problems that require attention.
- Identify possible influencing factors for people, product, procedure, policy, and performance.
- Prioritize ideas/problems; urgent ideas or problems are enacted upon first.
- Consensus of plan(s) for outcome.

Products of brainstorming encompass open discussion of clinical environment:
- What is the current status of the environment?
  - Staffing patterns: Professional staff, administrative staff, clinical support staff.
  - Patient population: General stratification of age groups, concentration of ethnic backgrounds, socio-economic variations (Fields & Glaser, 1997; Schroeder, 1994).
- What are the required clinical outcome measures needed for compliance?
  - Clinical outcome measurements:
    - ➤ Adequacy, anemia, hypertension, nutrition, diabetes mellitus, vascular access, bone and mineral metabolism (CMS, 2008b).
- Problems or situations related to the physical environment:
  - Materials, physical structural, impact on delivery of care.
- What are we doing that needs to be improved?
  - Processes not meeting clinical and organizational guidelines and protocols.
  - Options or possibilities for evaluation.
- Which components of the process, practice, or the evidence need to be addressed?
  - Breakdown the variables into specific data points (flow chart).
  - Identify the relationship between the data points (cause and effect diagram).
- How will the process, practice, or evidence be documented? Tools for data documentation may include:
  - Computerized medical record.
  - Documentation of patient events and clinical performance measures.
  - Regulated documents for the delivery of care.
  - Manual documented reports.
  - Physical observations and assessments of the data source.

- How will the process, practice, or evidence be collected? Physical collection tools can include automated reports such as:
  - Laboratory data.
  - Computerized dialysis treatment machine downloads.
  - Computerized query reporting.
  - Tally sheets/check lists.
  - Logs.
  - Surveys/questionnaires.
  - Interviews.
- How will the process, practice, or evidence be measured? Established clinical measurement tools can be used to accomplish this.
  - Measures Assessment Tool (MAT) (CMS, 2008a, 2008b).
  - Association for the Advancement of Medical Instrumentation (AAMI) RD47 (AAMI, 2003).
  - NKF Kidney Disease Outcomes Quality Initiative™ (KDOQI) (see Sidebar) (NKF, 2000, 2002, 2003, 2004, 2006a, 2006b, 2006c, 2006d, 2007).
  - CMS *Conditions for Coverage* (CMS, 2008b).
- Where in the process, practice, or evidence is there a variation from the expected goal? Explore the following:
  - People.
  - Process.
  - Procedure.
  - Policy.
  - Product (Cofer et al., 1994; Fields & Glaser, 1997; Peacock et al., 1995; Schroeder, 1994).

Tools for Data Collection

Data are not always available when needed, reinforcing the need to use data collection tools. Objective, data-driven tools foster the opportunity to avoid the omnipresent potential for bias or distortion.

- Data sheets provide a means to record data and require processes for analysis and interpretation.
- Check sheets permit data recording for direct data interpretation. Data events can be recorded or tallied to identify problems and causes to determine what action may be required.
- Survey forms are effective in getting input from a large group of people. Surveys are commonly used to determine patients' perceived needs or satisfaction in a facility. Survey results require analysis to be meaningful.
- An interview is an open-ended discussion to acquire input regarding targeted information and will require qualitative data analysis for interpretation (Brassard & Ritter, 1994; Schroeder, 1994).

Table 2-1 displays a laboratory value report that was used to collect patient data for evaluating the adequacy of dialysis. Columns listing Patient, Desired Kt/V, and Actual Kt/V were used to create the run chart titled "KT/V Values for October" (see Figure 2-6).

The check sheet tool can be used to collect information about situations or items that might indicate the frequency of an event or item. Table 2-2 represents a check sheet tool, and in this case, the auditor is looking for the number of the type

Table 2-1
Data Sheet

October Laboratory Results for Adequacy		
Patient	**Desired Kt/V**	**Actual Kt/V**
A	1.2	1.49
B	1.2	1.62
C	1.2	1.61
D	1.2	1.89
E	1.2	1.64
F	1.2	1.69
G	1.2	1.86
H	1.2	1.86
I	1.2	0.87
J	1.2	1.82
K	1.2	1.98
L	1.2	1.44
M	1.2	1.47
N	1.2	1.70
O	1.2	1.57
P	1.2	1.01
Q	1.2	1.38

Source: Used with permission from Joan Camarro Simard.

NKF References

KDOQI Hemodialysis Adequacy (NKF, 2006a)
KDOQI Hypertension and Anti-Hypertension Agents in CKD (BP) (NKF, 2004)
KDOQI Peritoneal Dialysis Adequacy (NKF 2006b)
KDOQI Nutrition (NKF, 2000)
KDOQI Chronic Kidney Disease (NKF, 2002)
KDOQI Bone Metabolism and Disease (NKF, 2003)
KDOQI Anemia (NKF, 2006c, 2007)
KDOQI Vascular Assess (NKF, 2006d)
Measures Assessment Tool (CMS 2008a)

---

of vascular access and percentages for the patient population (Brassard & Ritter, 1994; Kelly & Johnson, 2006; Schroeder, 1994).

Tools for Data Processes and Evaluations

Tools for data processing and evaluations are available in a variety of forms for charting processes and data evaluation. Tools for process descriptions are used to:
- Define the total process.
- Expose rework and complexity.
- Assist in data collection.
- Reduce document variations.

Table 2-2
Check Sheet

Problem to be Evaluated	Number of Occurrences	Total	Sample Size *n*	%
Patients with AVF/Right Arm	IIIII IIIII IIIII IIIII II	22	71	31%
Patients with AVF/Left Arm	IIIII IIIII IIIII IIIII IIIII IIIII II	32	71	45%
Tunneled Catheters RIJ	IIIII IIIII	10	71	14%
Tunneled Catheters LIJ	IIIII II	7	71	10%

Source: Used with permission from Joan Camarro Simard.

Flow Chart Diagram

A flow chart diagram graphically displays the steps that are performed in a specific process so:
- The process flow is understood.
- The current process is correctly delineated.
- Redundancies, inefficiencies, and misunderstandings are identified.
- Processes are streamlined and improved.
- Final documentation and education is provided.
- Advantages are ultimately available (Brassard & Ritter, 1994; Fields & Glaser, 1997; Joint Commission on Accreditation of Health Organizations [JACHO],1992; Peacock et al., 1995; Schroeder, 1994).

Flow charts are pictures of the process displayed through a variety of shapes, symbols, and action points (see Figure 2-3) (Brassard & Ritter, 1994; Fields & Glaser, 1997; Schroeder, 1994).
- Starting and ending points can be displayed by a rounded rectangle.
- A parallelogram can represent data elements.
- The rectangle is used to show a task or action that is part of the process under review. There may be multiple connecting points originating or terminating into it displayed by arrow connectors.
- A diamond represents a decision point or a yes/no answer (Brassard & Ritter, 1994; Fields & Glaser, 1997; Schroeder, 1994).
- Arrows show the direction or flow of the process.
- Be consistent, with "yes" choices branching down and "no" choices branching to the side.
- Additional shapes may be included to demonstrate:
  ○ Completed reports.
  ○ Computer data entry.
  ○ Delayed action points.
  ○ Continuation of the chart elsewhere (Brassard & Ritter, 1994; Fields & Glaser, 1997; Schroeder, 1994).

The flow chart in Figure 2-4 was designed to map out the evaluation process of a reprocessing program.

Cause and Effect Diagram

Cause and effect, or fishbone, diagrams display the structural components of a process or a brainstorming idea designed by the interdisciplinary team to investigate a problem-

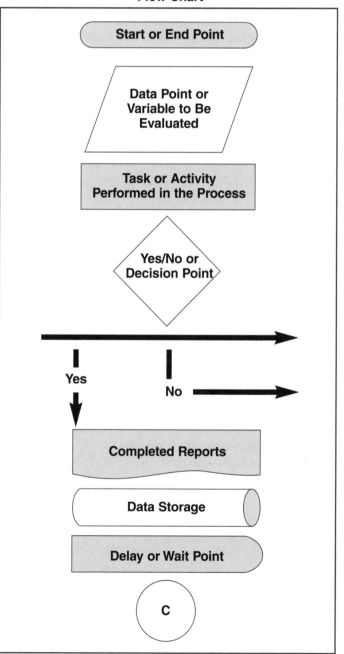

Figure 2-3
Flow Chart

Source: Used with permission from Joan Camarro Simard.

Figure 2-4
Flow Chart for Review of Reprocessing Program

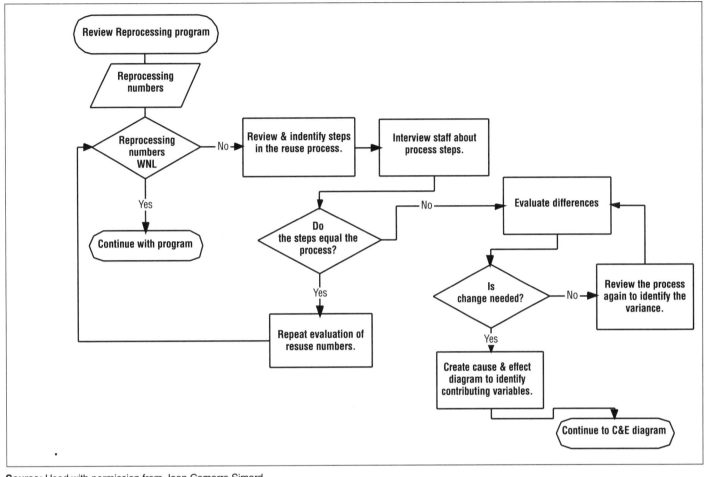

Source: Used with permission from Joan Camarro Simard.

atic concern. The design of the diagram is based on the Ishikawa diagram, which is commonly referred to as a "fishbone" diagram (Brassard & Ritter, 1994; Fields & Glaser, 1997; JCAHO, 1992; Peacock et al., 1995; Schroeder, 1994). Figure 2-5 is an example of a cause and effect diagram.

The cause and effect or fishbone diagram is used to visualize the possible causes related to a process or condition under review. The team is able to focus on specific contributing factors that can be classified as part of the processes (Brassard & Ritter, 1994; Fields & Glaser, 1997; Kelly & Johnson, 2006; Peacock et al., 1995). Team members can be assigned to investigate one of the branches. This can be helpful, especially if the team member is not directly involved in the process. The reviewer should not have any preconceived ideas of the process and what is to be expected.

Components or categories in the cause and effect diagram can be classified with the People, Process, Procedure, Policy, and Product branches, or as determined by the CQI team. Under each branch, additional branches are made with variables related to the process for evaluation (Brassard & Ritterr, 1994; Fields & Glaser, 1997; Kelly & Johnson, 2006; Peacock et al., 1995; Schroeder, 1994). Figure 2-5 represents possible components and subcomponents that might be evalu-

ated for a quality patient care process that involves patient adequacy.

Run Charts

A run chart is a simple, plotted chart that displays the progress of a process over a timeline. Trends, shifts, or changes can become apparent once data are collected in an organized form. Time and the number of occurrences are a part of the measurement process. Table 2-1 is a representation of data collected to monitor adequacy, and the information can then be displayed in a run chart (see Figure 2-6).

Run charts display data trends over a specific timeline. In this example, 1 month of Kt/V values have been compared with the KDOQI minimum goal of 1.2. Data points for each patient were plotted along the X axis, and measurement of the variables were plotted along the Y axis. This data representation indicated the patients' Kt/V range from less than the desired goal to exceptional values.

Control Charts

Control charts can be used to display data deviations based on mean/median data calculations that will determine an upper and lower control limits. Data values should fall within

Figure 2-5
Cause and Effect Diagram for Quality Patient Care Adequacy

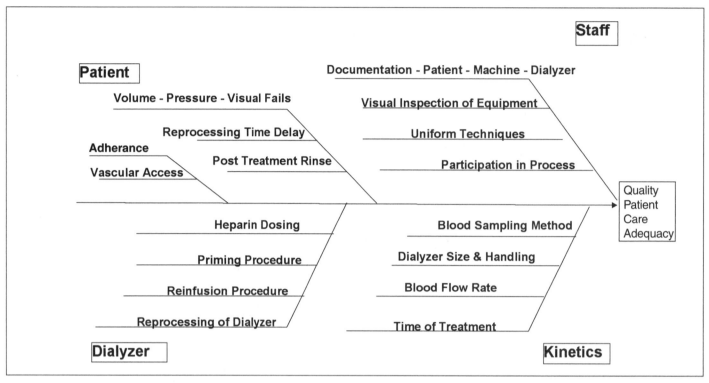

Source: Used with permission from Joan Camarro Simard.

Figure 2-6
KT/V Values for October

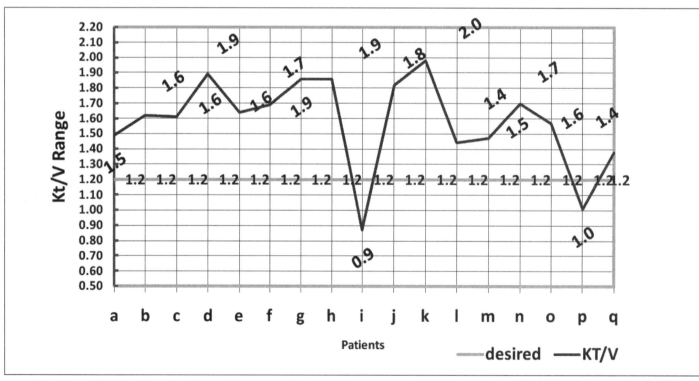

Note: The values within the graph are not placed at their exact value point and are shown as an example only.
Source: Used with permission from Joan Camarro Simard.

Figure 2-7
Plotted Data

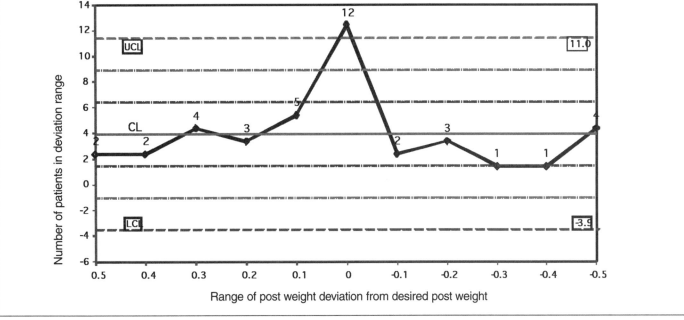

Source: Used with permission from Joan Camarro Simard.

the control limits (Brassard & Ritter, 1994; Fields & Glaser, 1997; Hoggard-Green & Daines, 1990; Kelly & Johnson, 2006; Schroeder, 1994).

Figure 2-7 displays plotted data of the ultrafiltration goals that were reached by patients in a 1-day time frame. Figure 2-7 informs the reader that 12 patients achieved the desired post-dialysis weight, 2 patients had a goal that was more than 0.5 kg over the goal, and 4 patients had post-weights more than 0.5 kg less than the desired goal.

Statistical Formats

Histogram and Pareto charts both provide ways to display the frequency distribution of data as it occurs.

Histogram

A histogram is a bar graph display of data over time and is used to identify problems or changes in a system or process. Raw data are used and will be displayed in the order they were obtained. Check sheets can usually organize data for graphing with a histogram. An example of a check sheet is seen in Table 2-3. Histograms:
- Identify data that may need further investigation of information collected over time.
- Graphically present the frequency distribution of data in bar form.
- Display large amounts of data that might be difficult to interpret in tabular form.
- Show relative frequency of occurrence of the various data.
- Display centering, variation, and shape of data (Brassard & Ritter, 1994; Hoggard-Green & Daines, 1990; Roth, 2002).

Figure 2-8 displays a histogram that calculated the average number of dialyzer reuses for a dialyzer reprocessing program.

Table 2-3 and Figure 2-8 represent the number of treatments delivered to a patient census of 59 during a one month period. Sixteen of the 59 patients received 210 dialysis treatments using reprocessed dialyzers during the designated month. A total of 801 treatments were delivered to all 59 patients for the month. The program goal is to obtain 25 reuses per the life of each dialyzer. The data in Table 2-3 display the number of reuses for each reprocessed dialyzer.

The histogram diagram shown in Figure 2-8 lists data values in order of occurrences. The numbers of dialyzers used are represented on the Y axis, and the number of reuses are displayed on the X axis. The data demonstrate a reverse bell curve.

Pareto Chart

Pareto charts graph data over time and can display results in a plotted order from highest to lowest, highlighting the frequency of data events. Pareto charts:
- Sort data for relative importance of a problem from highest to lowest values.
- Identify the measure that requires improvement or further investigation (Stimel, 2003).

Data in Table 2-4 sorted the same number of reuses for each reprocessed dialyzer. Results were sorted into cumulative values. The Pareto diagram will list the values in order of occurrences, with the greatest number of reuses plotted against the number of dialyzers (Brassard & Ritter, 1994; Fields & Glaser, 1997; Hoggard-Green & Daines, 1990; Kelly & Johnson, 2006; Schroeder, 1994).

Using the same reuse data as the histogram, the Pareto chart helps direct the attention of the team to review the reuse

Figure 2-8
Histogram Chart for Reprocessed Dialyzer Numbers

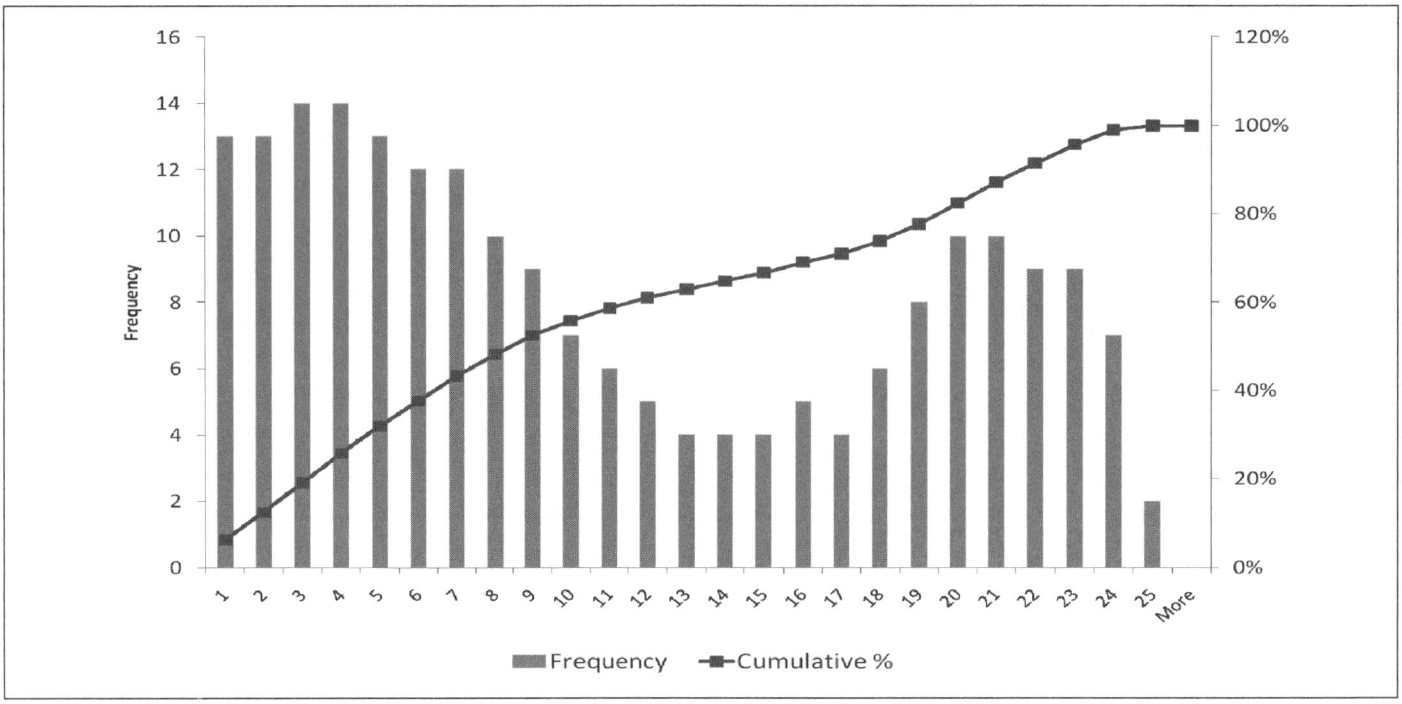

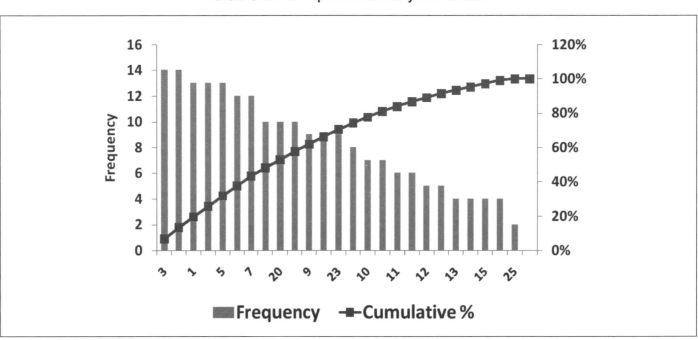

Source: Used with permission from Joan Camarro Simard.

Figure 2-9
Pareto Chart of Reprocessed Dialyzer Numbers

Source: Used with permission from Joan Camarro Simard.

Table 2-3
Histogram Data for Reprocessed Dialyzers

0	Frequency	Cumulative %
1	13	6%
2	13	12%
3	14	19%
4	14	26%
5	13	32%
6	12	38%
7	12	43%
8	10	48%
9	9	52%
10	7	56%
11	6	59%
12	5	61%
13	4	63%
14	4	65%
15	4	67%
16	5	69%
17	4	71%
18	6	74%
19	8	78%
20	10	82%
21	10	87%
22	9	91%
23	9	96%
24	7	99%
25	2	100%
More	0	100%
	210	

Source: Used with permission from Joan Camarro Simard.

Table 2-4
Data Sheet for Pareto Chart

0	Frequency	Cumulative %	0	Frequency	Cumulative %
1	13	6%	3	14	7%
2	13	12%	4	14	13%
3	14	19%	1	13	20%
4	14	26%	2	13	26%
5	13	32%	5	13	32%
6	12	38%	6	12	38%
7	12	43%	7	12	43%
8	10	48%	8	10	48%
9	9	52%	20	10	53%
10	7	56%	21	10	58%
11	6	59%	9	9	62%
12	5	61%	22	9	66%
13	4	63%	23	9	70%
14	4	65%	19	8	74%
15	4	67%	10	7	78%
16	5	69%	24	7	81%
17	4	71%	11	6	84%
18	6	74%	18	6	87%
19	8	78%	12	5	89%
20	10	82%	16	5	91%
21	10	87%	13	4	93%
22	9	91%	14	4	95%
23	9	96%	15	4	97%
24	7	99%	17	4	99%
25	2	100%	25	2	100%
More	0	100%	More	0	100%
				210	

Source: Used with permission from Joan Camarro Simard.

process, since 58% of reused dialyzers were processed fewer than 10 times (see Figure 2-9).

Conclusion

Tools for CQI programs provide team members with a mechanism to collect, sort, calculate, and analyze data elements. Once constructed, combined, and brought to the interdisciplinary team, tools can improve the team's understanding of the processes and procedures that are part of their delivery of care programs. Obtaining and maintaining a quality program today continues to require the use of tools and processes to provide for the ongoing need for quality assessment and performance improvement.

References

Association for the Advancement of Medical Instrumentation (AAMI) (2003). *AAMI standards and recommended practices: Dialysis.* Arlington, VA: Author.

Benner, P. (1982). From novice to expert. *American Journal of Nursing, 82*(3). 402-407.

Brassard, M., & Ritter, D. (1994). *The Memory Jogger™ II: A pocket guide of tools for continuous improvement and effective planning.* Salem, NH: GOAL/QPC.

Burrows-Hudson, S., & Prowant, B.F. (2005). Standards of care. In *Nephrology nursing standards of practice and guidelines for care* (pp. 7-10). Pitman, NJ: American Nephrology Nurses' Association.

Centers for Medicare and Medicaid Services (CMS). (2008a). *Center for Medicaid and State Operations/Survey & Certification Group.* Retrieved March 5, 2009, from http://www.cms.hhs.gov/ SurveyCertificationGenInfo/downloads/SCLetter08-21.pdf

Centers for Medicare and Medicaid Services (CMS). (2008b). *Conditions for coverage for end stage renal disease facilities*. Washington, DC: Federal Register.

Cofer, J.I., Greeley, H.P., & Coburn, J. (1994). The documentation improvement project. In *Information management: A guide to the JCAHO standards* (2nd ed., pp. 43-51). Marblehead, MA: Opus Communications, Inc.

Donabedian, A. (2003). *An introduction to quality assurance in health care*. New York, NY: Oxford University Press, Inc.

Education Portal. (2009). *Masters degree social work*. Retrieved March 5, 2009, from http://education-portal.com/masters_degree_social_work.html

Fields, W.L., & Glaser, D. (1997). Using statistical process control tools in the quality process. In C. G. Meisenheimer (Ed.), *Improving quality: A guide to effective programs* (2nd ed., pp. 237-258). Gaithersburg, MD: Aspen Publishers, Inc.

Hoggard-Green, J., & Daines, L. (1990). *Continuous quality improvement syllabus*. Salt Lake City, UT: Intermountain Healthcare.

Joint Commission on Accreditation of Healthcare Organizations (JCAHO). (1992). Tools of CQI. In *Educational program. Quality improvement in special care units*. Oakbrook, IL: Author.

Kelly, D.L., & Johnson, S.P. (2006). Measurement and statistical analysis in CQI. In C.P. McLaughlin & A.D. Kaluzny (Eds.), *Continuous quality improvement in health care. Theory, implementations and applications* (3rd ed., pp. 95-130). Sudbury, MA: Jones and Bartlett Publishers.

MSN Encarta Online Dictionary. (2009a). *Qualitative*. Retrieved January 9, 2009, from http://encarta.msn.com/dictionary_/qualitative.html

MSN Encarta Online Dictionary. (2009b). *Quantitative*. Retrieved January 9, 2009, from http://encarta.msn.com/dictionary_/quantitative.html

National Kidney Foundation (NKF). (2000). *KDOQI Clinical practice guidelines for nutrition in clinical renal failure*. Retrieved March 24, 2009, from http://www.kidney.org/professionals/KDOQI/guidelines_updates/doqi_nut.html

National Kidney Foundation (NKF). (2002). *KDOQI clinical practice guidelines for chronic kidney disease: Evaluation, classification, and stratification*. Retrieved February 28, 2009, from http://www.kidney.org/professionals/KDOQI/guidelines_ckd/toc.htm

National Kidney Foundation (NKF). (2003). *KDOQI clinical practice guidelines for bone metabolism and disease in chronic kidney disease*. Retrieved January 9, 2009, from http://www.kidney.org/professionals/KDOQI/guidelines_bone/index.htm

National Kidney Foundation (NKF). (2004). *KDOQI clinical practice guidelines on hypertension and antihypertensive agents in chronic kidney disease*. Retrieved January 9, 2009, from http://www.kidney.org/professionals/KDOQI/guidelines_bp/index.htm

National Kidney Foundation (NKF). (2006a). *KDOQI clinical practice guidelines and clinical practice recommendations 2006 update: Hemodialysis adequacy*. Retrieved January 9, 2009, from http://www.kidney.org/professionals/KDOQI/guideline_upHD_PD_VA/index.htm

National Kidney Foundation (NKF). (2006b). *KDOQI clinical practice guidelines and clinical practice recommendations 2006 update: Peritoneal dialysis adequacy*. Retrieved January 9, 2009, from http://www.kidney.org/professionals/KDOQI/guideline_upHD_PD_VA/index.htm

National Kidney Foundation (NKF). (2006c). *KDOQI clinical practice guidelines and clinical practice recommendations for anemia in chronic kidney disease*. Retrieved January 9, 2009, from http://www.kidney.org/professionals/KDOQI/guidelines_anemia/index.htm

National Kidney Foundation (NKF). (2006d). *KDOQI clinical practice guidelines and clinical practice recommendations 2006 Update: Vascular access*. Retrieved January 9, 2009, from http://www.kidney.org/professionals/KDOQI/guideline_upHD_PD_VA/index.htm

National Kidney Foundation (NKF). (2007). *KDOQI clinical practice guidelines and clinical practice recommendations for anemia in chronic kidney disease: 2007 Update of hemoglobon target*. Retrieved January 9, 2009, from http://www.kidney.org/professionals/KDOQI/guidelines_anemiaUP/index.htm

Nightingale, F. (1860). *Notes on nursing* (1960 printing). New York: Dover Publishers, Inc.

Peacock, E., Sims, T., & Bednar, B. (1995). The tools of continuous quality improvement (CQI). In G.S. Wick, & E. Peacock (Eds.), *American Nephrology Nurses' Association continuous quality improvement: From concept to reality* (pp. 41-51). Pitman, NJ: American Nephrology Nurses' Association.

Roth, G. (2002). *iSixSigma dictionary: Histogram*. Retrieved January 30, 2009, from http://www.isixsigma.com/404.asp?404:http://www.isixsigma.com:80/dictionary/histogram-19.htm

Schroeder, P. (Ed.). (1994). *Improving quality and performance: Concepts, programs, and techniques*. St.Louis, MI: Mosby-Year Book.

Stimel, A. (2003). *iSixSigma dictionary: Pareto*. Retrieved January 30, 2009, from http://www.isixsigma.com/404.asp?404;http://isixsigma.com:80/dictionary/pareto-60.htm

University of California San Francisco School of Medicine. (2009). *Competency-based advancement*. Retrieved January 4, 2009, from http://medschool.ucsf.edu/curriculum/competencies/

Weber State University. (n.d.). *Nutrition curriculum*. Retrieved January 4, 2009, from http://programs.weber.edu/nutrition/Curriculum.htm

Additional Reading

Meisenheimer, C.G. (1997). *Improving Quality, A guide to effective programs*. 2nd Edition. Gaithersburg, MD: Aspen Publishers, Inc.

| Chapter 2 | **CONTINUING NURSING EDUCATION EVALUATION FORM** | **1.1 Contact Hours** |

Using Continuous Quality Improvement Tools

ANNP0902

Applying Continuous Quality Improvement in Clinical Practice contains 22 chapters of educational content. Individual learners may apply for continuing nursing education credit by reading a chapter and completing the Continuing Nursing Education Evaluation Form for that chapter. Learners may apply for continuing nursing education credit for any or all chapters.

Please photocopy this test page, complete, and return to ANNA.
You can also download this form from www.annanurse.org (choose Education - CNE Activities - Publications)
Receive continuing nursing education credit (CNE) immediately by completing the CNE evaluation process in ANNA's Online Library. Go to www.annanurse.org, and click on the Online Library icon for more information.
Name: _____
Address: _____
City: _____ State: _____ Zip: _____
E-mail:_____ Preferred telephone: ☐ Home ☐ Work _____
State where licensed and license number: _____

CNE application fees are based upon the number of contact hours provided by the individual section. CNE fees per contact hour for ANNA members are as follows: 1.0-1.9 – $15; 2.0-2.9 – $20; 3.0-3.9 – $25; 4.0 and higher – $30. Fees for nonmembers are $10 higher.
CNE application fee for Chapter 2: ANNA member $15   Nonmember $25
ANNA Member: ☐ Yes ☐ No   ☐ Member # (if available) _____
☐ Check or money order enclosed   ☐ American Express   ☐ Visa   ☐ MasterCard
Total amount submitted:_____
Credit card number _____ Exp. Date _____
Name as it appears on the card: _____
NOTE: Your evaluation form can be processed in 1 week for an additional rush charge of $5.00
☐ **Yes, I would like this evaluation form rush processed. I have included an additional fee of $5.00 for rush processing.**

Instructions
1. To receive continuing nursing education credit for an individual study after reading the chapter, complete this evaluation form.
2. Detach, photocopy, or download (www.annanurse.org) the evaluation form and send along with a check or money order payable to **American Nephrology Nurses' Assocation** to: ANNA, East Holly Avenue Box 56, Pitman, NJ 08071-0056.
3. Test returns must be postmarked by **April 30, 2011.** Upon completion of the answer/evaluation form, a certificate will be sent to you.

This section was reviewed and formatted for contact hour credit by Sally S. Russell, MN, CMSRN, ANNA Director of Education Services.

> **CNE Application Fee for Chapter 2**
> **ANNA member = $15**
> **Nonmember = $25**

1. I verify that I have read this chapter and completed this education activity. _____Date _____
   Signature
2. What would be different in your practice if you applied what you have learned from this activity? (Please use additional paper if necessary.)
   _____
   _____
   _____
   _____

	Strongly disagree				Strongly agree
3. The activity met the stated objectives.					
a. Discuss strategies for using tools in a CQI/QAPI program.	1	2	3	4	5
b. Describe tools that can be used in a CQI/QAPI program.	1	2	3	4	5
c. Present examples of tools used for clinical performance measurements.	1	2	3	4	5
d. Describe tools that can be used in the evaluation process.	1	2	3	4	5
4. The content was current and relevant.	1	2	3	4	5
5. The content was presented clearly.	1	2	3	4	5
6. The content was covered adequately.	1	2	3	4	5

7. How would you rate your ability to apply your learning to practice?   ☐ diminished ability   ☐ no change   ☐ enhanced ability

Comments _____
_____

8. Time required to read the chapter and complete this form: _____ minutes

Root Cause Analysis in Quality Improvement

Leonor P. Ponferrada, BSN, RN, CNN

Objectives

Study of the information presented in this chapter will enable the learner to:
1. Define root cause analysis (RCA).
2. Identify 5 basic elements of a process.
3. List 3 general principles of root cause analysis.
4. Describe 5 steps in conducting a root cause analysis.
5. Illustrate causal factor charting.

Overview

Root cause analysis (RCA) is a systematic investigation that looks into an identified event or undesirable outcome. This allows the investigator(s) and other involved parties to "dig deeper" in order to better understand the fundamental or "root cause" of the problem. The purpose of RCA is to determine what happened, how it happened, why it happened, and what actions can be implemented to reduce the likelihood of a recurrence.

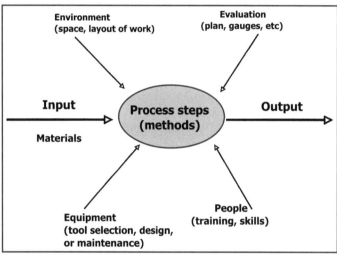

**Figure 3-1
Components of Process**

Source: Used with permission from Leonor Ponferrada.

Introduction

Root cause analysis (RCA) is an analysis framework adapted in health care to determine systemic causes of adverse events and to prevent recurrences (Percapio, Watts, & Weeks, 2008). It was originally developed in industrial psychology and systems engineering (Wu, Lipshutz, & Pronovost, 2008) and was widely applied in the nuclear branch of the United States Navy to set a high standard of performance for operational systems and personnel (Dew 2003a). Bagian and colleagues from the U.S. Department of Veterans Affairs (VA) and Croteau at the Joint Commission first introduced RCA to the medical community in the mid-1990s (Bagian et al., 2002). The Joint Commission now mandates the use of RCA of reported sentinel events in accredited hospitals. The VA system and its facilities are required to submit RCA reports for serious adverse events to the National Center for Patient Safety (Wu et al., 2008). End stage renal disease (ESRD) programs and facilities not affiliated with accredited hospitals or the VA System are not mandated to perform RCA on adverse events. It is, however, a system that can be applied in dialysis facilities to prevent recurrence or to decrease the incidence of these events. Identifying the true cause of a problem is a critical step in the continuous quality improvement process and paves the way to effective and lasting corrective actions.

What Is a Root Cause?

The underlying reason(s) for an undesirable outcome can be part of a process that is not performing as expected (Rummler & Brache, 1990). These authors promote focusing on the organization's processes if one wants to understand, improve, and manage the way work gets done (see Figure 3-1). The basic elements of a process generating an outcome include:
- The people involved.
- The machines and/or equipment, if applicable.
- The environment where the process occurs.
- The methods of performing the tasks in the process (Rummler & Brache, 1990).

When all process components are performing as expected, this typically produces desired outcomes with consistency. Undesirable events or outcomes are symptoms of a process that is not performing as planned. They are indications that one or more components of the process are not performing at the desired level, and RCA is one method to analyze the undesired events or outcomes.

Application of RCA

An organization that adapts the RCA framework should use common terminologies in order to facilitate improved understanding and communication among the team members conducting the investigation. The outcome of the RCA will produce a hierarchy of causes (NASA Safety Training Center Course, 2003). These are:

Table 3-1
Problem Assessment Chart

Method	Problem Origin	Consideration
Trouble shooting, problem-solving, or rework	Known	Problem or outcome seen before; the organization can live with the impact if it recurs.
Root cause analysis	Unknown	Problems or outcomes are symptoms of a process that is not performing as expected.
Crisis intervention	Unknown	Consider only as a temporary fix; action taken may be on the wrong process.

Source: Used with permission from Leonor Ponferrada.

Table 3-2
Determining When to Do Root Cause Analysis

Situations that:
Have serious outcomes.
Origin is unknown.
Are recurring with greatest frequency.
Consume the greatest resources to correct.

Source: Used with permission from Leonor Ponferrada.

Table 3-3
Examples of Events Where Root Cause Analysis May Be Utilized in a Dialysis Facility

Needle sticks/sharps exposure
Falls
Death(s) in the dialysis unit
Patient or staff injury
Medication errors

Source: Used with permission from Leonor Ponferrada.

- Direct or proximal causes.
- Intermediate causes.
- Root causes.

When an undesirable outcome occurs, it is necessary to look at more than just the immediately visible causes of the problem. These are known as the direct or proximate causes and are considered as such because they are the causes that appear immediately before the undesired outcome (NASA Safety Training Center Course, 2003). For example, poor preventive maintenance may be the direct or proximal cause of a faulty dialysis machine, but may not necessarily be the root cause.

"A root cause is the most basic causal factor, or factors, which if corrected or removed, will prevent recurrence of a situation" (Dew, 2003b, p. 60). It is usually one of multiple factors. These could be events, conditions, or organizational factors that contributed to or created the direct cause and subsequent undesired outcome. When a root cause is modified, corrected, or eliminated, recurrence of a situation is prevented or minimized. Intermediate causes are those between the proximate and root causes (NASA Safety Training Center Course, 2003).

Outcomes are also largely due to organizational factors. These factors include any operational or management systems in place that control and oversee the process implementation at any stage. These include but are not limited to the system's concept development, design, operation, and maintenance (NASA Safety Training Center Course, 2003). Examples include management decisions, organization policies (including content, implementation, and accountability), and organization resources (such as budgets, staffing, and training).

Do All Problems Require RCA?

RCA principles can be effectively applied to all problem-solving situations and activities. RCA does, however, have limitations. RCA is a retrospective investigation of events. Because accidents are highly unpredictable, it is impossible to know if the root cause established by the analysis is the cause of the accident (Reason, 1990). RCA can also be subject to investigators' bias, and it can be very time-consuming and labor-intensive (Wald & Shojania, 2001). Table 3-1 describes considerations that may need to be assessed to determine the method to use in correcting and eliminating problems. Simple trouble shooting or problem solving may be the most acceptable method to use when the origin of an event is known. For example, frequent infiltrations from needle sticks associated with a specific staff member may immediately be corrected with simple problem solving by retraining that staff member. RCA will be beneficial to the organization:

- When the origin of an event has serious outcomes.
- When the origin of an event is unknown.
- If the problem recurs with great frequency.
- If the problem consumes a great deal of resources to fix (see Table 3-2).

Applying quick solutions to such events that require in-depth investigation may provide only a temporary fix. If there is a recurrence, the action implemented was likely based upon the wrong process. Table 3-3 provides examples of events where RCA can be utilized in a dialysis facility.

Who Should Perform RCA?

In a dialysis facility, RCA will be more effective if there is full participation from team members who are chosen because of their proximity to the event. Teams that work together effectively can foster a real sense of being part of the solution rather than just part of the problem (Latino & Latino, 2006). All RCA investigations should be facilitated by a trained and unbiased member of the staff. This will ensure that all causal and influencing factors are identified and effective solutions are considered (McDonald & Leyhane, 2005). A facility should have a core team whose membership stays as consistent as possible, though ad-hoc team members may be necessary when exploring new or specific areas. For example, a group of nurses working in the dialysis unit may be chosen to participate as team members when exploring the process of medication administration.

Root Cause Analysis (RCA)

Specifically, the purpose of RCA is to determine three things:
- What happened.
- Why it happened.
- What can be done to reduce the likelihood of recurrence (Wichman & Greenall, 2006).

The method of conducting RCA requires a structured questioning process that enables investigators to recognize and discuss the underlying beliefs and practices that result in poor quality in an organization (Dew, 2003a). The primary aim is to ultimately implement recommendations that will prevent recurrence of the problem or decrease the frequency or the severity of the outcome. Many clinicians believe that because of many years of experience, they are quite adept at identifying solutions to problems. When dealing with complex problems, however, solutions may not actually address the root of the problem, and therefore, the same problem keeps coming back.

RCA goes beyond brainstorming or problem solving. The process requires a trained, unbiased facilitator and a team of subject matter experts to investigate the cause and effect relationships of an undesirable outcome (Latino & Latino, 2006). This proof takes the form of physical evidence related to the event. It is used to prove or disprove hypotheses developed during the exploration process of determining why things went wrong. RCA will typically "dig down deeper" and identify all possible causes, including physical, human, and latent root causes (McDonald & Leyhane, 2005).

Wald and Shojania (2001) maintain that to be credible, the RCA requires the application of established qualitative techniques that include data collection. That data, when analyzed, will supply evidence as to what happened. The analysis incorporates examining the sequence of actions and activities contributing to the event. This is concluded by a report summarizing the underlying causes and contributing factors leading to the event accompanied by recommendations to prevent or minimize recurrence.

The RCA Process

Prior to conducting the RCA, it is important to determine whether a risk to patients or employees exists, if it requires immediate action, and what appropriate actions should be taken (McDonald & Leyhane, 2005). In many healthcare organizations, this is accomplished through a team effort and may include stopping processes, taking equipment out of service, or performing other actions to ensure a safe environment.

Dialysis facilities have responsibilities to report to regulatory and healthcare safety organizations if an event is classified as a preventable, serious adverse event. Leaders of these facilities must be familiar with individual state regulations, laws, processes, and expectations. They need to know the expected timeframe for reporting and understand that timely reporting is critical.

Prior to conducting the RCA, it is also prudent to define the role of leaders and facilitators. As stated previously, an effective RCA requires involving a interdisciplinary staff at all levels who are closest to the event and those with decision-making authority. The team must have the flexibility to meet as often as necessary and be provided with the dedicated resources and time. The team must be empowered to complete its assessment and make recommendations for change while working with policy-driven established tools, structure, and timelines (McDonald & Leyhane, 2005). A policy to this effect must be developed, including the structure and timeline of the committee, and how RCA will be reported when it is completed. It should address tracking and monitoring of the implemented recommendations. Unit/facility policy must support consistent implementation of the recommended changes to reduce the likelihood of the event recurring.

Rooney and Vanden Heuvel (2004) describe a four-step process for conducting RCA: data collection, causal factor charting, root cause identification, and generating recommendations. They add a fifth step, preceding data collection, to emphasize the importance of clearly defining the problem prior to the investigation.

RCA Step 1: Clearly State and Define the Undesired Outcome

In most cases, undesired outcomes and events are straightforward. However, when there is a question, it may be necessary to review the organization standard at the time and compare it with the event that occurred. When there is a gap between them, a problem exists. Examples of undesired events include a patient fall, recurrence of the same dialysis machine alarms, or an employee who sustains a needle stick following treatment termination.

RCA Step 2: Data Collection

Complete information will help the RCA team understand the event and the factors associated with it. This is the most time-intensive step. Much of the information will come from documentation or through interviews with involved staff. They may be able to critically assess the contributing factors because of their proximity or involvement. In the case of interviews, it must begin immediately so the facts of the events will still be fresh. Questions that may be asked in order to identify the facts surrounding the undesired outcome may include:
- When did the event occur?
- Where did it occur?
- What conditions were present prior to its occurrence?
- What controls or barriers could have prevented its occurrence?
- What are all the potential causes?
- What actions can prevent recurrence?

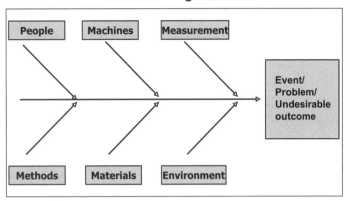

Figure 3-2
Fishbone Diagram Tool

Source: Ishikawa, 1985.
Adapted and used with permission from Leonor Ponferrada.

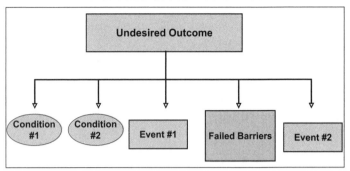

Figure 3-3
Event and Causal Factor Tree

Source: NASA Safety Training Center Course, 2003.

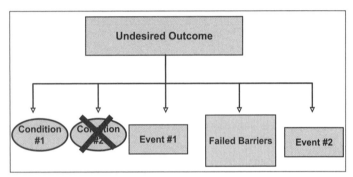

Figure 3-4
Event and Causal Factor Tree

Source: NASA Safety Training Center Course, 2003.

Table 3-4
Root Cause Investigation Plan and Results

Potential Causes	Priority	Evidence	Results

Source: Used with permission from Leonor Ponferrada.

The time frame for data collected should start at a date prior to the actual adverse event and must start at a time sufficient to add confidence that all the environmental and contributing factors are described and recognized (McDonald & Leyhane, 2005).

RCA Step 3: Create an Event and Causal Factor Chart

Causal factors are those contributors (human errors, and system and process failures) that if eliminated, would have either prevented the occurrence or reduced its severity. Charting causal factors provides a structure for investigators to organize and analyze the information gathered during the investigation, and to identify gaps and deficiencies in knowledge as the investigation progresses.

A tool that can be helpful at this stage is the fishbone diagram (Ishikawa, 1985). A fishbone diagram, also called a cause and effect diagram, is an effective tool to use in RCA. It is simple and helps the team identify factors related to the event. It addresses both system and process causes on one page. One starts out with a skeleton fishbone (see Figure 3-2), with the "head" labeled as the undesired outcome. Major branches are labeled with pertinent process factors, such as people,

machines, methods, and materials. The fishbone process must involve brainstorming and plotting of all possible causes by employees who are closest to the process. One must remember, however, that the cause and effect diagram is a list of *potential* root causes. This may include probable causes and root causes, as well as guesses. Each cause, therefore, must be reviewed and supported with data. All possible causes must be prioritized as to their possible contribution to the problem or event, and a hypothesis test must be performed to evaluate each potential cause (see Table 3-4).

Another tool that can be used during this step is to create a causal factor tree (NASA Safety Training Center Course, 2003). When using this tool, one starts by placing the undesired outcome at the top of the tree. All events, conditions, and exceeded or failed barriers that occurred immediately before the undesired outcome that might have contributed to it are added (see Figure 3-3).

- Events are real-time occurrences describing one discreet action, typically an error, failure, or malfunction. For example, a patient is dialyzed with the wrong dialysate.
- A condition is any state that may or may not result from an event and may have safety, health, quality, security, operational, or environmental implications. A patient developing

arrhythmias because of the wrong dialysate is a condition.

- A barrier may be a physical device or an administrative control used to reduce the risk of the undesired outcome to an acceptable level. Barriers can provide physical intervention (such as a guardrail) or procedural separation in time and space. An example of a barrier is to prevent the adverse event of dialyzing a patient on the wrong dialyzer by requiring two staff members to check a reprocessed dialyzer for the correct patient identification and information prior to treatment initiation.

The causal factor tree is a sequence diagram that describes the events leading up to an occurrence, the conditions surrounding it, and exceeded or failed barriers. Using this tool should begin as soon as investigators start to collect information about the occurrence. It should continue to be modified as long as relevant facts are uncovered and until such time when the investigators are satisfied with the thoroughness of the investigation. For example, if solid data indicate that one of the possible causes is not applicable, it can be eliminated from the tree (see Figure 3-4). Because of the complexity in health care, it is rare that undesired outcomes are the results of a single causal factor (McDonald & Leyhane, 2005). Events are usually the result of a combination of multiple contributors, and when only one causal factor is addressed, the recommendations will likely not be sufficient to prevent the recurrence.

When all possible causes have been identified, one of the

Table 3-5
How to Complete the "5-Whys"

Write down a potential cause.
Ask why the problem happens and write the answer down below the problem.
If the answer does not identify the root cause in step 2, ask why again and write down that answer.
Repeat step 3 until the investigation team is in agreement that the problem's root cause is identified.
Review preceding data collection.

Source: Williams, 2001.
Adapted and used with permission from Leonor Ponferrada.

Table 3-6
Increase in Peritonitis Rate

Potential Cause: Ineffective Patient Education
Why #1 – 72% staff turnover, one-third of staff have less than 1 year of experience.
Why #2 – Ineffective staff education.
Why #3 – Nurse manager on extended family leave (root cause).

Source: Used with permission from Leonor Ponferrada.

Figure 3-5
Event and Causal Factor Tree

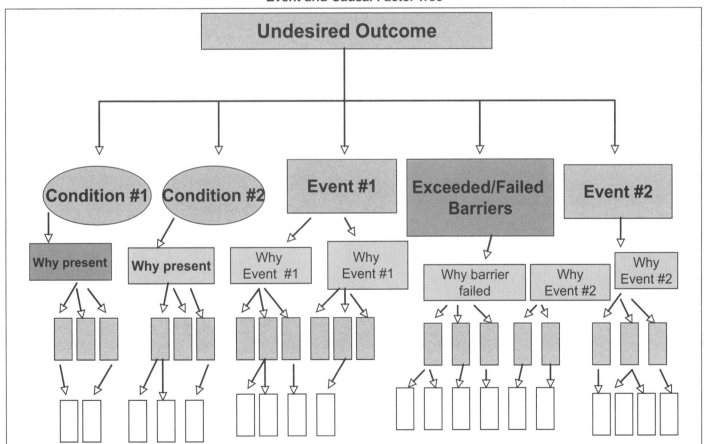

Source: NASA Safety Training Center Course, 2003

Figure 3-6
Event and Causal Factor Tree

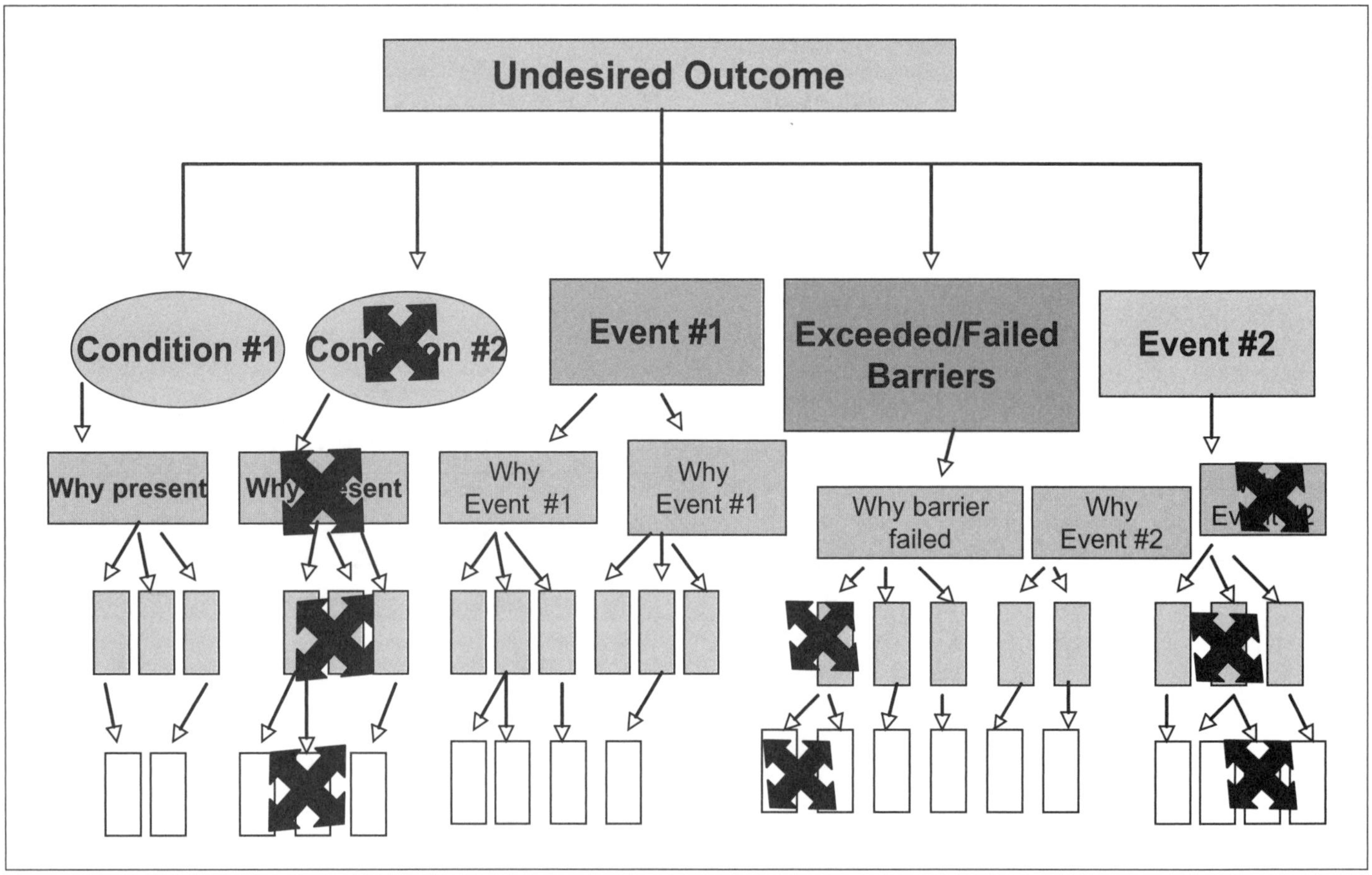

Source: NASA Safety Training Center Course, 2003.

Table 3-7
Root Cause Summary Event/Problem Description

Root Cause #1	Path Through Root Cause	Recommendations
Root cause #2	Path Through Root Cause	Recommendations
Root cause #3	Path through root cause	Recommendations

Source: Adapted from Rooney & Vanden Heuvel, 2004.
Used with permission from Leonor Ponferrada.

tests to determine the root cause is the 5-why analysis (see Table 3-5). It is a simple technique used by repeatedly asking "why" did each possible cause happen (Williams, 2001). The "why" question will need to be asked until the root cause(s) is/are reached. This includes all organizational factors that exert control over the undesired outcome. For any identified cause, the "5 why" is complete or discontinued when:
• Root cause is identified.

• Data are insufficient to continue.
• You reach a point when you decide that the problem is not correctable.

Theoretically, these decisions will be obvious by the 5th "why;" however, all "5 whys" are not necessarily required to drill down to the root causes. Each level must show logical relationship response to the one that preceded it. The "why" process stops when the team has enough information to identify the root cause. Again, each level of cause must be confirmed by data that had been collected. The 5-why technique is most helpful when problems involve human factors or interactions. Table 3-5 describes the steps to complete the 5 whys. This technique should be applied on a single cause factor at a time, and questions must be focused on the original issue. The resultant tree of questions and answers should lead to a comprehensive picture of potential causes for the undesired outcome. Table 3-6 shows an example of 5-Why technique. This example only requires 3 "whys" to get to the root cause of the problem.

RCA Step 4: Root Cause Identification

This step may involve the use of a decision diagram (see Figure 3-5) to identify the underlying reason(s) for each causal factor (NASA Safety Training Center Course, 2003). This is

Figure 3-7
Root Cause Identification

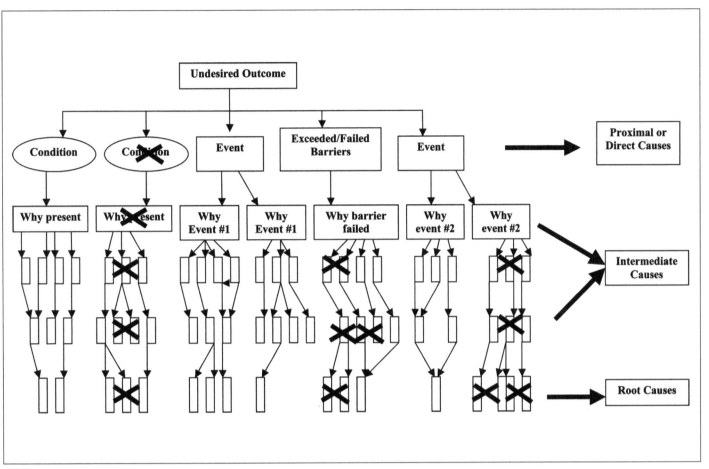

Source: NASA Safety Training Center Course, 2003.

where logic or the use of the 5-why analysis is helpful and why it is important to back the investigation with data. Digging down to the root cause of a problem can sometimes be difficult and uncomfortable for the RCA team and for management; however, long-term benefits and patient care outcomes must outweigh the discomfort (McDonald & Leyhane, 2005). The test is to ask if the event, condition, or barrier in question:

• Was corrected.
• Was eliminated or avoided.

Could the undesired outcome have been prevented or avoided? If the answer is yes, then it is a root cause and it should be kept in the tree. If the answer is no, then it should be eliminated from the tree (see Figure 3-6).

In some situations, it may be difficult to be 100% certain that an event or condition is a cause because the data necessary to provide certainty may not be available or are incomplete. In these situations, the RCA team can use the term "probable" to describe the cause and consider it as a reasonable cause, having more evidence for it than against (NASA Safety Training Center Course, 2003). These probable causes should remain on the tree until disproved. The remaining items on the tree are the causes necessary to produce the undesired outcome and can be categorized as proximate, intermediate, and root causes (see Figure 3-7).

RCA 5th and Final Step: Presentation Of Recommendations Generated From the Investigation

At a minimum, corrective actions should be generated to eliminate proximate causes and eliminate or mitigate the negative effects of root causes. In situations when multiple causes exist and there is limited budget, a quantitative analysis can be used to determine the total contribution of each cause to the undesirable outcome (NASA Safety Training Center Course, 2003). Analysis of the cause and effect diagram will help in setting priorities to arrange causes in order of importance. Those causes that contribute most to the undesirable outcome should be a focus for elimination, or the negative effects should be alleviated to minimize the risk. Presentation of results may be done in various ways. Table 3-7 shows one example of a root cause summary showing each root cause, the paths through root cause map associated with the causal factor, and recommendations to address each root cause identified (Rooney & Vanden Heuvel, 2004).

Recommendations for corrective actions must include timelines for implementation, monitoring strategies, and outcome measures (McDonald & Leyhane, 2005). In some situations, the RCA team may not be involved in the implementation of recommendations suggested, but they must be involved in the monitoring and review of outcomes. If the recommendations suggested are not implemented, the time and effort expended in the investigation and analysis are wasted, and the undesired outcome will likely recur. This will certainly discourage participation from employees in future RCA investigations. Recurrence of similar events are costly for the organization, and in situations where events compromise patient safety and/or violates compliance to imposed regulations, it may result in significant monetary fines or suspension of clinical operations. Organizations need to ensure that recommendations are tracked to completion.

Conclusion

Root cause analysis is an essential process for any organization that wants to continue to improve and is willing to engage in serious introspection and analysis (Dew, 2003b). RCA is a valuable management tool that can be readily learned by managers as well as frontline personnel. A review of the literature by Percapio and colleagues (2008) revealed that although there is still limited evidence of its effectiveness in health care, there is anecdotal evidence that RCA improves safety. The approach has been helpful in making meaningful changes and has helped organizations develop protocols that set the stage for reducing errors and preventing recurrence of adverse events.

There are several tools that are useful in performing RCA. These tools can be used alone or in combination during an RCA investigation. There are also a number of private businesses and consultants that provide services and assistance to help organizations in performance improvement. They can provide specialized training programs and suggest RCA tools to help organizations that are interested in their services. RCA can be conducted at several levels of depth and complexity. It is moving beyond simply telling employees "to be more careful in the future" as a consequence to an undesired event (Williams, 2001). The results of RCA can lead to lasting corrective actions that will improve outcomes and patient safety in a dialysis or other facility.

References

Bagian, J.P., Gosbee, J., Lee, C.Z., Williams, L., McKnight, S.D., & Mannos, D.M. (2002). The Veterans Affairs root cause analysis system in action. *Joint Commission Journal Quality Improvement*, 28, 531-545.

Dew, J.R. (2003a). *Using root cause analysis to make the patient care system safe*. Retrieved February 24, 2009, from http://bama.ua.edu/~st497/UsingRootCauseAnalysis%20.htm

Dew, J. (2003b). The seven deadly sins of quality management. *Quality Progress, 36*(9), 59-65.

Ishikawa, K. (1985). *What is total quality control? The Japanese way.* Englewood Cliffs, NJ; Prentice Hall.

Latino, R.J., & Latino, K.C. (2006). *Improving performance for bottom-line results.* (3rd ed.). Boca Raton, FL: CRC Press.

McDonald, A., & Leyhane, T. (2005). Drill down with root cause analysis. *Nursing Management, 36*(10), 26-32.

NASA Safety Training Center Course. (2003). *Root cause analysis: Overview.* Retrieved February 24, 2009, from http://www.hq.nasa.gov/office/codeq/rca/rootcauseppt.pdf

Percapio, K.B., Watts, B.V., & Weeks, W.B. (2008). The effectiveness of root cause analysis: What does the literature tell us? *The Joint Commission Journal on Quality and Patient Safety, 34*(7), 391-398.

Reason, J.T. (1990). *Human error*. New York: Cambridge University Press.

Rooney, J., & Vanden Heuvel, L. (2004). *Root cause analysis for beginners. Quality progress.* Milwaukee, WI; American Society for Quality.

Rummler, G., & Brache, A. (1990). *Improving performance: How to manage the white space on the organization chart.* San Francisco: Josey Bass, Inc.

Wald, H., & Shojania, K. (2001). Root cause analysis. In K.G. Shojania, B.W. Duncan, K.M. MacDonald, & R.M. Wachter (Eds.), *Making health care safer: A critical analysis of patient safety practices.* Retrieved February 25, 2009, from http://www.ahrq.gov/clinic/ptsafety/

Wichman, K., & Greenall, J. (2006). Using root cause analysis to determine the system-based causes of error. *Canadian Pharmaceutical Journal, 139*(3), 63-65.

Williams, P.M. (2001). Techniques for root cause analysis. *Baylor University Medical Center Proceedings, 14*(2), 154-157.

Wu, A.W., Lipshutz, A.K., & Pronovost, P.J. (2008). Effectiveness and efficiency of root cause analysis in medicine. *Journal of American Medical Association, 299*(6), 685-687.

Additional Readings

Institute of Medicine. (1999). *To err is human: Building a safer health system*. Washington, DC: National Academy Press.

The Joint Commission on the Accreditation of Healthcare Organizations. (2007). *Sentinel event policy and procedures.* Retrieved January 21, 2009, from www.jointcommission.org/SentinelEvents/PolicyandProcedures.htm

| Chapter 3 | CONTINUING NURSING EDUCATION EVALUATION FORM | 1.1 Contact Hours |

ANNP0903

Root Cause Analysis in Quality Improvement

Applying Continuous Quality Improvement in Clinical Practice contains 22 chapters of educational content. Individual learners may apply for continuing nursing education credit by reading a chapter and completing the Continuing Nursing Education Evaluation Form for that chapter. Learners may apply for continuing nursing education credit for any or all chapters.

Please photocopy this test page, complete, and return to ANNA.
You can also download this form from www.annanurse.org (choose Education - CNE Activities - Publications)
Receive continuing nursing education credit (CNE) immediately by completing the CNE evaluation process in ANNA's Online Library. Go to www.annanurse.org, and click on the Online Library icon for more information.

Name: _____

Address: _____

City: _____ State: _____ Zip: _____

E-mail:_____ Preferred telephone: ☐ Home ☐ Work_____

State where licensed and license number: _____

CNE application fees are based upon the number of contact hours provided by the individual section. CNE fees per contact hour for ANNA members are as follows: 1.0-1.9 – $15; 2.0-2.9 – $20; 3.0-3.9 – $25; 4.0 and higher – $30. Fees for nonmembers are $10 higher.

CNE application fee for Chapter 3: ANNA member $15   Nonmember $25

ANNA Member: ☐ Yes ☐ No   ☐ Member # (if available) _____

☐ Check or money order enclosed   ☐ American Express   ☐ Visa   ☐ MasterCard

Total amount submitted:_____

Credit card number _____ Exp. Date _____

Name as it appears on the card: _____

NOTE: Your evaluation form can be processed in 1 week for an additional rush charge of $5.00.

☐ **Yes, I would like this evaluation form rush processed. I have included an additional fee of $5.00 for rush processing.**

Instructions

1. To receive continuing nursing education credit for an individual study after reading the chapter, complete this evaluation form.

2. Detach, photocopy, or download (www.annanurse.org) the evaluation form and send along with a check or money order payable to **American Nephrology Nurses' Assocation** to: ANNA, East Holly Avenue Box 56, Pitman, NJ 08071-0056.

3. Test returns must be postmarked by **April 30, 2011**. Upon completion of the answer/evaluation form, a certificate will be sent to you.

This section was reviewed and formatted for contact hour credit by Sally S. Russell, MN, CMSRN, ANNA Director of Education Services.

> **CNE Application Fee for Chapter 3**
> **ANNA member = $15**
> **Nonmember = $25**

1. I verify that I have read this chapter and completed this education activity. _____ Date _____
   Signature

2. What would be different in your practice if you applied what you have learned from this activity? (Please use additional paper if necessary.)
   _____
   _____
   _____
   _____

	Strongly disagree				Strongly agree
3. The activity met the stated objectives.					
a. Define root cause analysis (RCA).	1	2	3	4	5
b. Identify 5 basic elements of a process.	1	2	3	4	5
c. List 3 general principles of root cause analysis.	1	2	3	4	5
d. Describe 5 steps in conducting a root cause analysis.	1	2	3	4	5
e. Illustrate causal factor charting.	1	2	3	4	5
4. The content was current and relevant.	1	2	3	4	5
5. The content was presented clearly.	1	2	3	4	5
6. The content was covered adequately.	1	2	3	4	5

7. How would you rate your ability to apply your learning to practice?   ☐ diminished ability   ☐ no change   ☐ enhanced ability

Comments _____
_____

8. Time required to read the chapter and complete this form: _____ minutes

Introduction to Six Sigma™

Billie Axley, MS, RN, CNN
Jackie Miller, BS, RN, CNN, CPHQ

Objectives

Study of the information presented in this chapter will enable the learner to:
1. Describe Six Sigma™ as referring to an operational philosophy, focusing on continuous improvement by decreasing the amount of variation that occurs in a process.
2. Compare two similarities and differences between continuous quality improvement methodology and Six Sigma.
3. List the steps in DMAIC methodology of Six Sigma.

Introduction

As with Dr. Edward Deming's work with the scientific method of solving problems through application of the Plan-Do-Check-Act (PDCA) cycle for continuous quality improvement (CQI), Six Sigma™ methodology uses work teams for problem solving and process improvement efforts that are data-driven. As an operational philosophy, Six Sigma focuses on continuous improvement, looking to decrease the amount of variation that occurs in a process.

What Is Six Sigma?

The term *Sigma* as a statistical concept represents the amount of "variation around the average of any process" (Brassard & Ritter, 2001, p. 4). To achieve Six Sigma, a process must not produce more than 3.4 defects per million opportunities (Brassard & Ritter, 2001). Six Sigma is used by organizations as a process improvement methodology to ensure it is improving its key process. It first identifies the key processes that would benefit most from improvement, defines and addresses a process with defects, and then provides information about what changes are working and which changes are not having an expected result (Brassard & Ritter, 2001).

Similarities in Six Sigma and CQI

In practice, Six Sigma and CQI methodologies are related. Six Sigma utilizes concepts of improvement, and many of the tools are similar to those used for CQI. For example, the PDCA remains as a part of the process for improvement (Brassard & Ritter, 2001). The improvement cycle has been translated as a six-step approach, or sub-methodology. The DMAIC methodology of Six Sigma is *Define, Measure, Analyze, Improve, and Control* (see Figure 1) (Brassard & Ritter, 2001).

Differences Between Six Sigma and CQI

Six Sigma differs from CQI, with an emphasis on more rigorous statistical methods, an aggressive schedule for the pace of improvement, and dedicated teams with dedicated projects. Full-time, dedicated employees may guide these projects (Brassard & Ritter, 2001). The employees who act as the experts in the improvement processes have formally progressed in training programs through defined levels of expertise. For example, a manager trained in the basics of Six Sigma has achieved a Green Belt level. A portion of time is generally dedicated to the support of Six Sigma initiatives working as

Figure 4-1
The DMAIC Methodology of Six Sigma

Define
- Equivalent to *Check* in PDCA.
- Find a process in need of improvement and define the problem, select the work team, and define the desired outcomes or goals of the project.

Measure
- Gain information about the process, also a part of *Check* in PDCA.
- Gather baseline data and develop the problem statement.

Analyze
- Examine the causes of the problem.
- Determine the root causes of the problem:
  - Example: Using a cause and effect diagram to identify barriers to completing intake forms within a one-week time frame.

Improve
- Equivalent to *Act* in PDCA.
- Identify actions that will reduce defects and variation created by the problem's root cause(s).
- Plan the implementation of the determined actions for improvement.

Implement
- Equivalent to *Do* in PDCA.
- Doing the changes, carrying out the plan, and measuring the results of the actions.
- As in Deming's CQI method, the question is asked, "Was there improvement?"
  - If improvement is not evident from the data, the Six Sigma team returns to step one of the cycle.

Control
- Equivalent to *Act* in PDCA.
- Incorporate successful changes into the everyday work culture of the organization.
- Involves reporting data:
  - Brassard and Ritter (2001) suggest using an updated scorecard tool to visually demonstrate the impact of the project's actions to those involved in the process and within the organization.
- Sets monitors to assure the improvements are permanent.

Source: Brassard & Ritter, 2001.
Adapted by Billie Axley. Used with permission from Billie Axley.

project team leaders. An employee at a Black Belt level would typically be a "full-time person intensively trained in quality management systems and advanced statistical tools and methods" (Brassard & Ritter, 2001, p. 5), dedicated to working on critical problems/opportunities alone or within teams (Brassard & Ritter, 2001). This individual would also be responsible for teaching, mentoring, and reviewing the work of other quality staff and managing large-scale improvement projects for the organization (Brassard & Ritter, 2001). In his work with CQI, Deming concluded that quality can be improved only if top management is part of the solution and participates in the quality improvement program. Deming advocated for CQI to be spread through organization-wide learning. Following the education process, the expectation of CQI is empowerment of all employees at all levels to lead in improvement processes (Tortorella, 1995).

Other differences may include the structure of the work team. The CQI team is selected from the organization's members on a basis of interest, expertise, and willingness. In Six Sigma, being part of an improvement team is more formal (Waddick, 2008), with a team charter developed which includes:

- "Business Case – What are the compelling business reasons for the project?" Is the project linked to key business goals and objectives? (p. 2).
- "Problem Statement – What specifically is the problem?" (p. 2).
- "Goal Statement – What is the goal or target of the improvement team's project? Meeting the SMART criteria (specific, measurable, attainable, relevant, and time-bound)" (p. 2).
- "Roles and Responsibilities" – Articulate for each team member and leadership where roles and responsibilities are documented (p. 3).
- "Project Scope – What are the boundaries of the project's scope?" What are the start and end points? How does the project manager ensure against "scope creep?" "What constraints might have an impact on the team?" (p. 3).
- "Milestones" – What is the project start date and estimated completion date? Is the project on schedule? Is there a project plan developed, and how did the project manager receive input to the development of the plan? What are the estimated completion dates of each activity? (p. 3).
- "Communication Plan" – What critical content must be communicated to whom, when, where, and how? Who receives the meeting minutes? Keep subject matter experts in the loop (p. 3).

Another difference between Six Sigma and traditional CQI may be found in conceptual time frames. For implementation, Dr. Deming's work in CQI included the need for systematic approach and the education of employees in the concepts of CQI and usage of tools. With CQI, each member of the organization continuously looks for opportunities for improvement and leads improvement projects. Emergent situations requiring immediate improvement projects may be conducted over as little as 24 to 48 hours to several days. Less emergent improvements may occur over 3 to 6 months, and based upon the specific project's needs, a CQI improvement project may occasionally span a time frame of a year.

Six Sigma seeks to create a culture that "demands perfection" (Brassard & Ritter 2001, p. 1). A "disciplined methodology" is taught by trained employees and "seems to work best when it is mandated from senior leadership" (Brassard & Ritter 2001, p. 9). For a complete Six Sigma program, Brassard and Ritter (2001) indicate that the pace of implementation varies depending upon the size of the organization, the number of people recruited and trained in Six Sigma, the competitiveness of the business environment, available financial resources, and the commitment of leadership. A "typical" implementation schedule is described by Brassard & Ritter (2001) for a mid-to-large size company, and although the actual size and complexity of the organization is not specifically indicated, it may be as follows:

- "Diagnose and plan: 0 to 6 months."
- "Introduce and build a solid foundation: 6 to 12 months."
- "Expand: 12 to 24 months."
- "Improve: 24 or more months" (Brassard & Ritter 2001, p.12).

Tools Used in Six Sigma

Common to both CQI and Six Sigma is the use of the run chart, Pareto chart, fishbone diagram (cause and effect), and flowcharts. Several tools may be considered for frequent use in the Six Sigma DMAIC methodology (Brassard & Ritter, 2001), including:

- Affinity diagram – "A graphic tool that organizes a large number of the team's ideas on an issue" (p. 192).
- Cause and effect diagram – "A graphic tool used to identify and organize all possible causes that influence an outcome" (p. 192).
- Control charts – Graphic chart that monitors "whether the process is stable or in control" (p. 192).
- Histogram – "A bar graph showing the frequency distribution of the process output, including centering and variation" (p. 192).
- Pareto chart – A bar chart which ranks identified causes.
- Scatter diagram – A graphic chart looking at the relationship between two variables.
- Tree diagram – A detailed list of "assignable tasks necessary to accomplish a broad goal" (p. 192).
- Failure Mode and Effects Analysis (FMEA) (Rath & Strong 2003):
  ○ Used most frequently in *Measure* and *Improve* phases.
  ○ A method to identify, estimate, and evaluate the risk associated with each potential defect or failure.
  ○ Identification of the effect for each potential failure on customer requirements.
  ○ Allows the team to focus resources on the greatest risk first. The goal with this tool is failure prevention.
- Cycle time:
  ○ A tool to identify the time required for each process step and total time for completion of product or service.
- "SIPOC":
  ○ High level process map that includes identification of:
    ➤ Suppliers.
    ➤ Inputs.
    ➤ Processes.
    ➤ Outputs.
    ➤ Customers.

Table 4-1
Intake Data Form Completion Table

	Initial Data	Form Standardization and Training	Scope of Practice – Training and Control
% Intake Form Complete	87%	100%	96%
% Intake Form Timely	48%	76%	86%
% MSP Complete	61%	67%	90%
% MSP Timely	42%	46%	79%
Sigma	1.81	2.26	3.03
P Value			0.004
Comment	Intake form completion required follow up from intake to facility.	Intake form completion required follow up from intake to facilty.	Form completion did not require follow up.

Source: Used with permission from Billie Axley and Jackie Miller.

Clinical Application of Six Sigma: New Patient Registration (Intake) Process Six Sigma Project

A project scope covered the registration and insurance review process for multiple state dialysis programs. The project team included three representatives from social services, two from the intake department, two from management, and one from the quality team. The regional vice president was champion and sponsor. Each dialysis facility received a new patient referral and completed intake forms with patient demographics and insurance information, such as Medicare-required Medicare Secondary Payer (MSP) and 2728 forms. The intake department verified coverage, entered the patient into an electronic medical record system, and set up billing with the appropriate provider. The senior management team approved this project as the percentage of patients without secondary coverage was trending upward. The accurate, timely flow of information to the intake department has an impact on the percentage of patients without secondary coverage.

Define, Measure, Analyze, Improve, Control (DMAIC) Methodology

Initial data collection results (see Table 4-1) showed 87% compliance with intake form completion, while 48% were timely. The secondary payer form completion was 61% in compliance, and 42% were timely. Data collection barriers included a variety of intake forms and faxes used by the facilities. The initial forms reviewed included hospital fact sheets and outdated forms that did not contain the required data elements. The completion of the intake forms required follow up calls to the facility for required information. Initial Sigma was calculated at 1.81.

Phase 1 – Quick Hit: Standardization of Forms

Results improved to 100% intake form completion, although follow-up calls were required from the intake department staff to complete the required data fields. Timeliness and completion of the MSP form showed slight improvement. Sigma level was calculated to be 2.26.

Cause and Effect Matrix Completed by Team

The Cause and Effect Matrix identified three critical defects in the intake process:

- Lack of standard operating procedure (SOP).
- Inconsistent data collection from the patient referral source, both hospital and physician office. Data included insurance, demographic, and contact information.
- Availability of staff trained on the intake process and paperwork on all patient shifts.

The team completed data collection on error type on each form submitted to the intake department, which were ranked on a Pareto chart. The tools identified the most frequent errors as incorrect form, omission of nephrologist's name, missing treatment start date, and illegible forms. The team implemented solutions and completed the statistical review with control charts and one-way ANOVA (see Figure 4-2 and Table 4-2). The ANOVA test validates the changes in processes resulted in statistically significant improvements. The control chart (see Table 4-2) identifies changes in percentage of patients without secondary coverage at each phase of the project.

Solutions

Form standardization was the quick hit.

- Delays were caused by back order of packets containing the required forms and obtaining approval to use the form throughout the area, as required by the organization's regional billing offices.
- The team learned the intake process existed but was not available in the facilities.
- The team updated the SOP, and copies were sent to facilities. Training on the use of forms and an SOP was completed via conference calls.
- As the project continued, the team discovered that a second

Figure 4-2
Individual – Moving Range Control Chart

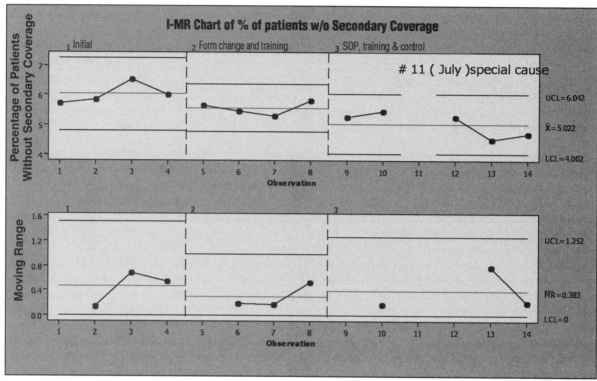

Source: Used with permission from Jackie Miller.

round of training was necessary. The facilities could not assure that a trained social worker, facility manager, or administrative assistant would be available on all shifts to cover new patients starting therapy.

- Management met with the referral source to assure the availability of the necessary patient registration information prior to accepting a patient into the outpatient facility.

Project Results

The project goal was to decrease the number of patients without secondary coverage to 5% and have 100% of forms completed in an accurate and timely framework. The control chart illustrates improvement in the percentage of patients without secondary insurance (see Figure 4-2). The July data were excluded as special cause variation, which is an unusual event that has an impact on a product or service. In this project, the number of new patients starting in July was an outlier, with greater than 60 patients starting dialysis. Special cause variation is reviewed and corrected independently. Results showed 3.86% patients without secondary coverage at the conclusion of the project.

The financial impact of the project was estimated and shared with the management team. An unintended consequence of the project was the reassignment of one of the intake coordinators as rework decreased. In the control phase, reports were developed to identify where patients were in the process of obtaining secondary insurance. These reports are

valuable to the facility managers in assuring that appropriate interventions are in place to obtain secondary coverage. Total project time was 12 months.

Lessons Learned

In this example of the registration process, utilizing Six Sigma methodologies to improve a process required the use of tools that would validate process change. This project demonstrated a statistically significant improvement in a process but did not reach the Six Sigma level or 3.4 defects per million opportunities. The Six Sigma tool set is very valuable in improving an existing process in healthcare setting.

Conclusion

Similar to CQI, Six Sigma engenders creating a culture of improvement, and the core principles of Six Sigma according to Brassard and Ritter (2001, p. 4) should be followed. These are:

- "Focus on customer satisfaction."
- "Increase revenue and reduce costs."
- "Improve performance project-by-project."
- "Priority of projects are based on their impact on the business."
- "Manage the organization as a system of connected process."
- "Apply the scientific approach – Plan-Do-Check-Act (PDCA)."
- "Pursue near perfection."
- "Use the full range of statistical tools for analyzing and solving problems."

Table 4-2
One-Way ANOVA
(Without July Initial and Control Only)

Source	DF	SS	MS	F	P
C14	1	2.314	2.314	13.36	0.008
Error	7	1.213	0.173		
Total	8	1.527			

Notes: S = 0.4162; R-Sq = 65.62%; R-Sq(adj) = 60.71%
July data not included in calculation as it was identified as an outlier.
Table reflects reporting in the control phase of DMAIC methodology.
Source: Used with permission from Jackie Miller.

Individual 95% CIs for Mean Based on Pooled Standard Deviation

Level	N	Mean	SD	Scale
1	4	6.0225	0.3661	5.00
3	5	5.0020	0.4501	5.50
				6.00
				6.50

Note: CI = confidence intervals.
Source: Used with permission from Jackie Miller.

- "Respect and build upon the knowledge, experience, and dedication of individuals throughout the organization."

It is important to ensure that every person is aware of the organization's commitment to its mission and vision. Keeping values in every aspect of the organization's foundation is core to both CQI and Six Sigma methodologies.

References

Brassard, M., & Ritter, D. (2001). *Sailing through Six Sigma: How the power of people can perfect processes and drive down costs.* Marietta, GA; Brassard & Ritter, LLC.

Rath & Strong. (2003). *Rath & Strong's Six Sigma pocket guide.* Lexington, MA; Rath & Strong Management Consultants.

Tortorella, M.J. (1995). The three careers of W. Edwards Deming. *Siam News.* Retrieved December 12, 2008, from http://deming.org/index.cfm?content=652

Waddick, P. (2008). *Six Sigma DMAIC quick reference – Define phase.* Retrieved December 12, 2008, from http://www.isixsigma.com/library/content/six_sigma_dmaic_quickref_define.asp

| **Chapter 4** | **CONTINUING NURSING EDUCATION EVALUATION FORM** | **1.2 Contact Hours** |

Introduction to Six Sigma™

ANNP0904

Applying Continuous Quality Improvement in Clinical Practice contains 22 chapters of educational content. Individual learners may apply for continuing nursing education credit by reading a chapter and completing the Continuing Nursing Education Evaluation Form for that chapter. Learners may apply for continuing nursing education credit for any or all chapters.

Please photocopy this test page, complete, and return to ANNA.
You can also download this form from www.annanurse.org (choose Education - CNE Activities - Publications)
Receive continuing nursing education credit (CNE) immediately by completing the CNE evaluation process in ANNA's Online Library. Go to www.annanurse.org, and click on the Online Library icon for more information.

Name: _____

Address: _____

City: _____ State: _____ Zip: _____

E-mail:_____ Preferred telephone: ☐ Home ☐ Work _____

State where licensed and license number: _____

CNE application fees are based upon the number of contact hours provided by the individual section. CNE fees per contact hour for ANNA members are as follows: 1.0-1.9 – $15; 2.0-2.9 – $20; 3.0-3.9 – $25; 4.0 and higher – $30. Fees for nonmembers are $10 higher.

CNE application fee for Chapter 4: ANNA member $15   Nonmember $25

ANNA Member: ☐ Yes ☐ No   ☐ Member # (if available) _____

☐ Check or money order enclosed   ☐ American Express   ☐ Visa   ☐ MasterCard

Total amount submitted:_____

Credit card number _____ Exp. Date _____

Name as it appears on the card: _____

NOTE: Your evaluation form can be processed in 1 week for an additional rush charge of $5.00.

☐ **Yes, I would like this evaluation form rush processed. I have included an additional fee of $5.00 for rush processing.**

Instructions

1. To receive continuing nursing education credit for an individual study after reading the chapter, complete this evaluation form.

2. Detach, photocopy, or download (www.annanurse.org) the evaluation form and send along with a check or money order payable to **American Nephrology Nurses' Assocation** to: ANNA, East Holly Avenue Box 56, Pitman, NJ 08071-0056.

3. Test returns must be postmarked by **April 30, 2011**. Upon completion of the answer/evaluation form, a certificate will be sent to you.

This section was reviewed and formatted for contact hour credit by Sally S. Russell, MN, CMSRN, ANNA Director of Education Services.

CNE Application Fee for Chapter 4
ANNA member = $15
Nonmember = $25

1. I verify that I have read this chapter and completed this education activity. _____ Date _____
   Signature

2. What would be different in your practice if you applied what you have learned from this activity? (Please use additional paper if necessary.)
   _____
   _____
   _____
   _____

	Strongly disagree				Strongly agree
3. The activity met the stated objectives.					
a. Describe Six Sigma™ as referring to an operational philosophy, focusing on continuous improvement by decreasing the amount of variation that occurs in a process.	1	2	3	4	5
b. Compare two similarities and differences between continuous quality improvement methodology and Six Sigma.	1	2	3	4	5
c. List the steps in DMAIC methodology of Six Sigma.	1	2	3	4	5
4. The content was current and relevant.	1	2	3	4	5
5. The content was presented clearly.	1	2	3	4	5
6. The content was covered adequately.	1	2	3	4	5

7. How would you rate your ability to apply your learning to practice?   ☐ diminished ability   ☐ no change   ☐ enhanced ability

Comments _____
_____

8. Time required to read the chapter and complete this form: _____ minutes

This educational activity is provided by the American Nephrology Nurses' Association (ANNA).
ANNA is accredited as a provider of continuing nursing education (CNE) by the American Nurses Credentialing Center's Commission on Accreditation (ANCC-COA).
ANNA is a provider approved of continuing nursing education by the California Board of Registered Nursing, provider number CEP 00910.
This CNE offering meets the Nephrology Nursing Certification Commission's (NNCC's) continuing nursing education requirements for certification and recertification.

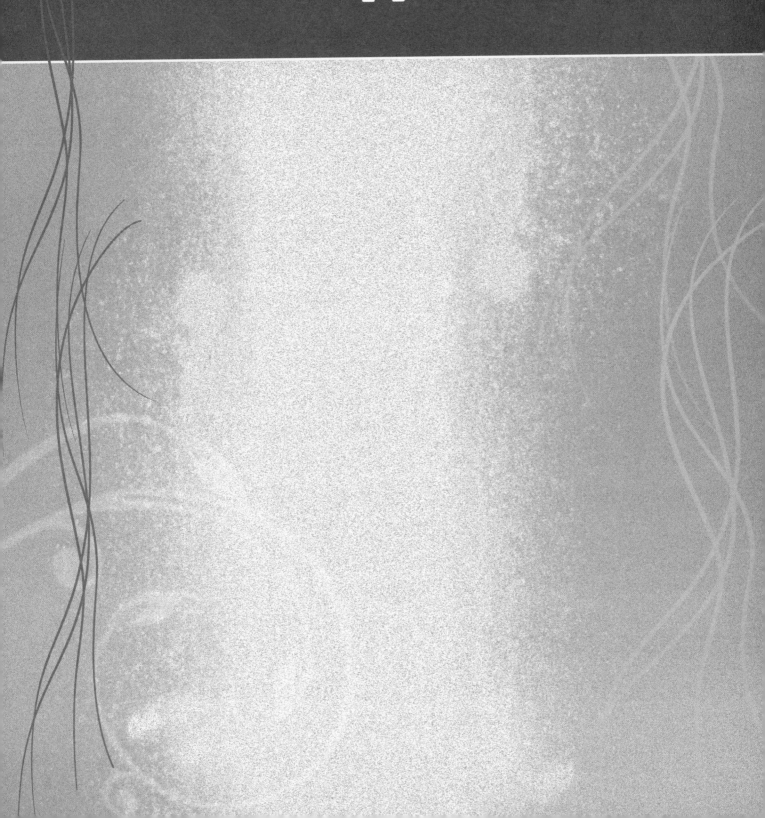

Section 2:
Clinical Applications

Clinical Application:
CQI in Anemia and Iron Management

Gail Wick, MHSA, BSN, RN, CNN

Objectives

Study of the information presented in this chapter will enable the learner to:
1. Explain how anemia and iron management are interrelated.
2. Describe the Check-Plan-Do-Check-Act cycle as related to iron management and patients with anemia.

Introduction

Providing adequate treatment for anemia and iron issues in a patient with renal dysfunction is dependent on numerous factors, ranging from co-morbid conditions and erythropoietin stimulating agent (ESA) dosing to having adequate iron available for erythropoiesis.

Iron management goes hand-in-hand with anemia management because two of the most common issues of hyporesponse to ESA therapy are iron deficiency and iron-restricted erythropoiesis. Common reasons are 1) failure to replenish iron from blood loss, 2) failure to replenish iron used for erythropoiesis, and 3) lack of iron availability due to infection/inflammation. Because of the interrelatedness of anemia and iron outcomes, they are considered together throughout this chapter.

Basic responsibilities of caregivers in managing anemia and iron outcomes include:
- Ongoing assessment of the patient and his or her treatment regimen.
- Timely and appropriate evaluation and intervention when issues arise.
- Clear, specific, and regular documentation of data; processes being used; interventions undertaken; and outcomes.
- Practice based on current standards and research.

Check-Plan-Do-Check-Act Cycle

To most effectively manage anemia and iron, use a formal continuous quality improvement (CQI) process. The CQI model used in this chapter is the Check-Plan-Do-Check-Act (CPDCA) cycle outlined in Chapter 1, "Concepts and Principles of Quality Management."

Chapter Guide

This chapter on anemia and iron management contains tools that can be used during the CQI process. Numerous quality improvement tools for adaptation or adoption into CQI programs, as well as case studies, are provided. Keep in mind that the goals of all actions are to provide high-quality patient care and to be a "Best-Practice" facility in anemia/iron management (see Figure 5-1).

Chapter Contents
Case Studies (Items 1 and 2)

A case study, which shows how a quality improvement team identifies infection as a root cause of hyporesponse in a

Figure 5-1
A Best-Practice Facility

- Sets and achieves anemia/iron management goals based on current science and consensus.
- Consistently follows physician-approved "state-of-the-art" anemia/iron management protocols, algorithms, or clinical practice guidelines (if in place) within the framework of a formal CQI program.
- Monitors hemoglobin (Hb) trends at least every 4 weeks depending on dosing changes and laboratory values.
- Maintains anemia/iron laboratory values based on current community standards.
- Evaluates hyporesponse factors in patients who fail to achieve or maintain target Hb and trends the hyporesponse factors within the facility.
- Analyzes and records data at least monthly to benchmark the facility's quality progress.
- Documents patient outcomes and changes in treatment plans, as well as quality improvements.
- Documents overall facility efforts to improve and maintain quality goals.

Source: Used with permission from Gail Wick.

patient, is included (Item 1). Additionally, a case study of a unit-wide quality improvement project is provided (Item 2).

Tip Chart for Anemia/Iron Issues (Item 3)

This chart describes changes in hematological and iron indices. Use it with the "Hyporesponse to the ESA Therapy Tool" discussed below to guide your assessments.

Iron-Related Considerations in ESA Hyporesponse (Item 4)

This chart outlines laboratory value changes that can occur with absolute iron deficiency and iron restricted erythropoiesis –functional iron deficiency and infection/inflammatory iron block. Use it with the "Hyporesponse to ESA Therapy Documentation Tool" (Item 12) discussed later in this chapter to guide your assessments.

Data Reports (Item 5)

Ongoing data collection is an important part of the

"Check" in the CPDCA cycle. Laboratory reports used to assess anemia/iron quality-related issues should include 3 to 6 months of laboratory data to include hemoglobin, TIBC, TSAT, serum ferritin, reticulocyte percent, PTH, and albumin. The laboratory values should be compared and trended to identify quality outcome issues as well as response to therapy. If at all possible, automate reports to make data collection more efficient. A sample report layout is shown (Item 5).

Anemia-Related Cause and Effect (Fishbone) Diagrams (Items 6, 7 and 8)

Three anemia-related cause and effect (root cause) diagrams are included. The "Anemia and Iron Management: Success in Reaching Targets" diagram highlights the factors that must be in place for an anemia and iron management program to succeed. The "Response to ESA Therapy" diagram lists the most common reasons why a patient does not respond to ESA therapy. It provides a broad overview of what must be considered if a patient's hemoglobin (Hb) is not within the target range. The "Response to ESA Therapy: Iron-Related Factors" diagram lists what must be considered for iron-related issues.

ESA IV Dosing Protocols (Items 9 and 10)

The Epogen® and Aranesp® IV Dosing Protocols samples illustrate guiding principles for dosing, a math helper, and a step-by-step guide to dosing ESAs based on laboratory values. These should be modified as needed to match the clinical practice philosophy of the treating physicians as well as current research and best practice. A protocol must be approved and signed by the physician prior to use with patients.

Sample IV Iron Dosing Protocol (Item 11)

This sample protocol illustrates factors to be considered in IV iron dosing.

Hyporesponse to ESA Therapy Documentation Tool (Item 12)

This documentation tool provides a checklist format to document that the common reasons for failure to obtain hemoglobin target goals have been explored, and hopefully, identified. It serves as the basis for the CQI action plan.

Anemia/Iron Assessment and Root Cause Trending Tool (Item 13)

Once you have identified the root causes of failure to respond to ESA therapy on each patient, trend them on this tool. The tool will assist you in determining the root causes that are most prevalent in your unit. With this knowledge, you can put systems and processes in place to prevent the most common causes of failure to obtain or sustain anemia and iron goals.

CQI Project Action Plan (Items 14 and 15)

Two sample action plans are provided – one for patient-specific action in the care planning process and one for unit-wide action. A written plan should be done for all patient-specific and unit-specific CQI projects and filed. For patients, this is often called an anemia/iron management care plan.

Resource Articles

Journal articles that discuss various aspects of anemia and iron management are listed in the Additional Readings section.

Steps for a CQI Approach to Anemia/Iron Management

Using the CPDCA Cycle for a Unit-Wide Anemia/Iron Issue

Failure to meet hemoglobin targets signals a need for an important CQI project. The CPDCA cycle is a good model to follow for a project such as this.

Check

- Check hemoglobins and iron values regularly to track and trend response to ESA and iron therapy. Follow unit policy for frequency.
- Identify and document patients who are not responding appropriately to ESA and iron therapy.

Plan

- If the unit is not meeting hemoglobin and iron targets, select a quality improvement project team to include MDs, RNs, dialysis technicians, dietitians, and social workers.
- Utilize the "Cause and Effect (Fishbone) Diagrams" (Items 6, 7, and 8) and the "Hyporesponse to ESA Therapy Documentation Tool" (Item 12) to identify common reasons or root causes for individual patient's failure to reach targets. Complete the "Hyporesponse to ESA Therapy Documentation Tool" (Item 12) for each patient to determine the root cause(s) contributing to their suboptimal response to ESA therapy.
- Use the "Tip Chart for Anemia/Iron Issues" (Item 3) and "Iron Values in Anemia and Iron Management Issues" (Item 4), as well as related journal articles, in the assessment process.
- Compile the root causes identified in step 2 on the "Anemia and Iron Assessment and Trending Worksheet" (Item 13) to identify root causes related to overall facility practice when anemia goals are not consistently achieved. Identification of common root causes will serve as the basis for developing a unit-wide action plan to improve anemia/iron outcomes.
- Develop an anemia/iron management action plan based on the most common root causes (Item 12). Should protocols be needed as part of the action plan, samples are provided in the "Sample Epogen Dosing Protocol" (Item 9) and the "Sample Aranesp Dosing Protocol" (Item 10). Additionally, a sample "Unit-Wide CQI Anemia/Iron CQI Project Action Plan" is shown as Item 15.

Do

- Educate patients, physicians, nurses, dialysis technicians, dietitians, and social workers about anemia/iron management and the specific quality improvement activities being undertaken.
- Ensure that communication has occurred with all necessary people to avoid confusion or misunderstandings.
- Implement the plan.

Check
- Check laboratory values per unit policy to track hemoglobin and iron parameters.
- Observe practices and processes as needed.

Act
- If outcomes improve, continue to follow the processes implemented in the action plan.
- If outcomes do not improve, re-evaluate the plan and implement.
- Document CQI projects in the appropriate records as well as in the unit's CQI book. Document patient care activities in the patient's chart.
- Repeat the CPDCA cycle, tracking and evaluating data regularly.

Steps for a Patient-Specific CQI Approach to Anemia/Iron Management

Using the CPDCA for a Patient-Specific Anemia/Iron Issue

Failure to meet hemoglobin targets signals a need for an important CQI project. The CPDCA cycle is a good model to consistently follow for anemia management.

Check
- Check the patient's hemoglobin regularly to track and trend response to ESA and iron therapy. Follow unit policy for testing frequency.
- Trend the patient's laboratory values and response to ESA and iron therapy.

Plan
- If a patient's hemoglobin or iron values are not within target range, either select a patient-specific quality improvement project team or a care planning team to include MDs, RNs, dialysis technicians, dietitians, and social workers.
- "Utilize the Cause and Effect (Fishbone) Diagrams" (Items 6, 7, and 8) and the "Hyporesponse to ESA Therapy Documentation Tool" (Item 12) to review and identify common reasons or root causes for why the patient is not responding appropriately to ESA therapy.
  Note: If the Hb is > 12 Gm/dL, evaluate ESA dosing for body weight. Ensure that if an ESA IV Dosing Protocol is being used, it is being consistently followed and ESA doses titrated per protocol.
- Complete the "Hyporesponse to ESA Therapy Documentation Tool" (Item 12) for each patient failing to achieve goals to document the root cause(s) contributing to hyporesponse in individual patients.
- Use the "Tip Chart for Anemia/Iron Issues" (Item 3) and "Iron Values in Anemia and Iron Management Issues" (Item 4), as well related journal articles, in the assessment process.
- Work with the multidisciplinary team to address the correctable causes for failure to respond to ESA. If adjustments in ESA or iron therapy dosing are needed, ESA and iron dosing protocols can be used to guide ESA dosing. Sample dosing protocols are provided (Items 9, 10, and 11).

- Develop an anemia/iron management action or care plan for each patient. A sample is provided as Item 14. A unit-wide CQI plan (a sample is provided as Item 15) should be developed if anemia/iron management is a unit-wide issue (in contrast to a specific patient).

Do
- Educate patients, physicians, nurses, dialysis technicians, dietitians, and social workers about anemia management and the specific quality improvement activities to be undertaken.
- Implement the plan(s).

Check
- Check hemoglobins per policy to track and trend response to the action plan(s).
- Document which patients respond to the CQI intervention and those who fail to respond using anemia and iron reports.

Act
- For patients who respond, follow ESA and IV Iron Dosing Protocols (samples in Items 9, 10, and 11) for routine dosing to encourage consistency.
- For patients who continue to fail to respond to ESA therapy, refer to the "Hyporesponse to ESA Therapy Documentation Tool" (Item 12) to continue to assess for correctable causes of hyporesponse to ESA therapy.
- Document CQI projects and care plans in the appropriate records.
- Implement routine practice guidelines to prevent hyporesponse in the future. Track data and causes monthly.
- Repeat the CPDCA Cycle.

These tools are provided as samples only and are not intended to suggest or direct specific unit practices or patient care.

Additional Readings

Bowe, D., & Ammel, D. (2005). Using CQI strategies to improve and simplify IV iron and anemia management: A dialysis facility's experience. *Nephrology Nursing Journal, 32*(5), 535-543.

Breiterman-White, R. (2007). Hemoglobin variability: Managing the higher end of the target range. *Nephrology Nursing Journal, 34*(2), 201-204, 213.

Easom, A. (2006). The challenges of using serum ferritin to guide IV iron treatment practices in patients on hemodialysis with anemia. *Nephrology Nursing Journal, 33*(5), 543-551.

McCarley, P. (2006). The KDOQI clinical practice guidelines and clinical practice recommendation for treating anemia in patients with chronic kidney disease: Implications for nurses. *Nephrology Nursing Journal, 33*(4), 423-427,445.

National Kidney Foundation (NKF). (2006). *KDOQI clinical practice guidelines and clinical practice recommendations for anemia in chronic kidney disease.* Retrieved April 4, 2009, from http://www.kidney.org/professionals/KDOQI/guidelines_anemia/cpr32.htm

Pruett, B., Johnson, S. & O'Keefe, N. (2007). Improving IV iron and anemia management in the hemodialysis setting: A collaborative CQI approach. *Nephrology Nursing Journal, 34*(2), 206-213.

Item 1
CQI at Work: Patient-Specific Anemia/Iron Management CQI Case Study

Problem Statement: Decreased response to ESA therapy.

CHECK – Monitor Data, Symptoms, Conditions, and Circumstances to Identify Areas for Improvement

Hemoglobins are routinely monitored monthly unless ESA therapy dose changes are in effect or laboratory values are out of target. It is noted that Mr. Johnson's hemoglobin (Hb) is below the target set by the unit. The CQI process is initiated.

PLAN – Select a Team and Analyze the Situation

A quality improvement/care planning team is formed. It consists of a nephrologist, RN team leader (primary nurse), dialysis technician, social worker, and dietitian.

Data are collected. These include laboratory work, physical examination, and review of the patient's current health history and circumstances. The review reveals laboratory values as follows:

- Hb 10% (has slowly trended downward from 11.5 g/dL over 3 months).
- Serum iron 35 ug/dL.
- Serum ferritin 650 ng/mL and trending up for two months.
- Transferrin saturation (TSAT) 18% (has trended downward from 25% over 2 months).
- WBC 12,000/mm^3.
- Calcium 9.0 mg/dL.
- Phosphorus 5.0 mg/dL.
- PTH 260 pg/dL.

CQI tools used by the team included:
- Interview.
- Brainstorming.
- Trend analyses.
- Hyporesponse to ESA Therapy Documentation tool.
- CQI Action/Care Plan.
- Anemia/Iron Assessment and Trending Worksheet.

Root cause identified:
- Current health status – Infected toe around the nailbed.

Action/care plan:
- Treat the infection.
- Teach daily diabetic foot care to Mr. Johnson and his wife.
- Arrange for daily visit by a home health nurse.
- Maintain Epoetin alfa dosage at 6,000 units thrice weekly (TIW).
- Continue IV iron therapy once active infection has been resolved.
- Monitor hemoglobin every 2 weeks and iron indices at 4 and 8 weeks after initiating the treatment plan.
- Evaluate response to therapy at 4 and 8 weeks after initiating the treatment plan.

DO – Implement the Plan after Education and Communication

The plan is implemented after communicating the plan to all parties involved, including the caregivers, patient and patient's family.

CHECK – Assess Outcomes
- Laboratory work.
- Status of infection.

Follow-up laboratory test results were as follows:

Time Interval	Hemoglobin	Transferrin Saturation	Ferritin
2 weeks	10 g/dL		
3 weeks	10.5 g/dL		
4 weeks	11 g/dL	22%	480 ng/mL
8 weeks	11.5 g/dL	24%	360 ng/mL

ACT – Sustain the Gain

Within a few weeks, physical examination revealed no evidence of infection in the toe. To prevent future problems, more frequent reviews of the patient's diabetes management and foot care were added to his care plan. Because of the number of patients with diabetes in the unit, routine foot checks were added to the care plans of all patients.

The patient's anemia and iron management regimen was continued.

Note: This tool is provided as a sample only and is not intended to suggest or direct specific unit practices or patient care.
Source: Used with permission from Gail Wick.

Item 2
CQI at Work: Unit-Wide Anemia/Iron Management CQI Case Study

Problem Statement: Anemia management target outcomes are not being met.

CHECK – Monitor Data, Symptoms, Conditions, and Circumstances to Identify Areas for Improvement

- Hemoglobins (Hb) are routinely monitored monthly unless ESA therapy dose changes are in effect or laboratory values are out of target. The Quality Improvement (QI) or Quality Assessment and Performance Improvement (QAPI) Committee reviews anemia and IV iron management parameters monthly at the meeting. The primary care team that regularly cares for the patients also monitors the laboratory data as well as clinical occurrences for specific patients.
- Using a trending report of the last 3 months of labs, the Committee notes that the unit's hemoglobin targets have not been met for the last 2 months.
- Many patients have elevated serum ferritin levels and low TSAT levels.
- A decision is made to initiate a unit-wide CQI project to address anemia and IV iron management issues.
- The CQI process is initiated.

PLAN – Select a Team and Analyze the Situation

- They organize a team consisting of a physician, nurse, dialysis technician, social worker, and dietitian to analyze the current situation.

Tools used include:
- Cause-and-effect diagrams for response to ESA and iron deficiency.
- Data collection tools.
- Anemia and iron management protocols or algorithms.

Root causes identified included:
- Majority of patients with serum ferritin greater than 500 ng/mL are on iron hold, as directed by the current protocol.
- The caregivers are not proactively identifying patients with inflammation.

An action plan is developed and includes:
- Track and compile new information on IV iron and anemia management to include:
  - KDOQI guidelines on hemoglobin, TSAT, and serum ferritin.
  - Recent studies for treatment of patients with hemoglobin below target.
- Develop and implement assessment tools for identification of iron-restricted erythropoiesis and causes of inflammation.
- Update the IV iron management protocol.
- Set up educational programs for staff.
- Communicate CQI activities to caregivers, patient, and patient's family.

DO – Implement the Plan after Educating and Communicating

- The plan is implemented.
- The caregivers consistently follow the plan.

CHECK – Assess Outcomes

- TSAT and serum ferritin values are checked per MD order until the hemoglobin and iron levels are stable. Once stable, the TSAT is checked monthly and serum ferritin is checked quarterly.
- Using the fishbone (cause and effect) diagram as a guide, the direct care staff monitors patients' general health status for anything that may impact anemia and iron status.
- The QI committee reviews the data at the QI monthly meeting.
  - A greater number of patients are achieving target hemoglobin levels, which may be due to aggressive treatment of inflammatory processes that if unresolved, can lead to ESA hyporesponse.
  - More patients are receiving maintenance IV iron.
  - More frequent treatment of iron-restricted erythropoiesis.
  - Overall number of units of ESA used has decreased.

ACT – Sustain the Gain

- The doctors and staff adopt the updated anemia and iron management protocols (Proactive).
- All new patients are assessed for risk factors for anemia and iron problems (Proactive).
- The literature is reviewed regularly to ensure that protocols are current.
- The project is documented and put in the CQI book.

Note: This tool is provided as a sample only and is not intended to suggest or direct specific unit practices or patient care.
Source: Used with permission from Gail Wick.

Item 3
Tip Chart for Anemia/Iron Issues

Test	Target/Normal	Considerations in Anemia/Iron Management - CKD
Hemoglobin	10 – 12 or 11 – 12 gm/dL depending on reference source (target range)	Target range is normally achieved when erythropoietic stimulating agent (ESA) and iron therapy are balanced and factors for hyporesponse are eliminated or minimized. ESA doses should be based on product insert. When doses greater than those recommended are needed to maintain target hemoglobin levels, consider factors in hyporesponse to ESA therapy.
Reticulocytes	0.5 – 2.0% (normal)	When > normal, consider increased erythropoiesis from ESA therapy, blood loss and/or hemolysis. When below normal, consider: inadequate erythropoiesis, inadequate bone marrow response due to secondary hyperparathyroidism (SPHT), medication suppression or infection.
C-reactive Protein (CRP)	Normal: < 3 mg/dL, >1 mg/dL is clinically significant and 3 – 10 mg/dL indicates inflammation. Patient on dialysis often 10 - 20 mg/dL, > 15 - 20 mg/dL indicates inflammation.	CRP is an acute phase reactant and as such, reflects the presence and severity of an infection. The general population has a lower "normal" range than patients with CKD stage 5 because of a number of factors. When CRP is > 15 - 20 mg/dL, suspect infection or inflammation and evaluate along with other indicators, such as TSAT, serum ferritin and WBC/differential.
White Blood Cells (WBC)	5 – 10x 10^3/mm (normal)	The WBC is the gross count of every cell in a blood sample that is not red, regardless of its cell type. A high WBC generally points to infectious process(es) but there are exceptions. When assessing the possibility of infection as a cause for elevated serum ferritin, an elevated WBC *may* indicate the possibility of infection; a differential may provide a more detailed analysis.
Transferrin Saturation (TSAT)	>20% (target)	When > 20%, indicates adequate iron in circulation for erythropoiesis. When < 20%, inadequate iron is available for erythropoiesis as a result of absolute iron deficiency or iron-restricted erythropoiesis. Evaluate TSAT with other indicators, e.g. serum ferritin, TIBC, hemoglobin, etc. When > 50%, suggests excess iron in the body and IV iron administration is often withheld. Always determine when iron was last given if TSAT is significantly elevated since last testing to ensure that IV iron has not been given within last 5 – 7 days (will falsely elevate results).
Serum Ferritin	>200 ng/mL (HD) >100 ng/mL (PD) (targets)	An indirect indicator of iron stores in the body; a good indicator of iron deficiency when < 200 mg/mL in patients on HD or < 100 mg/dL in patients on PD. Indicates adequate iron stores when > 200 mg/dL in patients on HD and >100 mg/dL in patients on PD. In addition to being an indicator of iron stores, it is also an acute phase reactant. Levels increase with inflammation and infection, liver disease, malnutrition and malignancy. When assessing serum ferritin levels > 500 mg/dL, evaluate other indicators for such underlying issues as inflammation/infection, liver disease, malnutrition and/or malignancy to determine cause.
Total Iron Binding Capacity (TIBC)	240 – 450 μ/dL (normal)	Indicates the transferrin receptors available to bind with iron; it is decreased in malnutrition and chronic disease. It is important to look at the TIBC to see if it is <200 ng/mL as the TSAT may be falsely elevated (it is calculated based upon the TIBC) and therefore is lower than indicated by the lab test result..
Mean Corpuscular Volume (MCV)	89 – 95 mm (normal)	Is the first index reported on a CBC and is a measure of red blood cell (RBC) size. May be normocytic, indicating normal RBC size. Microcytosis (low MCV) may indicate iron deficiency, thalassemia, lead poisoning with normal iron ferritin or aluminum toxicity. Macrocytosis (high MCV) can be caused by numerous conditions, but the three most common are chronic alcohol abuse, B12 deficiency and folate deficiency.
Albumin	3.5 – 5.0 g/dL (normal)	When within normal range, generally indicates adequate dietary protein. Levels below normal are often found in inadequate nutrition, infection, inflammation and with certain medications. Elevated albumin levels may be found with dehydration and the use of certain medications. Serum ferritin may be an indicator of malnutrition; when levels are elevated, evaluate to determine if malnutrition is a factor. TIBC is evaluated along with albumin because TIBC, a negative phase reactant, is decreased in malnutrition.
Parathyroid Hormone (PTH)	150 – 300 pg/mL (target range)	When the PTH is < 150 pg/mL, evaluate for adynamic bone disease, aluminum toxicity and chronic calcium loading. PTH > 300 pg/ml is suggestive of secondary hyperparathyroidism. Prolonged elevated PTH can damage bone marrow and diminish response to ESA therapy.
URR or Kt/V	>65% or > 1.2 (target)	Lower target levels indicate inadequate dialysis. This may be a factor in failure to respond to ESA therapy and should be evaluated if hemoglobin does not respond to therapeutic doses of ESA.

Note: This tool is provided as a sample only and is not intended to suggest or direct specific unit practices or patient care.
Source: Used with permission from Gail Wick.

Item 4
Iron Values in Anemia and Iron Management Issues

	Absolute Iron Deficiency	Functional Iron Deficiency/Iron Restricted Erythropoiesis	RE Blockade
Transferrin	↑	↑	↓
Serum Iron	↓	↓	↓
Total Iron Binding Capacity (TIBC)	↑	↑	↓
Transferrin Saturation (TSAT)	↓	↓	↓
Serum Ferritin	↓	Normal or ↑	Blocked
Iron	Blood loss or ↓ iron	Iron supply outstripped	↑ Ferritin
Response to Iron Therapy	↑ Hb	↓ Hb	None
Response to ESA Therapy	↑ Hb	↓ Ferritin	
Sedimentation Rate/CRP			↓

Note: This tool is provided as a sample only and is not intended to suggest or direct specific unit practices or patient care.
Source: Used with permission from Trish McCarley.

Item 5
Anemia and Iron Management Report

Patient Name	Draw Date	Hb	TIBC	Iron	TSAT	Ferritin	Alb, Serum	Ret%	PTH, Intact	ESA Dose	Iron Dose
Patient 1											
Patient 1											
Patient 1											
Patient 2											
Patient 2											
Patient 2											
Patient 3											
Patient 3											
Patient 3											

Note: This tool is provided as a sample only and is not intended to suggest or direct specific unit practices or patient care.
Source: Used with permission from Gail Wick.

Item 6
Anemia and Iron Management: Success in Reaching Targets

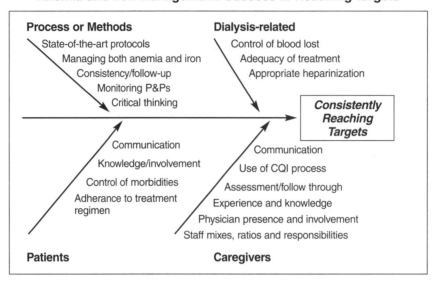

Note: This tool is provided as a sample only and is not intended to suggest or direct specific unit practices or patient care.
Source: Used with permission from Gail Wick.

Item 7
Response to ESA Therapy Cause and Effect Diagram

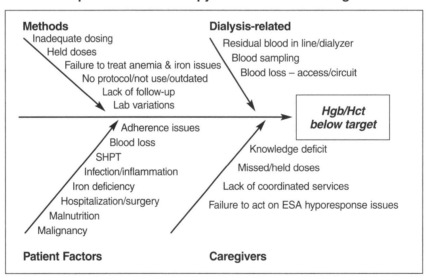

Note: SHPT = secondary hyperparathyroidism.
Note: This tool is provided as a sample only and is not intended to suggest or direct specific unit practices or patient care.
Source: Used with permission from Gail Wick.

Item 8
Response to ESA Therapy:
Iron-Related Factors Cause and Effect Dialgram

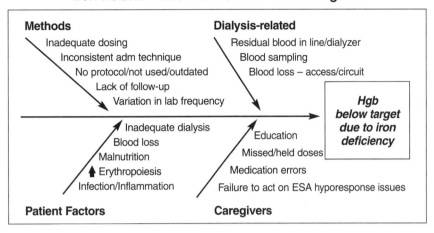

Note: This tool is provided as a sample only and is not intended to suggest or direct specific unit practices or patient care.
Source: Used with permission from Watson Pharma, Inc.

Item 9
SAMPLE Epogen® IV Dosing Protocol

Guiding Principles in the Epogen® IV Dosing Protocol:
- The target for anemia management in this unit is a hemoglobin (Hb) of 11 to 12 g/dL.
- Initiate Epogen® IV therapy when the patient's Hb is < 10. Obtain UIBC, CBC and differential, reticulocyte count and iron indices: TSAT, serum ferritin, iron and TIBC. Obtain stool guaiac as needed.
- Manage anemia and iron together. All patients should have adequate iron stores to maintain erythropoiesis. Ensure that the patient has adequate iron stores before increasing ESA dose.
- This protocol is based on 3x/week dosing.
- Base decisions for EPO dose changes on trends in laboratory values rather than a single value.
- Change Epogen® doses no more than once per month unless clinically indicated and specifically ordered by a doctor because it takes 4 to 6 weeks to respond to EPO dose changes.
- Epogen® doses > 20,000 units require the anemia manager to consult with the physician and to consider factors for hyporesponse.
- The maximum allowed Epogen® dose is 30,500 U per treatment or 400,000 U per month (no reimbursement exceptions).
- Reduce the Epogen® dose by 25% when the Hb is > 12.5g/dl and maintain in response to the hemoglobin level.
- The frequency of Hb monitoring in patients treated with ESA should be at least monthly.
- Hold the Epogen® dose when the Hb is > 13.5g/dl.
- Draw interim Hb levels on patients who were receiving Epogen®, but placed on hold because of a high Hb.
- Resume Epogen® on patients who were placed on hold when their Hb is <13 g/dl.
- The lowest Epogen® dose given every treatment is 100 units.

- Missed doses should be made up during the patient's next treatment. If the hemoglobin increases more than 1 g/dl in any 2-week period, decrease the Epogen® dose by 10%. If it is the result of a blood transfusion, do not decrease, but consult with doctor for specific medication order.

Notes:
- CMS policy requires the ESA dose be reduced (no specified amount) when the CMS reported Hb is >13 g/dl and the dose maintained in response to the hemoglobin level.
- CMS requires medical justification for routinely maintaining Hb levels >13 g/dl in patients on dialysis treated with an ESA.
- A trend is defined as 3 or more laboratory results that move in the same direction over a minimum of 2 months.

Definitions:
- Hb: Hemoglobin
- CMS-reported Hb: Last Hb drawn in the month.
- ESA: Erythropoiesis-stimulating agent.
- Interim Hb: Any Hb other than the last one of the month.

Math Helper:
Select the appropriate multiplier to calculate the dose change as indicated by the protocol.

Formula: Current dose x multiplier = new dose.

Multiplier Grid		
	10%	25%
Increase dose	X 1.1	X 1.25
Decrease	X 0.9	X 0.75

Note: This tool is provided as a sample only and is not intended to suggest or direct specific unit practices or patient care.
Note: See next page for Epogen® Dose Management.
Source: Used with permission from Gail Wick.

Item 9 (continued)
Epogen® (EPO) Dosing Adjustments Guidelines

New Patient Not on ESA Therapy		
Patient Hemoglobin	**Intervention**	**Clinical Notes and Comments**
< 10 g/dL	50 to 100 U/kg 3 times a week (TIW).	Epogen® is dosed based on weight. Recommended starting dose is 50 – 100 U/kg 3 times a week (TIW). Follow Guiding Principles.

Post-Hospitalization Patients		
For patients who have a hospital stay > 1 day, obtain the last H&H from the hospital and adjust ESA according to maintenance dosing protocol.		

Maintenance Dosing		
Patient Hemoglobin	**Intervention**	**Clinical Notes and Comments**
< 10 g/dL	Increase EPO by 25% rounded to higher 100 U. Notify the doctor during group rounds.	Follow guiding principles for all categories. If the Hb fails to achieve target Hb, check for factors for hyporesponse (see CQI program). Talk with the anemia manager and/or physician about addressing the factors. Complete patient specific CQI action/care plan.
10.0 to 10.9 g/dL	Increase EPO dose by 10% rounded to the next higher 100 U. Increase the EPO dose every 4 weeks (on a monthly basis), until the Hgb is 11 to 12 g/dL.	Complete the hyporesponse form to assess for factors for hyporesponse to ESA (see CQI program). Talk with the anemia manager and/or physician about addressing the factors. Complete patient specific CQI action/care plan.
11 to 12 g/dL	Maintain the EPO dose unless the Hb is trending upward and approaching 12 g/dL. In that case, decrease the dose by 10%, rounding to the next lower 100 U. If the Hb is trending downward and approaching 11 g/dL, increase the dose by 10% rounding to the next higher 100 U.	Note: An upward trend is defined as 3 or more consecutive labs over 2 or more months that have increased $\geq$ 0.5 g/dl and the Hb is $\geq$ 11.8 g/dl. A downward trend is defined as 3 or more consecutive labs over 2 or more months that have decreased $\geq$ 0.5 g/dl and the Hb is $\leq$ 11.3 g/dl. Note: Hbs that are trending up toward 12 g/dL or down toward 11 g/dL, require dose adjustments to try to keep the Hb within the target range of 11 to 12 g/dL.
12.1 to 12.5 g/dl	Decrease the EPO dose by 10% rounding to the next lower 100 U, every 4 weeks (on a monthly basis), until the Hb is 11 to 12 g/dL.	
12.6 to 13.5 g/dl	Reduce EPO dose by 25% rounding to the next lower 100U. Decrease every 4 weeks (on a monthly basis), per protocol until Hb is 11 to 12 g/dl.	
> 13.5 g/dl	Hold EPO dose and order interim Hb to be drawn in 2 weeks. When Hb < 13.0, immediately resume EPO at a 25% reduction from the previous dose rounding to the next lower 100 U. Notify the physician during group rounds.	Note: Monitor both monthly and interim labs, resume dose at a 25% reduction when first result is <13.0 g/dl.

Medical Director Signature: _____ Date:_____

Note: This tool is provided as a sample only and is not intended to suggest or direct specific unit practices or patient care.
Source: Used with permission from Gail Wick.

Item 10
SAMPLE Aranesp® IV Dosing Protocol

Guiding Principles in the Aranesp® IV Dosing Protocol:
- The target for anemia management in this unit is a hemoglobin (Hb) of 11 to 12 g/dL.
- Initiate Aranesp® IV therapy when the patient's Hb is < 10. Obtain UIBC, CBC, and differential, reticulocyte count and iron indices: TSAT, serum ferritin, iron, and TIBC. Obtain stool guaiac as needed.
- Manage anemia and iron together. All patients should have adequate iron stores to maintain erythropoiesis.
- Ensure that the patient has adequate iron stores before increasing ESA dose.
- This protocol is based on 1x/week dosing.
- Base decisions for Aranesp® dose changes trends in laboratory values rather than a single value.
- Aranesp® dose changes are done no more than once per month unless clinically indicated and specifically ordered by a doctor because it takes 4 to 6 weeks to respond to dose changes.
- Aranesp® doses > 240 mcg require the anemia manager to consult with the physician and to consider factors for hyporesponse.
- The maximum allowed Aranesp® dose is 240 mcg per treatment or 1,200 mcg per month with no more than six doses allowed in one month (no reimbursement exceptions).
- The policy is to reduce the Aranesp® dose by 25% when the Hb is > 12.5g/dL and maintain in response to the hemoglobin level.
- The frequency of Hb monitoring in patients treated with ESA should be at least monthly.
- Hold the Aranesp® dose when the Hb is ≥ 13.5g/dl.
- Draw an interim Hb level on patients who were receiving Aranesp® but placed on hold because of a high Hb.
- Missed doses should be made up during the patient's next treatment.

- If the Hb increases more than 1 g/dl in any 2-week period, decrease Aranesp® by 10%. If it is the result of a blood transfusion, do not decrease but consult with the doctor for a specific medication order.
- The lowest Aranesp® dose given is 5 mcg every other week.

Notes:
- CMS policy requires that the ESA dose be reduced (no specified amount) when the CMS reported Hb is >13 g/dL and the dose maintained in response to the hemoglobin level.
- CMS requires medical justification for routinely maintaining Hb levels > 13g/dL in patients on dialysis treated with an ESA.
- A trend is defined as 3 or more laboratory results that move in the same direction over a minimum of 2 months.

Definitions:
- Hb: Hemoglobin.
- CMS-reported Hb: Last Hb drawn in the month.
- ESA: Erythropoiesis-stimulating agent.
- Interim Hb: Any Hb other than the "monthly lab draw."

Math Helper:
Select the appropriate multiplier to calculate the dose change as indicated by the protocol.

Formula: Current dose x multiplier = new dose.

Multiplier Grid		
	10%	25%
Increase dose	X 1.1	X 1.25
Decrease	X 0.9	X 0.75

Note: This tool is provided as a sample only and is not intended to suggest or direct specific unit practices or patient care.
Note: See next page for Aranesp® Dose Management Guidelines.
Source: Used with permission from Gail Wick.

Item 10 (continued)
Aranesp® Dosing Adjustment Guidelines

New Dialysis Patient Not on ESA Therapy		
Patient Hemoglobin	**Intervention**	**Clinical Notes and Comments**
< 10 g/dL	0.45 mcg/kg once weekly	Aranesp® is dosed based on weight. Recommended starting dose is 0.45 mcg/kg once weekly. Follow Guiding Principles.

Post-Hospitalization Patients		
For patients who have a hospital stay > 1 day, obtain the last H&H from the hospital and adjust ESA according to maintenance dosing protocol.		

Maintenance Dosing		
Patient Hemoglobin	**Intervention**	**Clinical Notes and Comments**
< 10 g/dL	Increase Aranesp® by 25% rounded to higher 5 mcg. Notify the doctor during group rounds.	Follow Guiding Principles for all categories. If the Hb fails to achieve target, check for reasons for the hyporesponse (see CQI program). Talk with the anemia manager and/or physician about addressing the factors. Complete patient-specific action plan.
10.0 to 10.9 g/dL	Increase Aranesp® dose by 10% rounded to the next higher 5 mcg. Increase the Aranesp® dose every 4 weeks (on a monthly basis), until the Hb is 11 to 12 g/dL.	Complete the hyporesponse form to access for reasons for the hyporesponse to ESA (see CQI program). Talk with the anemia manager and/or physician about addressing the factors. Complete patient-specific action plan.
11 to 12 g/dL	Maintain the Aranesp® dose, unless the Hb is trending upward and approaching 12 g/dL. In that case, decrease the dose by 10%, rounding to the next lower 5 mcg. If the Hb is trending downward and approaching 11 g/dL, increase the dose by 10% rounding to the next higher 5 mcg.	Note: An upward trend is defined as 3 or more consecutive labs over 2 or more months that have increased $\geq$ 0.5 g/dl and the Hb is $\geq$11.8 g/dl. A downward trend is defined as 3 or more consecutive labs over 2 or more months that have decreased $\geq$ 0.5 g/dl and the Hb is $\leq$ 11.3 g/dl. Note: Hbs that are trending up toward 12 g/dL or down toward 11 g/dL, require dose adjustments to try to keep the Hb within the target range of 11 to 12 g/dL.
12.1 to 12.5 g/dl	Decrease the Aranesp® dose by 10% rounded to the next lower 5 mcg. Decrease every 4 weeks (on a monthly basis), until the Hb is 11 to 12 g/dL.	
12.6 to 13.5 g/dl	Reduce Aranesp® dose by 25% to the next lower 5 mcg. Decrease every 4 weeks (on a monthly basis), per protocol until Hb is 11 to 12 g/dl.	
> 13.5 g/dl	Hold Aranesp® dose, and order interim Hb to be drawn in 2 weeks. When Hb < 13 g/dl, immediately resume the Aranesp® dose at a 25% reduction from the previous dose rounding to the next lower 5 mcg. Notify the physician during group rounds.	Note: Monitor both monthly and interim labs, resume dose at a 25% reduction when first result is < 13.0 g/dl

Physician Signature: _____ Date:_____

Note: This tool is provided as a sample only and is not intended to suggest or direct specific unit practices or patient care.
Source: Used with permission from Gail Wick.

Item 11
Iron Management Protocol
SAMPLE

Labs	Action Steps
If Hemoglobin is < 11, consider the following:	
Repletion: TSAT ≤ 25% and Serum Ferritin < 200	Administer 125 mg Sodium Ferric Gluconate IVP over 10 minutes x 8 sessions (TOTAL 1 Gram) Draw labs 5 to 7 days post-iron course completion 　A. If still TSAT < 25% and serum ferritin < 200ng/mL, repeat repletion regimen 　B. If iron replete, see action steps below If not iron replete after two rounds of iron repletion therapy, notify anemia manager or doctor for further patient assessment.
TSAT ≤ 25% and Serum Ferritin > 200 but < 1200	If no signs of active infection and ESA ≥ 22,500 U/week, administer 125 mg Sodium Ferric Gluconate IVP over 10 minutes x 8 sessions (TOTAL 1 gram). Draw labs next month.
If the Hemoglobin is >11, consider the following:	
Maintenance Iron Regimen: TSAT > 25% and Serum Ferritin > 200 but < 500	Administer 62.5 mg Sodium Ferric Gluconate IVP over 5 to 7 minutes weekly.
TSAT > 25% and Serum Ferritin > 500 but < 1200	Administer 62.5 mg Sodium Ferric Gluconate IVP over 5 to 7 minutes every other week.
TSAT > 25% and Ferritin > 1200	Hold iron for 1 month* and reorder serum ferritin and TSAT next month. When ferritin trends upward, assess for potential reasons.
TSAT > 50% Ferritin any level	Notify anemia manager or doctor for patient specific assessment.
*KDOQI recommends holding iron up to 3 months. It is recommended that when iron is being held, iron indices be monitored monthly.	

Physician Signature:_____ Date:_____

Note: This tool is provided as a sample only and is not intended to suggest or direct specific unit practices or patient care.
Source: National Kidney Foundation, 2006.
Source: Used with permission from Gail Wick.

Item 12
Root Cause Documentation Tool – Hyporesponse to ESA Therapy

The chart below lists the common potential root causes for failure to respond to ESA therapy. Starting in the left upper corner (inadequate ESA dose), assess the patient for the presence of one or more of these as part of the CQI process. Anemia/iron, nutrition and MBD lab values for 3 - 6 months should be used as part of this process. Document actions taken on the CQI action/care plan.

Last 3 Hgb/dates: _____ g/dL on _____; _____ g/dL on _____; _____ g/dL on _____

☐ **Inadequate ESA dose:** ☐ Low dose for weight: wt _____; ESA _____ U TIW or other _____ ☐ Held doses _____ in past month ☐ Frequent dose changes _____ /month ☐ Missed treatments/doses _____ /month	☐ **Patient was been hospitalized in past month** ☐ Known blood loss ☐ Known to miss ESA while hospitalized ☐ ESA not started upon return from hospital Hospitalization dates: _____ Returned to facility: _____	☐ **Iron Deficiency** ☐ Serum ferritin < 200 ng/dL for hemodialysis _____ ng/mL ☐ Serum ferritin < 100 ng/dL for CKD/PD _____ ng/dL ☐ TSAT < 20% _____ % ☐ MCV < 180 μm^3/RBC _____ μm^3/RBC ☐ Not on iron therapy Current iron orders:
☐ **Possible infection or inflammation** ☐ ↑ Ferritin _____; _____; _____ ng/mL ☐ ↓ TSAT _____; _____; _____ ng/mL ☐ ↑ WBC _____ μL ☐ ↑ CRP _____ mg/dL Acute or chronic infection present (note what/where:	☐ **Blood loss** ☐ GI bleed or recent surgery (circle) ☐ Positive stool - occult blood ☐ System leak, separation or clotting ☐ Venous line not clear upon rinse ☐ Excessive bleeding at access sites ☐ Menses or abnormal uterine bleeding	☐ **SHPT** ☐ Documented disease ☐ Bone changes ☐ PTH 300 pg/mL _____ pg/mL
☐ **Co-morbidities/Meds** ☐ Cancer ☐ Hematologic disorder _____ ☐ AIDS ☐ Chemo ☐ On analgesics or antibiotics (Circle) ☐ Other: _____	☐ **Inadequate Dialysis** ☐ Missed or shortened treatment _____ /mo ☐ URR < 65% _____ % ☐ Kt/V < 1.2	☐ **Malnutrition** ☐ Protein intake below recommended levels ☐ ↓ albumin or prealbumin ☐ ↓ NPNA
☐ **Vitamin Deficiency** ☐ Change in MCV ☐ B12 < 140 pg/mL ☐ Folic acid < 3 ng/mL ☐ B6 < 5 ng/mL	☐ **Hemolysis** ☐ Acute fall in Hgb after stabilization ☐ ↓ Haptoglobin ☐ ↓ LDH ☐ ↑ K+ ☐ Hemolysis of extracorporeal system ☐ On med that can cause hemolysis	☐ **Protocol Issues** ☐ No protocol(s) ☐ Protocol(s) are outdated ☐ Protocols are not consistently followed ☐ Anemia and iron protocols are incongruent

Signature: _____
Date: _____
Attach CQI action plan and trending tools

Hyporesponse to ESA Documentation tool
Gail Wick, 2007. Used with permission

Note: This tool is provided as a sample only and is not intended to suggest or direct specific unit practices or patient care.
Note: NPNA = normalization of the protein equivalent of nitrogen appearance, SHPT = secondary hyperparathyroidism.

Project Dates: From: ___ / ___ / ___   To: ___ / ___ / ___

Page: ___ of ___

Item 13
Anemia/Iron Assessment and Trending Worksheet
Purpose: To Identify and Trend Cause of Failure to Reach Targets

Column headers (worksheet grid):

- Patients' Names
- Hgb > 11 (insert value)
- Hgb > 13 (insert value)
- Absolute Iron Deficiency
- Iron-Restricted Erythropoiesis
- Ferritin > 1200 (insert value)
- Inadequate ESA Dose for Weight
- ESA > 150 U/kg or 4.5 mcg/kg
- Patient Factors – General
- ^ Recent Infection/Inflammation
- ** Blood Loss
- Recent Hospitalization
- Recent Surgery
- Kt/V < 1.2 and/or URR < 65%
- SHPT   PTH > 300
- Vitamin Deficiency
- Missed Tmts (#/mo)
- Shortened Tmts (min/mo)
- Missed ESA Dose (# in last mo)
- Meds that Impact RBCs
- Malnutrition
- ^^ Personnel-Method/Materials
- Total Factors

Form Instructions

1. Write in patient's name.
2. Place # of root cause(s) as appropriate. May have more than one root cause.
3. Check boxes for other root causes.
4. Include form as part of CQI assessment and trending.

Definitions:

Absolute Iron Deficiency
  Hgb < 11; TSAT < 20%; Serum Ferritin < 200

Iron-Restricted Erythropoiesis
  Hgb < 11; TSAT < 20%; Serum Ferritin > 200

*Patient Factors – General

1. Diabetes Type I
2. Diabetes Type 2
3. Hypertension/Cardiac
4. Arthritis
5. GI Bleeding/Other Hemorrhage
6. Hematological Disease
7. HIV/Aids
8. Malignancy
9. Smoking
10. Aluminum Toxicity
11. Other

**Blood Loss

12. Needle Sites
13. Clotted Dialyzer
14. Catheter Site
15. Greater Than 2/Month Blood Draws
16. +Stool, Occult blood
17. Recent Surgery
18. Menses/Abdominal Uterine Bleeding
19. Other

^ Infection/Inflammation

20. Catheter Access
21. Latent Graft/Fistula
22. Wounds/Ulcers
23. Cellulitis
24. URI/Flu/Pneumonia
25. Hepatitis
26. Dental Disease
27. Arthritis Exacerbation
28. Lupus Exacerbation
29. Failed Transplant
30. Positive Urine Culture
31. Sinusitis
32. Lupus Flare Up

^^ Personnel-Method/Materials

33. No Facility Protocol
34. Protocol Not Based on KDOQI
35. Inconsistent Use of Protocol
36. Inconsistent Practice
37. Poor Patient Input/Knowledge
38. Holding doses
39. ESA-Related Medication Error
40. Other

Comments (Specific Patient)

Note: This tool is provided as a sample only and is not intended to suggest or direct specific unit practices or patient care.

Source: Used with permission from Gail Wick and Kathy Spiegal.

Item 14
Continuous Quality Improvement Action Plan
Patient-Specific CQI/Care Plan

Patient Name:_____ Date Created: October 3, 2007 Updated: _____

PROBLEM STATEMENT: Hgb < target of 11g/dl
October 3: Hgb = 10.1
Serum ferritin = 431
TSAT = 18%

ROOT CAUSES:
- Recent hospitalization for viral gastritis on 9/18; now resolved.
- Functional Iron Deficiency (FID): TSAT = 18% and serum ferritin = 431

DATA REQUIRED: Hb, TSAT, serum ferritin, recent health history

---

SOLUTIONS TO IMPLEMENT: Goal: Increase Hb to target range of 11 to 12:
1. Trend lab data and ESA and iron dosing for past 6 months
2. Review recent health history and new issues, co-morbidities, circumstances
3. Physical assessment
4. Complete "Hyporesponse to ESA Therapy" tool
5. Ensure that ESA and iron protocols are being consistently followed

Action Plan (steps)	Responsible Team Member	Start Date	Estimated Completion Date	Checkpoint Dates	Date Completed	Comments (Status, outcomes, disposition, etc.)
Review ESA dosing and lab trends, recent health history, dialysis events and current situation	Team leader and care team	10-3	10-6		10-5	10-3 – Completed ESA dosing history, lab review, recent dialysis events, and recent health history.
Physical exam	CD	10-3	10-6		10-5	
Complete ESA hyporesponse tool to document root cause(s)	Team leader	10-3	10-6		10-5	Root causes determined – Recent hospitalization and FID/Iron-restricted Erythropoiesis
Audit patient records for protocol use	Nurse manager	10-3	10-6		10-5	ESA and iron dosing per protocol
Ongoing review of anemia data and application of anemia/iron management guidelines: • Hb (monthly or as indicated) • TSAT and serum ferritin monthly, then quarterly • ESA dosing – Review and follow ESA protocol • Iron dosing – Review and follow protocol	Team leader with review by CD		Dosing changes made based on monthly lab draws	Monthly	Ongoing	10-5 – Increased Aranesp dose by 10% per protocol to 25 mcg. Repletion round of iron initiated to treat FID/Iron-restricted erythropoiesis

Note: CD = clinic director.
Note: This tool is provided as a sample only and is not intended to suggest or direct specific unit practices or patient care.
Source: Used with permission from Gail Wick.

Item 15
SAMPLE
Continuous Quality Improvement Action Plan
Unit-Wide Anemia/Iron CQI Project

Original Date:_____ Date of plan update: _____

PROBLEM STATEMENT: < 80% of patients meet unit goal of hemoglobin $\geq$ 11 g/dL	

ROOT CAUSES:
- Inadequate or inconsistent ESA dosing.
- Time lags in changing ESA doses after monthly labs.
- Outdated protocol.
- Failure to resolve root causes of failure to respond to ESA therapy.

DATA REQUIRED:
- Monthly labs and dosing reports.
- Root causes of hyporesponse to ESA (see tool).

SOLUTIONS TO IMPLEMENT:
1. Updated protocol that is consistently followed.
2. Develop and implement trending tool for lab data.
3. Use ESA hyporesponse tools to identify patient-specific root causes and unit-wide root cause trends.

Action Plan (steps)	Responsible Team Leader	Start Date	Estimated Completion Date	Checkpoint Dates	Date Completed	Comments (Status, outcomes, disposition, etc.)
Establish and consistently follow an anemia protocol.	XYZ	Jan. 1	Feb. 1	Ongoing	Feb. 1	March 21, Update: New protocol in place as of February. Utilized for February and March ESA and iron dosing changes. xyz is taking lead on review of dosing changes with input by Dr. XYZ. To date, going well. Will monitor outcome improvement trends and report monthly.
Designate staff nurses as anemia managers for their specific patients. Train. Audit 25% of charts for 3 months.	XYZ	Feb. 1	May 31	Ongoing		March 21: Out of 25 chart audits, 3 patients treated "off protocol." Reasons justified. RNs following protocol appropriately. Hyporesponse forms for individual patients being completed and care plans/action plans developed and implemented. Root causes being trended.
Monitor anemia/iron labs and focus initially on patients with sub-xx Hb.	XYZ	Feb. 7	Ongoing	Ongoing		March 21 Update: Labs reviewed. 31% of patients have sub-xx hgb in March compared to 34% in February (3% improvement).
Use the XYZ Labs generated anemia/iron trending report.	XYZ	Feb.	Ongoing	Ongoing		March 21 Update: See attached report and CQI trending reports for February and March.
Train staff on principles of anemia/iron management.	XYZ	Mar. 1	April 1	Mar. 15		March 21 Update: All nurses, technicians, social workers and dietitians attended anemia/iron management 101 workshop. Anemia/iron management workshop 201 attended by all nurses. All staff nurses actively managing anemia/iron on their patients. Continue 25% of patients monthly audits for adherence to protocol.

Note: This tool is provided as a sample only and is not intended to suggest or direct specific unit practices or patient care.
Source: Used with permission from Gail Wick.

Chapter 5	CONTINUING NURSING EDUCATION EVALUATION FORM	1.2 Contact Hours

Clinical Application: CQI in Anemia and Iron Management **ANNP0905**

Applying Continuous Quality Improvement in Clinical Practice contains 22 chapters of educational content. Individual learners may apply for continuing nursing education credit by reading a chapter and completing the Continuing Nursing Education Evaluation Form for that chapter. Learners may apply for continuing nursing education credit for any or all chapters.

Please photocopy this test page, complete, and return to ANNA.
You can also download this form from www.annanurse.org (choose Education - CNE Activities - Publications)
Receive continuing nursing education credit (CNE) immediately by completing the CNE evaluation process in ANNA's Online Library. Go to www.annanurse.org, and click on the Online Library icon for more information.
Name: _____
Address: _____
City: _____ State: _____ Zip: _____
E-mail:_____ Preferred telephone: ☐ Home ☐ Work _____
State where licensed and license number: _____

CNE application fees are based upon the number of contact hours provided by the individual section. CNE fees per contact hour for ANNA members are as follows: 1.0-1.9 – $15; 2.0-2.9 – $20; 3.0-3.9 – $25; 4.0 and higher – $30. Fees for nonmembers are $10 higher.
CNE application fee for Chapter 5: ANNA member $15   Nonmember $25
ANNA Member: ☐ Yes ☐ No   ☐ Member # (if available) _____
☐ Check or money order enclosed   ☐ American Express   ☐ Visa   ☐ MasterCard
Total amount submitted:_____
Credit card number _____ Exp. Date _____
Name as it appears on the card: _____
NOTE: Your evaluation form can be processed in 1 week for an additional rush charge of $5.00.
☐ Yes, I would like this evaluation form rush processed. I have included an additional fee of $5.00 for rush processing.

Instructions
1. To receive continuing nursing education credit for an individual study after reading the chapter, complete this evaluation form.
2. Detach, photocopy, or download (www.annanurse.org) the evaluation form and send along with a check or money order payable to **American Nephrology Nurses' Assocation** to: ANNA, East Holly Avenue Box 56, Pitman, NJ 08071-0056.
3. Test returns must be postmarked by **April 30, 2011**. Upon completion of the answer/evaluation form, a certificate will be sent to you.

This chapter was reviewed and formatted for contact hour credit by Sally S. Russell, MN, CMSRN, ANNA Director of Education Services.

CNE Application Fee for Chapter 5
ANNA member = $15
Nonmember = $25

1. I verify that I have read this chapter and completed this education activity. _____ Date _____
   Signature
2. What would be different in your practice if you applied what you have learned from this activity? (Please use additional paper if necessary.)
   _____
   _____
   _____
   _____

	Strongly disagree				Strongly agree
3. The activity met the stated objectives.					
a. Explain how anemia and iron management are inter-related.	1	2	3	4	5
b. Describe the Check-Plan-Do-Check-Act cycle as related to iron management and patients with anemia.	1	2	3	4	5
4. The content was current and relevant.	1	2	3	4	5
5. The content was presented clearly.	1	2	3	4	5
6. The content was covered adequately.	1	2	3	4	5

7. How would you rate your ability to apply your learning to practice?   ☐ diminished ability   ☐ no change   ☐ enhanced ability

Comments _____
_____

8. Time required to read the chapter and complete this form: _____ minutes

This educational activity is provided by the American Nephrology Nurses' Association (ANNA).
ANNA is accredited as a provider of continuing nursing education (CNE) by the American Nurses Credentialing Center's Commission on Accreditation (ANCC-COA).
ANNA is a provider approved of continuing nursing education by the California Board of Registered Nursing, provider number CEP 00910.
This CNE offering meets the Nephrology Nursing Certification Commission's (NNCC's) continuing nursing education requirements for certification and recertification.

Clinical Application: CQI in Mineral and Bone Disorder Management:
A Multi-Phase Approach Grounded in Research

Rebecca Wingard, MSN, RN, CNN
MaryKay Shepherd, RD

Objectives

Study of the information presented in this chapter will enable the learner to:

1. Identify the risk of death for at least two elevated phosphorus ranges in the hemodialysis patient population.
2. Define the Pareto principle.
3. Discuss 3 principles of algorithm development.
4. Identify a CQI project goal other than a parathyroid hormone (PTH) algorithm to address another cause of high PTH or phosphorus levels.
5. Describe the impact the PTH cycle time can have on PTH outcomes.
6. Identify one reason based on research data why patients on dialysis may require vitamin D supplementation, regardless of PTH level.

Overview

1. High serum phosphorus is the bone metabolism parameter that is most strongly associated with increased mortality in patients on dialysis.
2. The basis for CQI projects directed at improving patient outcomes should be grounded in research.
3. Multiple factors can have an impact on an outcome, but per the Pareto principle, a focus on the factor with the biggest impact on the outcome is the best place to start.
4. Improvement in outcomes with multiple factors will require a multi-phase approach, for example, multiple and subsequent CQI projects that address each factor.
5. Cycle time is a measure of the time it takes to go through a defined activity or set of activities, and can influence patient outcomes.
6. Observations and measures obtained during a CQI project can be the basis for a subsequent project.

Introduction

The classic continuous quality improvement (CQI) question of "Can we do better?" is often perceived to require a complex answer to address mineral and bone disorders in patients on dialysis. The good news is that the nephrology community has "done better," and as research continues to reveal new information, the picture of how to manage mineral and bone disorders becomes clearer. Nephrology nurses can be confident in their ability to continue to improve the morbidity and mortality of patients on dialysis with mineral and bone disorders, leveraging the patient as the leader in managing his or her level of wellness. The goal of this chapter is to encourage nurses to embrace management of mineral and bone disorders as a multi-phase process within the total spectrum of care. The expertise of the entire team, using CQI principles, can open the road to success and thereby provide a bright future for patients.

Research-Based Approach

Parathyroid Hormone (PTH) Levels, Phosphorus, Calcium, and Calcium X Phosphorus Product

Upon which parameter do nurses focus, and how should the complex interactions among these measurements be managed? Managing all parameters is critical, but recent literature clearly points to phosphorus as the strongest independent risk factor for mortality. It has been shown that patients with elevated phosphorus levels (greater than 5.0 mg/dL) have an increased mortality risk (Block et al., 2004a). In a large hemodialysis population (greater than 40,000 patients), it has been shown that patients with serum phosphorus of 6.0 to 7.0 mg/dL had a 25% increased risk of death. This risk increased further for each higher level of phosphorus, up to twice the risk of death for serum phosphorus equal to or greater than 9.0 mg/dL (Block et al., 2004a). These authors also showed an increased risk of death for moderate to severe elevations of serum PTH; however, the risk was more modest when compared to phosphorus.

Nursing practice is evidence-based, so what does this tell us? The classic quality improvement concept set forth by Vilfredo Pareto helps place things in perspective. Pareto noted that things are not equally distributed, which can be applied to the idea that a problem (such as mortality) is not equally affected by all factors. The Pareto principle suggests that 80% of the problem comes from 20% of the causes, directing focus on the "vital few" (Breyfogle, 2003). Current information indicates that PTH and phosphorus can affect mortality, with phosphorus having the stronger association with higher mortality. The Pareto principle directs one to first address these two main factors of mineral and bone disorders that influence mortality.

In addition to phosphorus, recent research has spotlighted the role of vitamin D supplementation in persons with and without renal disease. There are vitamin D receptor sites in multiple tissues. Vitamin D deficiency is increasingly being linked to diseases, such as malignancy, diabetes, hypertension, and cardiovascular disease (CVD), in patients not on dialysis

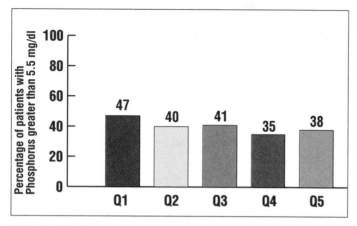

Figure 6-1
Reduction of Percent of Patients with Elevated Phosphorus Levels with Use of Algorithm

Note: Q = Number of quarters following algorithm implementation.
Source: Used with permission from MaryKay Shepherd.

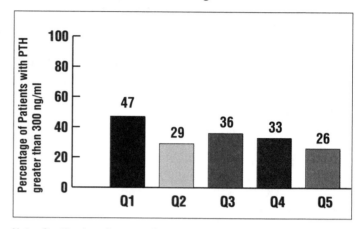

Figure 6-2
Reduction of Percent of Patients with Elevated PTH with Use of Algorithm

Note: Q = Number of quarters following algorithm implementation.
Source: Used with permission from MaryKay Shepherd.

(Holick, 2006). Data show improved mortality for patients on dialysis who are on vitamin D regardless of PTH level (see "Future Trends" section later in this chapter) (Teng et al., 2005).

Based on the importance of phosphorus control, PTH management, and the use of vitamin D, the following CQI project illustrates an approach to mineral and bone disorders. A PTH algorithm is the primary focus of the intervention, with a secondary effect on phosphorus levels.

The Challenge

This clinic recognized past successes in the management of mineral and bone disorders but also saw an opportunity for further improvement. At the start of the project, data for the most recent quarter showed that 47% of patients had serum phosphorus levels greater than 5.5 mg/dL, and similarly, 47% had a PTH greater than 300 ng/ml (see Figures 6-1 and 6-2). Both indicators exceeded target ranges. Per the National Kidney Foundation's (2003) Kidney Disease Outcomes Quality Initiative Guidelines (KDOQI), individual patient goals were set at phosphorus levels of 3.5 to 5.5 mg/dL, and PTH 150 to 300 ng/ml. With this in mind, a team was organized to begin the CQI process and established the primary goal to reduce the percent of patients above the target for PTH by at least 10% during the next 6 months. A secondary goal was established to reduce the percent of patients above the target phosphorus by at least 5%.

The CQI Team

A CQI team was formed, with the Medical Director selected as the project leader. The team included three dietitians, a nurse practitioner, and charge nurses at each of the three clinics involved. These clinics were selected from among 8 area clinics to implement change on a small scale. If project goals were met, the intent was to expand the project actions to the remaining facilities. The nephrologist and dietitians met each quarter to discuss the direction of the

project. As a team, they decided to focus on one primary action: implementation of a new vitamin D algorithm while maintaining other phosphorus management per usual clinic practices. A plan was developed with action steps assigned to specific CQI team members to be implemented over about six months. This algorithm would affect PTH but also have secondary effects on phosphorus, and it was expected that future projects would address phosphorus management with more direct approaches. This would be a multi-phase process of improvement.

Algorithm Development and Implementation

The algorithm was developed by the team with the following principles in mind: a) simplicity, b) patient goals of PTH 150 to 300 ng/ml and phosphorus 3.5 to 5.5 mg/dL, c) build on success with use of cinacalcet, and d) maximize the patient's opportunity for parenteral vitamin D dosing. An algorithm was developed, and patients were started on a low-dose vitamin D analog. This was implemented as initial therapy for patients whose PTH was elevated, when serum calcium (Ca) and calcium x phosphorus product (CxP) were in target range. It is important to note that in the algorithm, the team defined the CxP target range as equal to or less than 60. For those patients whose calcium was in range and whose PTH levels were resistant to low-dose vitamin D analog, vitamin D was maintained, and cinacalcet was added. As PTH returned to target range, cinacalcet was reduced and/or discontinued, while maintaining vitamin D as long as possible (see Table 6-1). Thus, vitamin D analog was the first drug used and the last drug removed to maximize the patient's exposure to it. While the CQI team used specific dosing in its algorithm, only general guidelines are provided in Table 6-1. This is to be used in consultation with a nephrologist to determine specific drug dosing and frequency of laboratory measurement.

The algorithm was implemented in the three clinics, and PTH and phosphorus results were tracked and recorded by

Table 6-1
Intravenous Vitamin D/Cinacalcet Algorithm Guidelines

Suggested Dosing for Initiation	Dose Change (low, medium, high*)
• iPTH is 250-300 and Ca equal to or less than 10.0 and CxP equal to or less than 60	Start at low dose of vitamin D; consider weekly or 2x/week dosing.
• iPTH is 301-400 and Ca is equal to or less than 10.0 and CxP equal to or less than 60	Start vitamin D at medium dose or increase frequency of current dose up to 3x/week.
• iPTH is greater than 400 and Ca is equal to or less than 10 and CxP equal to or less than 60	Start vitamin D at high dose.
• iPTH is greater than 300 and Ca is greater than 10.0 or CxP is greater than 60	Start low dose cinacalcet daily; check Ca and P in 1 week.
Maintenance Dosing	
• If iPTH is less than150	Reduce vitamin D to low dose; if PTH still too low, then discontinue cinacalcet. Consult physician before discontinuing vitamin D.
• iPTH is greater than 300 and no change or increased from previous iPTH	Adjust Vitamin D up to low dose maximum. Add low dose cinacalcet or increase cinacalcet to next dose level unless calcium is below target, or patient is non-adherent with cinacalcet.
• iPTH is greater than 300 and decreased from previous iPTH	If on Vitamin D, continue. If on cinacalcet only, increase dose to next level.
HOLD Guidelines	
• Hold Vitamin D for Ca above target; reduce Vitamin D each treatment for CxP above target x 2 lab draws.	
• Hold cinacalcet for Ca below target	

*For algorithm development, the physician must determine specific dosing levels. All algorithms must reflect individual physician orders.
Source: Used with permission from MaryKay Shepherd.

the medical director (project leader). Although the project was planned to conclude in 6 months, a plan for a full year of data collection was put in place to measure success of maintaining the project's results.

Results

PTH

After implementation of the vitamin D algorithm, the percentage of patients with PTH greater than 300 ng/ml was reduced from a baseline of 47% to 29% within one quarter (see Figure 6-2). The second quarter continued to show improvement compared to baseline data. The percentage of patients with PTH greater than 300 ng/ml, however, had worsened compared to the previous quarter (36% in Q3 vs. 29% in Q1). After reinforcement of consistent algorithm implementation, the following two quarters showed improvement from 36% in the third quarter to 33% and 26% respectively, during the fourth and fifth quarters of measurement.

Phosphorus

For the secondary target of phosphorus, the percentage of patients with phosphorus greater than 5.5 mg/dL showed

improvement. Phosphorous levels decreased during algorithm use from 47% at baseline to 40%, 41%, 35%, and 38% in the second, third, fourth, and fifth quarters, respectively (see Figure 6-1). This improvement in phosphorus control was thought to be a result of a greater number of patients for whom cinacalcet was prescribed (an increase from 10% to 30%), and the use of consistent and lower doses of vitamin D (the average vitamin D dose was reduced by 35%).

Cinacalcet is indicated for treating elevated parathyroid hormone levels but has also been shown to lower calcium and phosphorus levels in patients on dialysis (Block et al., 2004b). With the complexities of managing the nutritional status of patients and the challenges of finding ways to improve mortality, it is helpful for the interdisciplinary team to utilize an algorithm that can improve both PTH and phosphorus levels.

Spreading a Best Practice

The results showed that the project goals were met to improve PTH and phosphorus outcomes. It was learned that regular, consistent reinforcement and training of new dietitians regarding algorithm use was necessary to maintain

Figure 6-3
Control Chart of Clinic A PTH Cycle Time in Days

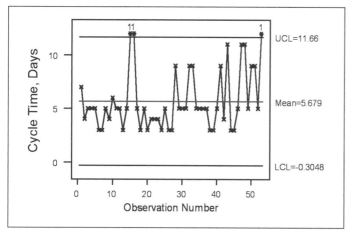

Note: UCL = upper control limit, LCL = lower control limit.
Source: Used with permission from MaryKay Shepherd.

Figure 6-4
Control Chart of Clinic B PTH Cycle Time in Days

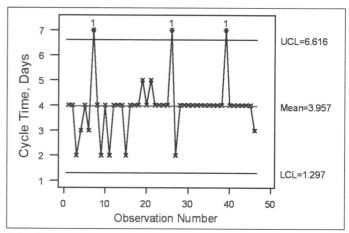

Note: UCL = upper control limit, LCL = lower control limit.
Source: Used with permission from MaryKay Shepherd.

improved outcomes. The analysis of project results were presented to area medical directors, and the decision was made to implement the algorithm in all 8 of the area's dialysis clinics. Dietitians were educated on executing the algorithm, and subsequently held meetings at each clinic to educate nurses and staff.

Next: Intensive Focus on Phosphorus And Cycle Time

What's next? This team had great success with improving PTH and phosphorus level management by implementing an evidence-based algorithm. To continue improvement specifically for phosphorus control, patient adherence with phosphorus binder medications was the next area of focus. To assist in the development of an effective patient teaching plan, a review of the literature to determine successful program approaches would be beneficial. This will illuminate the success others have had with motivational interviewing techniques to teach patients and involve patient care technicians in this team process (Karalis & Wiesen, 2007).

During the PTH algorithm implementation, the team noticed a high variation in cycle time days. Cycle time is a measure of the time it takes for a work activity (or activities) to be completed (Breyfogle, 2003). The quality manager had recently undergone Six Sigma™ green belt training in a subset of Six Sigma methodology and tools (see Chapter 4, "Introduction to Six Sigma," for information on this methodology). The manager volunteered to develop a control chart of cycle time days for two clinics to determine if this observation was a significant problem. PTH cycle time was defined as the number of days between the date the laboratory reported the PTH result to the clinic and the date a new vitamin D order change was recorded in the medical record, if indicated by the algorithm.

Cycle times were observed to have wide variation within and among clinics. Figures 6-3 and 6-4 show control charts

for Clinic A and Clinic B. A control chart is a CQI tool that measures variation of a process over time (Breyfogle, 2003). Data points are plotted over time, and the control chart indicates the deviation from the average for each data point. The extent of deviation from the average is indicated by statistically determined upper and lower control limits. A data point that lies within these limits falls within normal common cause variation limits (variation expected based on past performance of the process), indicating the performance of the process being measured is in control. A data point outside of the control limits indicates the process is out of control due to special causes (Breyfolge, 2003). This provides an opportunity to evaluate these causes and reduce the variation.

Clinic A had a mean cycle time of 5.679 days compared to Clinic B, with a cycle time of 3.957 days. These data suggest an opportunity for improvement for Clinic A to meet the standard established by Clinic B. Both clinics had data points outside the control limits, representing an opportunity for them both to reduce variation. A future focus on shortening and reducing variation in cycle time would assure treatment of abnormal PTH values as quickly and consistently as possible, potentially increasing the time that patients are in their target range.

Conclusion

Future Trends: Vitamin D Use For Patients within PTH Target?

Low levels of vitamin D pose potential health consequences for patients not on dialysis (Holick, 2006). Patients new to hemodialysis are profoundly deficient in both 25 vitamin D (inactive form) and 1,25 vitamin D (active form), even in patients with PTH less than 150 ng/ml (Wolf et al, 2007). These lower levels of vitamin D were associated with increased mortality compared to normal levels of 25 vitamin D. The risk of mortality with mild to moderate deficiency (10 to 30 ng/ml) increased by 30%, and for patients with severe deficiency of vitamin D (less than 10 ng/ml), mortality risk increased by 60%. These data apply to mortality from any cause as well as CVD mortality. Similar findings for 25 vitamin D were also seen for 1,25 vitamin D. Supplementation of 1,25 vitamin D was shown to reduce the risk of mortality in multiple categories, even for patients who received vitamin D with low levels of PTH (Teng et al., 2005). Finally, data have shown a 28% increased risk of death for patients on hemodialysis not on vitamin D, compared to those on any type of vitamin D (Tentori et al., 2006). This information raises questions, such as "How will the nephrology community guidelines for using vitamin D change in the future?" or "What new information will come to light regarding other factors for management of mineral and bone disorders, such as phosphorus?" A well-known anonymous quote assures, "Change is inevitable, improvement is optional." The CQI process is *continuous*. It requires the ability to stay informed about changes in knowledge and practice, and to revise processes to continually improve practice and processes for excellence in patient care.

References

Block, G.A., Klassen, P.S., Lazarus, J.M., Ofsthun, N., Lowrie, E.G., & Chertow, G.M. (2004a). Mineral metabolism, mortality, and morbidity in maintenance hemodialysis. *Journal of the American Society of Nephrology, 15*(8), 2208-2218.

Block, G.A., Martin K.J., de Francisco, A.L., Turner, S.A., Avram, M.M., Suranyi, M.G., et al. (2004b). Cinacalcet for secondary hyperparathyroidism in patients receiving hemodialysis. *New England Journal of Medicine, 350*(16), 1516-1525.

Breyfogle, F.W. (2003). *Implementing Six Sigma* (2nd ed.), Hoboken NJ: John Wiley & Sons, Inc.

Holick, M.F. (2006). High prevalence of vitamin D inadequacy and implications for health. *Mayo Clinic Proceedings, 81*(3), 353-373.

Karalis, M., & Wiesen, K. (2007). Motivational interviewing. *Nephrology Nursing Journal, 34*(3), 336-338.

National Kidney Foundation (NKF). (2003). K/DOQI clinical practice guidelines: Bone metabolism and disease in chronic kidney disease. *American Journal of Kidney Diseases, 42,* S1-S201.

Teng, M., Wolf, M., Ofsthun, M.N., Lazarus, J.M., Hernan, M.A., Camargo, C.A., et al. (2005). Activated injectable vitamin D and hemodialysis survival: A historical cohort study. *Journal of the American Society of Nephrology, 16*(4), 1115-25.

Tentori, F., Hunt, W.C., Stidley, C.A., Rohrscheib, M.R., Bedrick, E.J., Meyer, K.B., et al. (2006). Mortality risk among hemodialysis patients receiving different vitamin D analogs. *Kidney International, 70*(10), 1858-1865.

Wolf, M., Shah, A., Gutierrez, O., Ankers, E., Monroy, M., Tamez, H., et al. (2007). Vitamin D levels and early mortality among incident hemodialysis patients. *Kidney International, 72,* 1004-1013.

| Chapter 6 | CONTINUING NURSING EDUCATION EVALUATION FORM | 1.2 Contact Hours |

Clinical Application: CQI in Mineral and Bone Disorder Management: A Multi-Phase Approach Grounded in Research

ANNP0906

Applying Continuous Quality Improvement in Clinical Practice contains 22 chapters of educational content. Individual learners may apply for continuing nursing education credit by reading a chapter and completing the Continuing Nursing Education Evaluation Form for that chapter. Learners may apply for continuing nursing education credit for any or all chapters.

Please photocopy this test page, complete, and return to ANNA.
You can also download this form from www.annanurse.org (choose Education - CNE Activities - Publications)
Receive continuing nursing education credit (CNE) immediately by completing the CNE evaluation process in ANNA's Online Library. Go to www.annanurse.org, and click on the Online Library icon for more information.

Name: _____

Address: _____

City: _____ State: _____ Zip: _____

E-mail:_____ Preferred telephone: ☐ Home ☐ Work_____

State where licensed and license number: _____

CNE application fees are based upon the number of contact hours provided by the individual section. CNE fees per contact hour for ANNA members are as follows: 1.0-1.9 – $15; 2.0-2.9 – $20; 3.0-3.9 – $25; 4.0 and higher – $30. Fees for nonmembers are $10 higher.

CNE application fee for Chapter 6: ANNA member $15   Nonmember $25

ANNA Member: ☐ Yes ☐ No   ☐ Member # (if available) _____

☐ Check or money order enclosed   ☐ American Express   ☐ Visa   ☐ MasterCard

Total amount submitted:_____

Credit card number _____ Exp. Date _____

Name as it appears on the card: _____

NOTE: Your evaluation form can be processed in 1 week for an additional rush charge of $5.00.

☐ **Yes, I would like this evaluation form rush processed. I have included an additional fee of $5.00 for rush processing.**

INSTRUCTIONS

1. To receive continuing nursing education credit for an individual study after reading the chapter, complete this evaluation form.

2. Detach, photocopy, or download (www.annanurse.org) the evaluation form and send along with a check or money order payable to **American Nephrology Nurses' Assocation** to: ANNA, East Holly Avenue Box 56, Pitman, NJ 08071-0056.

3. Test returns must be postmarked by **April 30, 2011**. Upon completion of the answer/evaluation form, a certificate will be sent to you.

This section was reviewed and formatted for contact hour credit by Sally S. Russell, MN, CMSRN, ANNA Director of Education Services.

> **CNE Application Fee for Chapter 6**
> **ANNA member = $15**
> **Nonmember = $25**

1. I verify that I have read this chapter and completed this education activity. _____Date _____
                                                                    Signature

2. What would be different in your practice if you applied what you have learned from this activity? (Please use additional paper if necessary.)
_____
_____
_____
_____

	Strongly disagree				Strongly agree
3. The activity met the stated objectives.					
a. Identify the risk of death for at least two elevated phosphorus ranges in the hemodialysis patient population.	1	2	3	4	5
b. Define the Pareto principle.	1	2	3	4	5
c. Discuss three principles of algorithm development.	1	2	3	4	5
d. Identify a CQI project goal other than a parathyroid hormone (PTH) algorithm to address another cause of high PTH or phosphorus levels.	1	2	3	4	5
e. Describe the impact the PTH cycle time can have on PTH outcomes.	1	2	3	4	5
f. Identify one reason based on research data why patients on dialysis may require vitamin D supplementation, regardless of PTH level.	1	2	3	4	5
4. The content was current and relevant.	1	2	3	4	5
5. The content was presented clearly.	1	2	3	4	5
6. The content was covered adequately.	1	2	3	4	5
7. How would you rate your ability to apply your learning to practice?	☐ diminished ability		☐ no change		☐ enhanced ability

Comments _____
_____

This educational activity is provided by the American Nephrology Nurses' Association (ANNA).
ANNA is accredited as a provider of continuing nursing education (CNE) by the American Nurses Credentialing Center's Commission on Accreditation (ANCC-COA).
ANNA is a provider approved of continuing nursing education by the California Board of Registered Nursing, provider number CEP 00910.
This CNE offering meets the Nephrology Nursing Certification Commission's (NNCC's) continuing nursing education requirements for certification and recertification.

Clinical Application: Adequacy of Hemodialysis

Maggie Tatarek, RN, CNN

Objectives

Study of the information presented in this chapter will enable the learner to:
1. Describe the benefits of using urea kinetic modeling over urea reduction ratio to determine dialysis adequacy.
2. List methods for analyzing adequacy data in a continuous quality improvement project.

Overview

In the 1950s, the National Institute of Diabetes and Digestive and Kidney Diseases (NIDDK) was established as part of the National Institutes of Health (NIH). In the 1960s, NIDDK supported research that would advance dialysis technology from the bulky plate and frame dialyzers requiring rebuilding after each use to the hollow-fiber dialyzer membrane being used today (Lysaght, 1996). Moving on to 1993, the NIDDK sponsored a conference on the morbidity and mortality of patients on dialysis. Subject matter experts developed, among other recommendations, a quantitative evaluation of dialysis dose and adequacy. The reduction of urea, the chief nitrogenous constituent of urine and the final product of protein metabolism in the body, was chosen for the evaluation of how effectively a dialysis treatment removed waste products from the patient's body (NIH, 1993).

Introduction to Hemodialysis Adequacy

How does the nephrology community currently measure hemodialysis (HD) treatment adequacy? Two blood samples, a pre-dialysis blood urea nitrogen (BUN) and a post-dialysis BUN, are drawn and placed into a formula for calculating the percentage of BUN removed by dialysis, yielding a urea reduction ratio (URR). For minimally adequate dialysis, the National Kidney Foundation (NKF) – Kidney Disease Outcomes Quality Initiative™ (KDOQI) Guideline 4.2 recommends a target dose for patients on HD with residual function less than 2 mL/minute should be a spKt/V of 1.4 per dialysis (3 times per week) or a URR of 70% (NKF, 2006). There are some limitations to using URR as a measure of HD adequacy. It does not account for the contribution of ultrafiltration to the final dose of delivered Kt/V. URR does not support calculation of normalized protein catabolic rate (NPCR) that provides an estimate of the dietary protein intake in steady-state. Finally, URR does not take into account for the patient's residual kidney function to urea clearance, which can be significant at the onset of ESRD. Therefore, KDOQI Clinical Practice Guideline 2 (NKF, 2006) recommended that the delivered dose for patients on HD should be measured using formal urea kinetic modeling (UKM). UKM is a "formal" mathematical analysis of both pre and post-dialysis BUN concentrations. It uses documented treatment information, such as time of dialysis, actual blood flow and dialysate flow rates, accurate fluid lost during dialysis, and the ultrafiltration coefficient (KoA) of the dialyzer used (King, 2008). Formal UKM can be used to prescribe individualized hemodialysis treatment parameters and computes the adequacy of the delivery of the dialysis prescription (the desired Kt/V) on the day pre and post-BUN samples are drawn.

What Is Kt/V?

K indicates clearance by the dialyzer expressed in milliliters per minute (mL/minute) as provided by the manufacturer (typically derived in aqueous solution in vitro). Time is indicated by t, both minutes of HD and number of treatments per week. The volume of urea distribution in total body water is represented by V. Kinetic modeling also accounts for urea generated by the body during dialysis and between treatments, and solute transfer as indicated by urea removed with excess fluid removal. Patients with larger amounts of fluid to be removed may experience more urea removal because of convective transport. With formal UKM, utilizing computational software is necessary to compute Kt/V and can be used to calculate the exact treatment time required to deliver a particular HD dose at a known blood and dialysate flow rate on a particular dialyzer. The volume of urea distribution is derived from a mathematical iteration of two formulas, the first providing the end dialysis volume (Vt) and the second calculating the urea generation rate (G) between consecutive HD treatments; this is the prescribed Kt/V (King, 2008).

Single Pool (spKt/V) or Equilibrated or Double Pool (eKt/V)

Single pool refers to the removal of urea from one space, the vascular system, from which dialysis occurs. Urea is distributed across body water presenting in intracellular, extracellular, and the vascular spaces. Urea is removed from the blood during HD through the principle of diffusion (for example, solutes moving from high concentration to low concentration). This continues to occur until the urea has equalized or equilibrated across all three spaces after HD has ceased, called urea rebound. When monitoring the delivery of the HD dose, it is important to include urea rebound in the calculation, which can vary greatly among adult patients. This occurs 15 minutes after the end of the HD treatment for the majority of patients to 60 minutes for small-stature patients who experience intradialytic hypotensive episodes (Jean, Charra, Chazot, & Laurent, 1999). Formal UKM (from the spKt/V) calculates the eKt/V; on average, the eKt/V is 0.2 units less than the spKt/V but can be significantly higher in the smaller-stature patients mentioned above (NKF, 2006).

Standard for Dialysis Adequacy

How does your facility measure adequacy? It is important for all patients receiving HD in the same facility to measure the delivered dose of therapy using the same method. Pre and post-HD blood samples for the measurement of BUN levels must be drawn during the same HD treatment. The pre-BUN should be drawn immediately prior to initiation of the HD treatment using a method that avoids dilution of the blood sample with saline or heparin. Consistency within the facility must be employed in the method for drawing post-BUN samples. According to KDOQI Guideline 4, target dose for adequacy for patients receiving HD 3 times per week with a residual clearance (Kr) less then 2 mL/min/1.73 m² is a spKt/V of 1.4 per dialysis or URR of 70%. The eKtdr/V, double pool, residual function target would be 1.2 (NKF, 2006).

Interdisciplinary Team Approach to Adequacy As a CQI Process

The interdisciplinary team consists of the medical director, clinical manager, RNs, patient care technicians, dietitians, social workers, and the patient. One might ask, "Why is it so important that the team monitors and takes action for dialysis adequacy?" Research shows that the impact of missing even one treatment a month carries a greater risk of death than the patient whose fluid gains are greater than 5.7% of their body weight, a patient whose phosphorus is greater than 7.5 mg/dL, or the patient whose potassium is greater than 6 mKq/L (Saran et al., 2003).

The Quality Assessment Performance Improvement (QAPI) team should discuss the target Kt/V at the facility level and then review data on its current performance in achieving the desired patient outcomes. The QAPI team is expected to address improvement initiatives with action plans, implementing plans, checking outcomes, and incorporating successful actions into the facility's routine (Centers for Medicare and Medicaid Services [CMS], 2008). A resource for a facility working with the CQI process is the End Stage Renal Disease (ESRD) Networks, which assist dialysis facilities with improving the quality of patient care. The ESRD Networks conduct quality improvement projects, provide technical assistance to facilities, investigate and resolve patient complaints, validate facility and patient data, sponsor outreach and educational activities for patients and providers, and provide technical and educational materials to patients and providers (Medicare, n.d.) This is an opportune time to begin a CQI process if one is not already in place.

Tools for Collecting and Analyzing Data

Collecting individual and facility adequacy reports is one way to measure and collect baseline data for a CQI project. One suggestion is to generate a report that provides each patient's prescribed treatment time in minutes compared to how many minutes the patient was actually dialyzed on each treatment.
- Identify those patients who are meeting their prescribed

treatment time but are not achieving the adequacy target.
- Identify patients who are not receiving their prescribed treatment time.

These data will assist the team in considering what action steps will help promote a behavior change – either with the patient, the staff, or both. Does your team provide a patient report card or routinely review dialysis adequacy results with patients? Does your team routinely share adequacy outcome reports to the clinic staff?

Some methods for analyzing data include:
- *Force field analysis* to identify driving and restraining forces.
- *Fishbone diagram* to identify root causes contributing to the problem.
- *Flow charts* to create a common understanding of a process, or to identify misplaced steps or unnecessary complexity in a process.
- *A run chart* provides a snapshot of frequency over time; it is a simple way to visually examine data over a period of time.
- *Pareto chart* to visually recognize where the majority of the problems (opportunities for improvement) lie.

Using a "Fishbone Diagram" to Determine Root Causes

First, the team identifies categories for brainstorming possible root causes of the problem. Using the fishbone diagram, the team lists its categories and again brainstorms to identify root causes (see Figure 7-1). Examples of categories for brainstorming root causes include:
- Clinical practice.
- Staff-related.
- Treatment-related.
- Patient-related.
- Access-related.
- Kt/V assessment.

Plan-Do-Check-Act

The CQI tool, the Plan-Do-Check-Act cycle, can be used to begin a focus on improving adequacy.

Plan
- Gather data:
  ○ Identify patients running their prescribed treatment time not meeting adequacy target.
  ○ Identify patients not running prescribed treatment time.
- Identify root causes to achieving adequacy and develop action plan:
  ○ Educate patients on the importance of receiving an adequate dose of dialysis.
  ○ Educate staff members on the importance of providing an adequate does of dialysis.
- Include the medical director/attending nephrologist(s) to support dialysis adequacy education for patients and staff members:
  ○ Review patient report cards or outcomes with patient.
  ○ Review monthly adequacy quality indicator data in QAPI committee; on-going evaluation of action plan for improving HD adequacy.

Figure 7-1
Fishbone Diagram to Determine Root Causes – Hemodialysis Adequacy

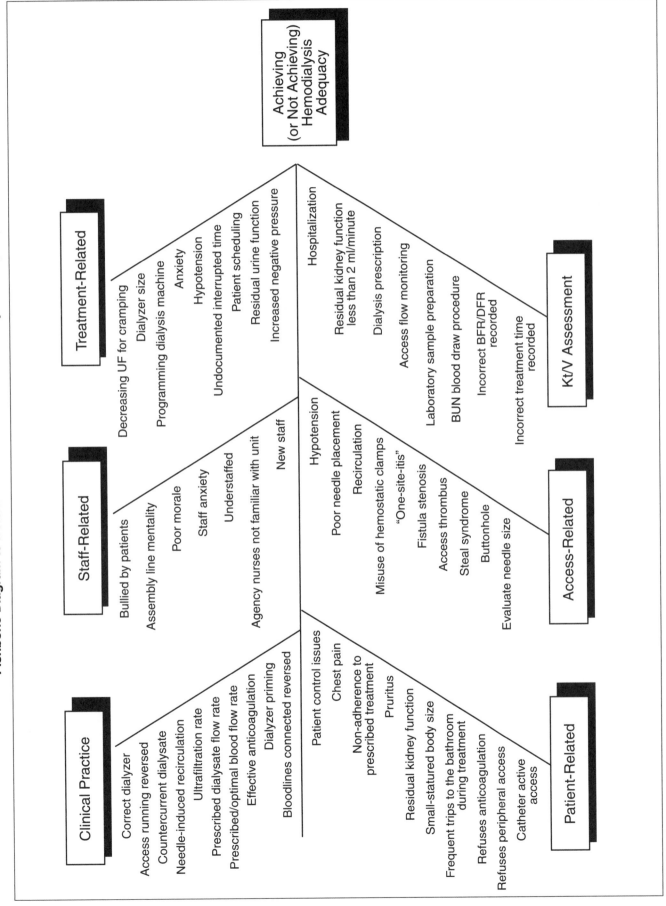

Source: Used with permission from Maggie Tatarek.

○ Identify a patient advocate to support education for adequacy for all patients. This is a key element for patients to understand their plans of care and the importance to achieve adequacy.

○ Include patients in developing their individualized "Plan of Care" addressing treatment adequacy.

Do

- Provide education and re-educate patients and staff on the "whys" to improve adequacy, treatment factors that have an impact on adequacy, and possible interventions.
- Collect residual kidney function samples for kinetic modeling.
- Ensure method for obtaining BUN samples is consistent throughout the facility.
- Schedule and provide education for staff to ensure awareness of facility policy and procedures related to adequacy of treatment.
- Review action plan(s) in monthly QAPI meetings with the interdisciplinary team.
- Develop a reporting method to inform staff members of facility outcomes (for example, a quality leader board in a common area, such as the break room).
- Document interventions implemented to improve treatment adequacy:
  ○ Example: Work with the patient to have him or her agree to remain on HD for the prescribed time for one month to see if improvement in the patient's well being is noticed by the patient.
  ○ Example: Explore potential access problems if an adequate blood flow is not delivered from the vascular access.
- Develop a patient mentor program with a patient advocate to support education for adequacy.
- Designate a team member to work with patient on plan of care for adequacy

Check

- CQI plan adopted and implemented by all staff.
- Interactive discussion between staff and patients on achieving adequacy goal.
- Encourage support among patients for improving adequacy.
- Update a quality leader board.
- Utilize an adequacy suggestion box for staff's input between CQI meetings.

Act

- Evaluate sustained improvement in patient adequacy.
- Positive reinforcement with patients for commitment to achieving adequacy.
- Positive reinforcement with staff for commitment to patients.
- Celebrate successes!

Conclusion

Achieving and sustaining adequate dialysis for patients is a team effort. The success begins with patients who have control over their dialysis experience. If your patients do not understand the ramifications of receiving less-than-adequate HD, they cannot begin to make behavior changes to address this challenge. It is your commitment, as part of the nephrology team, to know when there is a problem, how to address and resolve the problem, and always work toward a goal of optimal dialysis for every patient.

There are many valuable data collection tools available to assist you in identifying those patients who are not achieving adequacy goals and how they can adversely have an impact on treatment adequacy. The importance of achieving adequacy should be a daily topic for staff and patients. Nephrology nurses are the patients' facilitators to optimal living on dialysis.

References

Centers for Medicare and Medicaid Services (CMS). (2008). *Medicare program: Conditions for coverage for end-stage renal disease facilities.* Washington, DC: Federal Register.

Jean, G., Charra, B., Chazot, C., & Laurent, G. (1999). Quest for post dialysis urea rebound – Equilibrated Kt/V with only intradilaytic samples. *Kidney International, 56,* 1149-1153.

King, B., (2008). Principles of hemodialysis. In C.S. Counts (Ed.), *Core curriculum for nephrology nursing* (5th ed. pp. 662-681). Pitman, NJ; American Nephrology Nurses' Association.

Lysaght, M. J. (1996). Turning points: Hemodialysis membrane. *Dialysis & Transplantation.* 25(10), 657-662.

Medicare. (n.d.) *Dialysis facility compare: Concerns or complaints about quality of care.* Retrieved on July 18, 2008, from http://www.cms.hhs.gov/dialysisfacilitycompare

National Institute of Health (NIH). (1993). Morbidity and mortality of dialysis. *NIH Consensus Statement, 11*(2), 1-33.

National Kidney Foundation (NKF). (2006). KDOQI *Clinical practice guidelines and clinical practice recommendations: Hemodialysis adequacy, guideline 4, minimally adequate hemodialysis.* Retrieved December 4, 2008, from www.kidney.org/PROFESSIONALS/kdoqi/guideline_upHD_PD_VA/index.htm

Saran, R., Bragg-Gresham, J.L., Rayner, H.C., Goodkin, M.L., van Dijk, P., Kurokawa, K., et al. (2003). Nonadherence in hemodialysis: Associations with mortality, hospitalization, and practice patterns in the DOPPS. *Kidney International, 64,* 254-262.

Chapter 7 | CONTINUING NURSING EDUCATION EVALUATION FORM | 1.4 Contact Hours

Clinical Application: Adequacy of Hemodialysis   **ANNP0907**

Applying Continuous Quality Improvement in Clinical Practice contains 22 chapters of educational content. Individual learners may apply for continuing nursing education credit by reading a chapter and completing the Continuing Nursing Education Evaluation Form for that chapter. Learners may apply for continuing nursing education credit for any or all chapters.

Please photocopy this test page, complete, and return to ANNA.
You can also download this form from www.annanurse.org (choose Education - CNE Activities - Publications)
Receive continuing nursing education credit (CNE) immediately by completing the CNE evaluation process in ANNA's Online Library. Go to www.annanurse.org, and click on the Online Library icon for more information.

Name: _____

Address: _____

City: _____ State: _____ Zip: _____

E-mail: _____ Preferred telephone: ☐ Home ☐ Work _____

State where licensed and license number: _____

CNE application fees are based upon the number of contact hours provided by the individual section. CNE fees per contact hour for ANNA members are as follows: 1.0-1.9 – $15; 2.0-2.9 – $20; 3.0-3.9 – $25; 4.0 and higher – $30. Fees for nonmembers are $10 higher.

CNE application fee for Chapter 7: ANNA member $15   Nonmember $25

ANNA Member: ☐ Yes ☐ No   ☐ Member # (if available) _____

☐ Check or money order enclosed   ☐ American Express   ☐ Visa   ☐ MasterCard

Total amount submitted: _____

Credit card number _____ Exp. Date _____

Name as it appears on the card: _____
NOTE: Your evaluation form can be processed in 1 week for an additional rush charge of $5.00.
☐   **Yes, I would like this evaluation form rush processed. I have included an additional fee of $5.00 for rush processing.**

INSTRUCTIONS

1. To receive continuing nursing education credit for an individual study after reading the chapter, complete this evaluation form.

2. Detach, photocopy, or download (www.annanurse.org) the evaluation form and send along with a check or money order payable to **American Nephrology Nurses' Assocation** to: ANNA, East Holly Avenue Box 56, Pitman, NJ 08071-0056.

3. Test returns must be postmarked by **April 30, 2011**. Upon completion of the answer/evaluation form, a certificate will be sent to you.

This section was reviewed and formatted for contact hour credit by Sally S. Russell, MN, CMSRN, ANNA Director of Education Services.

CNE Application Fee for Chapter 7
ANNA member = $15
Nonmember = $25

---

1. I verify that I have read this chapter and completed this education activity. _____ Date _____
   Signature

2. What would be different in your practice if you applied what you have learned from this activity? (Please use additional paper if necessary.)
   _____
   _____
   _____
   _____

	Strongly disagree				Strongly agree
3. The activity met the stated objectives.					
a. Describe the benefits of using urea kinetic modeling over urea reduction ratio to determine dialysis adequacy.	1	2	3	4	5
b. List methods for analyzing data in a continuous quality improvement project.	1	2	3	4	5
4. The content was current and relevant.	1	2	3	4	5
5. The content was presented clearly.	1	2	3	4	5
6. The content was covered adequately.	1	2	3	4	5

7. How would you rate your ability to apply your learning to practice?   ☐ diminished ability   ☐ no change   ☐ enhanced ability

Comments _____
_____

8. Time required to read the chapter and complete this form: _____ minutes

This educational activity is provided by the American Nephrology Nurses' Association (ANNA).
ANNA is accredited as a provider of continuing nursing education (CNE) by the American Nurses Credentialing Center's Commission on Accreditation (ANCC-COA).
ANNA is a provider approved of continuing nursing education by the California Board of Registered Nursing, provider number CEP 00910.
This CNE offering meets the Nephrology Nursing Certification Commission's (NNCC's) continuing nursing education requirements for certification and recertification.

Clinical Application: CQI in Vascular Access Management

Lesley C. Dinwiddie, MSN, RN, FNP, CNN

Objectives

Study of the information presented in this chapter will enable the learner to:
1. State two reasons why continuous quality improvement (CQI) in vascular access for hemodialysis (VA/HD) is essential.
2. Relate the history of clinical performance measures (CPMs) designed to implement CQI for VA/HD nationally.
3. Describe a recent large-scale clinical application of CQI in VA/HD.
4. Describe the mandate for CQI and the use of a vascular access team (VAT) prescribed in the KDOQI™ update of 2006.
5. List the data necessary for comprehensive CQI for VA/HD.
6. List the actions of the VAT for accomplishing CQI for VA/HD.
7. Cite one vascular access-related CQI example in the HD setting and one vascular access-related CQI example in the chronic kidney disease setting.

Introduction

Hemodialysis (HD) cannot be performed without access to a blood vessel with high flow. Flow is the product of volume and velocity sufficient to allow for safe, efficient, and effective dialysis. Frequent, direct access to the vascular system for several hours per treatment, several times per week puts the patient who is at risk on a continuum for many complications. This continuum includes subclinical inflammation, bacterial endocarditis, vessel stenosis and occlusion, to major hemorrhage, air embolism, or systemic fulminant infection (Breiterman-White, 2006).

There are significant variations across the United States and around the globe in practice patterns regarding the establishment and maintenance of HD vascular accesses. Quality initiatives seek to inform the public about facility-specific quality of care and encourage providers to improve the care they provide. The literature is replete with data on the morbidity, mortality, and healthcare costs of vascular access for hemodialysis (VA/HD). Oversight by the patient's interdisciplinary care team has been mandated in the Centers for Medicare and Medicaid Services (CMS) *Conditions for Coverage* (CMS, 2008). This oversight for VA/HD is a critical activity that must be continuously monitored for improvement opportunities.

Continuous Quality Improvement Through Clinical Performance Measures

Clinical Performance Measures (CPMs) illustrate both the need for and the gains that can be made through continuous quality improvement (CQI). Implemented in 1998 as outcome measures for the original 1997 National Kidney Foundation Dialysis Outcomes Quality Initiative (DOQI) guidelines, there were four CPMs chosen for vascular access (NKF, 1997). Over time, they have effectively shown both the challenges and improvements that can be made when data are collected on a large scale (CMS, 2004). Four CPMs for vascular access were originally chosen to:
1. Quantify the number of arteriovenous fistulae (AVF) for both incident and prevalent patients to determine if the percentages approximated or exceeded the DOQI goals of 50% and 40%, respectively. The CPM data define incident patients with end stage renal disease (ESRD) as equal to or greater than 18 years of age who initiated their first maintenance course of HD for ESRD on or between January 1 and August 31, and who were alive on December 31, and who were on HD continuously between October 1 and December 31, inclusive. Prevalent patients with ESRD are equal to or greater than 18 years of age who were alive on December 31, and who were on HD continuously between October 1 and December 31, inclusive. Prevalent patients include patients incident between January 1 and August 31 (CMS, 1999, p. 19).
2. Quantify the number of catheters being utilized as the prevalent vascular access for a period of longer than 90 days, with the DOQI goal being less than 10% of all prevalent accesses.
3. Determine what percentage of patients with arteriovenous grafts (AVG) was being prospectively monitored for venous stenosis on a routine basis using a variety of DOQI-approved methods.
4. Determine the percentage of catheters inserted into the subclavian vein in comparison to the percentage inserted into the internal jugular vein (CMS, 1999). Data for this fourth CPM were never collected because it became readily apparent that facility documentation on the catheter insertion site was frequently incomplete based on lack of detail in the procedural notes. This awareness illustrated the need for focused education for HD personnel in the physical assessment of the catheter insertion site, tunnel, and exit site (Dinwiddie, 2000).

Ten years later, there are data from the remaining three CPMs that demonstrate practice patterns for vascular access nationwide. Neither the CPM data collected nor the revised 2001 Kidney Dialysis Outcomes Quality Initiative™ (K/DOQI) (NKF, 2001) significantly changed practice in the first five years (CMS, 2004).

A National CQI Project

While substantial progress had been made in other key indicators, such as dialysis adequacy, vascular access continued to present significant challenges (Institute for Healthcare Improvement [IHI], 2003). Despite the KDOQI guidelines, CPMs, and international consensus that creation and mainte-nance of AVF in the majority of patients on HD constitutes best practice, the percentages of both incident and prevalent AVFs exhibited insignificant growth, falling far short of the NKF-KDOQI recommendations. At the same time, catheter access increased rather than decreased (CMS, 2004). There were increasing numbers of patients receiving HD, with a con-comitant increase in incident catheter usage that led to a con-sequential increase in morbidity and mortality related to vascu-lar access. Through the ESRD Networks' quality improvement projects, CMS attempted to encourage better practices with focused education for those facilities consistently not meeting the KDOQI goals. This did not elicit significant nationwide change. As a result, CMS asked IHI to assist in developing the National Vascular Access Improvement Initiative (NVAII), an initiative that was launched in 2003 (IHI, 2003). The slogan "Fistula First" epitomized that effort, and 11 key clinical and organization changes were provided for increasing AV fistula use and improving HD patient outcomes (Fistula First, 2008b). Not coincidentally, the number-one change concept was for "routine CQI review of vascular access." This specific change concept provided (and continues to provide) recommended steps for placement, planning, and care of the patient's vascu-lar access, along with links to related literature and tools. One example of related tools provided in the routine CQI review change concept includes a "Monthly Performance Tracking Tool," a spreadsheet for tracking trends in data. A second tool provided is a "root cause analysis for patients with a hemodial-ysis catheter," which is designed to be completed for each patient with a catheter each month (Fistula First, 2008a).

It was not until CMS recognized that real improvement would not materialize without intensifying the resources and expectations throughout all related disciplines that the Fistula First Breakthrough Initiative (FFBI) was launched in 2005. This initiative accelerated and led to a dramatic change in the AVF percentages in both incident and prevalent patients. Within a relatively short period of time, the national AVF prevalence rate reached and exceeded the original DOQI goal for AVF prevalence (Fistula First, 2008b). As of 2006, 42% of patients on HD use AVFs, representing a 27% increase in AVF use rates since the initiative began in 2003 (Fistula First, 2008b).

CQI: Raising the Bar

As a result of the improvement in both incident and preva-lent AVF rates, new goals were developed in true CQI fashion. The goal for AVF creation was raised to 65%, with continued emphasis on minimizing central venous catheter access, in the 2006 major revision of the KDOQI guidelines (NKF, 2006). The FFBI group raised the goal to 66% of patients on HD with AVFs for 2009 (Fistula First, 2008b). The 2006 revised KDOQI guidelines recognized that reaching these goals would require the use of a formal CQI process. A team approach to care represents a best practices model for achieving these vas-cular access goals. The first statement in *Guideline 8: Clinical Outcomes Goals* states, "Each center should establish a data-base and CQI process to track the types of accesses created and the complication rates for these accesses" (NKF, 2006, p. S258). The guidelines were also specific in recommending that all patients on HD receive care from a vascular access team (VAT). The VAT was defined as "the patient and a group of professionals involved in management of vascular access that includes care-givers who construct, cannulate, monitor, detect problems in, and repair vascular accesses" (NKF, 2006, p. S182). Members of the VAT include nephrologists, nephrolo-gy nurses, patient care technicians, nurse practitioners, physi-cian assistants, interventionalists, surgeons, and the vascular access coordinator.

Making CQI for VA/HD a Reality

How can providers of HD and the VAT operationalize the recommendations of KDOQI and the FFBI to properly accom-plish CQI for VA/HD? The identified group first needs to truly operate as a team, not just a loose affiliation of professionals who are involved episodically in vascular access management. A useful description of team dynamics and the specific work of the VAT is detailed in an NKF publication on a team approach to caring for patients with chronic kidney disease (CKD) (NKF, 2008). According to Dinwiddie (2007), the CQI process for the VAT includes data collection and database management of:
- Vascular access history.
- Current access type and site.
- Average flow rates per treatment.
- Average blood volume processed.
- Average arterial and venous machine pressures.
- Access monitoring and surveillance data.
- Laboratory results associated with adequacy such as urea reduction rates and Kt/V.
- Number and type of cannulation events.
- Number and type of dysfunction events.
- Number and type of interventions to correct events such as:
  - Re-cannulation.
  - Catheter placement.
  - Referral to interventionalist or surgeon.
  - Instillation of lytic.
  - Prompt diagnosis of bacteremia by positive culture.
  - Antibiotic therapy.

Based upon an effective model of CQI, the VAT should communicate at least monthly to:
- Review individual and aggregate facility data.
- Identify root causes for events in both the individual and facility.
- Track, plan, and act upon trends and events that predict dysfunction.
- Evaluate interventions and their outcomes.
- Review current literature for vascular access associated research and recommendations.
- Set goals for individuals and the overall patient population to improve vascular access outcomes.
- Affirm the plan for each patient's next step if the current access becomes dysfunctional or fails.

An excellent example of this vascular access CQI in action

was described by Doss, Schiller, and Moran (2008) who, through data collection, detected the problem of buttonhole site and systemic infection both in an in-center and home HD populations. Evaluation of the individual cases led them to identify that the probable root cause of these infections was failing to follow proper cannulation procedure, specifically improper scab removal prior to cannulation. A new policy of access preparation was implemented, including cleaning the access before and after scab removal. It was recognized that re-education of patients and staff to the new policy was necessary, with ongoing education emphasizing the importance of aseptic technique. A plan to evaluate effectiveness of the procedure was stated; the problem was developed into a manuscript and published in a peer-reviewed nursing journal (*Nephrology Nursing Journal*) so that other CQI programs could learn from their experience.

The CQI process and example described above is for HD providers and the VAT caring for the patient with Stage 5 CKD in the chronic outpatient setting. CQI, however, should be ongoing for all patients with kidney disease in the CKD and acute settings. This continuum of care should be reflected in individual care and also in the creation of policies and procedures to implement best practice. An example of this continuum of care can be found in the author's personal communication with direct caregivers (M. Toplosky, personal communication, March 31, 2008). A CQI team developed the following protocol in response to peripherally inserted central catheter (PICC) placement as standard of care for all patients needing vascular access for long-term IV therapy regardless of co-morbid disease and the potential for HD/VA in the future.

PICC Placement Guideline

- If the patient's estimated glomerular filtration rate (eGFR) is between 30 and 60 mL/minute, first consider using a small bore tunneled IJ catheter. If a PICC is chosen, avoid using the non-dominant arm.
- Avoid PICC placement and place a tunneled, small bore internal jugular (IJ) catheter if the patient:
  - Has an eGFR less than 30mL/minute.
  - Is a recipient of a renal transplant or a candidate for transplant.
  - Is currently on peritoneal dialysis.

Conclusion

Vascular access care delivered by an interdisciplinary team set forth as part of the 2006 KDOQI guidelines has been mandated in the CMS regulations (CMS, 2008) as a component of the basic patient plan of care. Not only should the team evaluate the patient on HD for the most appropriate vascular access type, taking into consideration co-morbid conditions and other risk factors, it must also routinely monitor the patient's vascular access to prevent access failure. Clearly, this regulation can only be actualized through the CQI process, which for VA/HD, must be implemented in a deliberate and methodical fashion. Creativity is required to promote communication among team members who frequently practice in different locations, as well as other team dynamics essential to making integrated team work a reality.

Another potential barrier for the CQI process in VA/HD is that vascular access dysfunction is episodic. The team may become focused on those patients they see most frequently, while those with the most functional accesses may not receive the level of oversight necessary to prevent or diagnose dysfunction early, or equally, to recognize and appreciate what works well. Perhaps the greatest CQI tool the VAT can implement may be a dedicated vascular access coordinator to properly operationalize the team process and make CQI a reality.

References

Breiterman-White, R. (2006). Vascular access for hemodialysis. In A. Molzahn & E. Butera (Eds.) *Contemporary nephrology nursing: Principles and practice* (2nd ed.). Pitman, NJ; American Nephrology Nurses' Association.

Centers for Medicare and Medicaid Services (CMS). (1999). *ESRD special report: Developing clinical performance measures for the care of patients with end stage renal disease.* Retrieved February 25, 2009, from http://www.cms.hhs.gov/CPMProject/Down loads/ ESRDCPMDevelopmentProcessFinalReport.pdf

Centers for Medicare and Medicaid Services (CMS). (2004). *Annual report: End Stage Renal Disease Clinical Performance Measure Project.* Baltimore, MD: Department of Health and Human Services, Centers for Medicare & Medicaid Services, Office of Clinical Standards & Quality.

Centers for Medicare and Medicaid Services (CMS). (2008). *Conditions for coverage for end-stage renal disease facilities: Quality assessment and performance improvement.* Retrieved February 25, 2009, from http://www.cms.hhs.gov/apps/media/press/ fact sheet.asp?Counter=3028&intNumPerPage=10&checkDate=&che ckKey=&srchType=1&numDays=3500&srchOpt=0&srchData=& keywordType=All&chkNewsType=6&intPage=&showAll=&pYear =&year=&desc=false&cboOrder=date

Dinwiddie, L.C. (2000). Identifying the insertion site of a central vein catheter. *Nephrology Nursing Journal, 27*(3), 326.

Dinwiddie, L.C. (2007). Overview of the role of a vascular access nurse coordinator in the optimisation of access care for patients requiring haemodialysis. *Hong Kong Journal of Nephrology, 9*(2), 99-103.

Doss, S., Schiller, B., & Moran, J. (2008). Buttonhole cannulation – An unexpected outcome. *Nephrology Nursing Journal, 35*(4). 417-419.

Fistula First. (2008a). *Change concept #1: Routine CQI review of vascular access. Related tools.* Retrieved February 25, 2009, from http://www.fistulafirst.org/professionals/changes1.php

Fistula First. (2008b). *History of the Fistula First Project.* Retrieved February 17, 2009, from http://www.fistulafirst.org/about_us/ history.php

Institute for Healthcare Improvement (IHI). (2003). *National Vascular Access Improvement Initiative (NVAII).* Retrieved February 17, 2009, from http://www.fistulafirst.org/pdfs/NVAIIProjectDescrip tion.pdf

National Kidney Foundation (NKF). (1997). Dialysis Outcomes Quality Initiative (NKF-DOQI). Clinical practice guidelines for hemodialysis vascular access. *American Journal of Kidney Diseases,30*, 5154-5196.

National Kidney Foundation (NKF). (2001). Kidney Disease Outcomes Quality Initiative (NKF-K/DOQI). Clinical practice guidelines for vascular access. *American Journal of Kidney Diseases,37*(Suppl. 1), S137-S181.

National Kidney Foundation (NKF). (2006). KDOQI Clinical Practice Guidelines for Vascular Access, update 2006. *American Journal of Kidney Diseases,48*(1, Suppl.1), S176-S307.

National Kidney Foundation (NKF). (2008). *Elements of excellence: A team approach to chronic kidney disease care.* New York: Author.

Additional Readings

Burrows-Hudson S., & Prowant, B. (2005). *Nephrology nursing standards of practice and guidelines for care.* Pitman, NJ: American Nephrology Nurses' Association.

Centers for Medicare & Medicaid Services (CMS). (2005). *CMS launches breakthrough initiative for major improvement in care for kidney patients.* Retrieved February 25, 2009, from http://www.cms.hhs.gov/apps/media/press/release.asp?Counter=1386

Dinwiddie, L.C. (2008). Vascular access for hemodialysis. In C. Counts (Ed.), *Core curriculum for nephrology nursing* (5th ed., pp. 735-764). Pitman, NJ: American Nephrology Nurses' Association.

| **Chapter 8** | **CONTINUING NURSING EDUCATION EVALUATION FORM** | **1.1 Contact Hours** |

Clinical Application: Continuous Quality Improvement in Vascular Access Management **ANNP0908**

Applying Continuous Quality Improvement in Clinical Practice contains 22 chapters of educational content. Individual learners may apply for continuing nursing education credit by reading a chapter and completing the Continuing Nursing Education Evaluation Form for that chapter. Learners may apply for continuing nursing education credit for any or all chapters.

Please photocopy this test page, complete, and return to ANNA.
You can also download this form from www.annanurse.org (choose Education - CNE Activities - Publications)
Receive continuing nursing education credit (CNE) immediately by completing the CNE evaluation process in ANNA's Online Library. Go to www.annanurse.org, and click on the Online Library icon for more information.

Name: _____

Address: _____

City: _____ State: _____ Zip: _____

E-mail:_____ Preferred telephone: ☐ Home ☐ Work _____

State where licensed and license number: _____

CNE application fees are based upon the number of contact hours provided by the individual section. CNE fees per contact hour for ANNA members are as follows: 1.0-1.9 – $15; 2.0-2.9 – $20; 3.0-3.9 – $25; 4.0 and higher – $30. Fees for nonmembers are $10 higher.

CNE application fee for Chapter 8: ANNA member $15   Nonmember $25

ANNA Member: ☐ Yes ☐ No   ☐ Member # (if available) _____

☐ Check or money order enclosed   ☐ American Express   ☐ Visa   ☐ MasterCard

Total amount submitted:_____

Credit card number _____ Exp. Date _____

Name as it appears on the card: _____
NOTE: Your evaluation form can be processed in 1 week for an additional rush charge of $5.00.
☐ Yes, I would like this evaluation form rush processed. I have included an additional fee of $5.00 for rush processing.

Instructions
1. To receive continuing nursing education credit for an individual study after reading the chapter, complete this evaluation form.
2. Detach, photocopy, or download (www.annanurse.org) the evaluation form and send along with a check or money order payable to **American Nephrology Nurses' Association** to: ANNA, East Holly Avenue Box 56, Pitman, NJ 08071-0056.
3. Test returns must be postmarked by **April 30, 2011**. Upon completion of the answer/evaluation form, a certificate will be sent to you.

This section was reviewed and formatted for contact hour credit by Sally S. Russell, MN, CMSRN, ANNA Director of Education Services.

CNE Application Fee for Chapter 8
ANNA member = $15
Nonmember = $25

---

1. I verify that I have read this chapter and completed this education activity. _____ Date _____
   Signature
2. What would be different in your practice if you applied what you have learned from this activity? (Please use additional paper if necessary.)
   _____
   _____
   _____

	Strongly disagree				Strongly agree
3. The activity met the stated objectives.					
a. State two reasons why continuous quality improvement (CQI) in vascular access for hemodialysis (VA/HD) is essential.	1	2	3	4	5
b. Relate the history of clinical performance measures (CPMs) designed to implement CQI for VA/HD nationally.	1	2	3	4	5
c. Describe a recent large-scale clinical application of CQI in VA/HD.	1	2	3	4	5
d. Describe the mandate for CQI and the use of a vascular access team (VAT) prescribed in the KDOQI™ update of 2006.	1	2	3	4	5
e. List the data necessary for comprehensive CQI for VA/HD.	1	2	3	4	5
f. List the actions of the VAT for accomplishing CQI for VA/HD.	1	2	3	4	5
g. Cite one vascular access-related CQI example in the HD setting and one vascular access-related CQI example in the chronic kidney disease setting.	1	2	3	4	5
4. The content was current and relevant.	1	2	3	4	5
5. The content was presented clearly.	1	2	3	4	5
6. The content was covered adequately.	1	2	3	4	5

7. How would you rate your ability to apply your learning to practice?   ☐ diminished ability   ☐ no change   ☐ enhanced ability

Comments _____
_____

8. Time required to read the chapter and complete this form: _____ minutes

Clinical Application: CQI with Fluid Management in Hemodialysis

Diana Hlebovy, BSN, RN, CHN, CNN

Objectives

Study of the information presented in this chapter will enable the learner to:
1. Describe the importance of incorporating fluid management into the facility Quality Assessment and Performance Improvement Plan.
2. Discuss the occurrence rate of intradialytic morbidities (ischemic events) during hemodialysis.
3. List potential clinical performance measures.
4. Identify root causes of inaccurate fluid management.
5. Complete the Plan-Do-Check-Action-Cycle related to fluid management.

Introduction: Scope of Challenge

Cardiovascular morbidity and mortality remain unacceptably high in the hemodialysis (HD) population. This is a persistent challenge in spite of the nephrology community's emphasis on urea kinetic modeling for adequacy of treatment monitoring, more permeable and biocompatible dialyzer membranes, and renewed focus on improving nutrition and anemia management (Mees, 2004). The United States has the highest mortality rate for patients on dialysis of any country using modern dialysis techniques (Henning 2007). According to the U.S. Renal Data System (USRDS) *2008 Annual Data Report,* the annual adjusted mortality rate for prevalent dialysis patients in the U.S. is 201.2 deaths per 1000 patient-years (USRDS, 2008). A review of the literature reveals cardiovascular disease as the major cause of hospital admissions for patients on HD. Cardiovascular disease is responsible for 49% of chronic and 40% of acute admissions, while pulmonary edema remains the most common hospital-admitting diagnosis (Spiegal, Michelis, Panagopoulos, DeVita, & Schwimmer, 2005). Hypervolemia is the most common cause of hypertension and left ventricular hypertrophy, and cardiovascular disease affects the mortality rate of patients on HD (National Kidney Foundation [NKF], 2006). The individual patient's rate of physiological fluid shifts from interstitial tissues back to the intravascular system during HD, which creates a challenge for the nephrology team. Volume shifts and hypoxemia during HD result in stress to the myocardium. Myocardial ischemia has been reported in 22% of HD treatments (Bleyer, 2008).

Bleyer (2008) reports that in a representative U.S. dialysis center of 100 patients, there will be approximately 20 deaths per year, 5 of which will be from sudden death. "Sudden death is responsible for approximately 25% of all deaths in the dialysis population" (Bleyer, 2008, p.1). Sudden death can result from stress applied to a damaged myocardium, and dialysis is a remarkable cardiac stressor related to volume shifts, electrolyte changes, cardiac ischemia, and hypoxemia occurring during HD (Bleyer, 2008). These challenges present opportunities for performance improvement in clinical practice related to fluid management.

Current Knowledge Related to Challenge

The perfect HD treatment would be one in which the calculated goal of ultrafiltration (UF) would bring the patient to a normovolemic and normotensive status without intradialytic morbidities. According to the 2008 Centers for Medicare and Medicaid Services (CMS) *Conditions for Coverage,* this type of fluid volume management combined with the adequate clearance of toxins determines adequacy of dialysis (CMS, 2008a). Over-estimation of the estimated dry weight leading to hypervolemia has significant consequences, with up to 90% of patients on HD having hypertension despite taking an average of three different antihypertensive medications (NKF, 2006).

Data from the Dialysis Morbidity and Mortality Wave 2 Study found that congestive heart failure was present in 40% of patients with end stage renal disease (ESRD) (Bleyer, 2008). According to the 2006 NKF Kidney Disease Outcomes Quality Initiative™ (KDOQI) Clinical Practice Guidelines, 90% of patients with ESRD could be normotensive by achieving their dry weight. Studies have shown that blood pressure decreases and reaches a new steady state within approximately 6 weeks after achieving a true dry weight and will not increase with increasing body mass (NKF, 2006). Control of dry weight equates to control of blood pressure, and thus, an increase in survival rates, a correlation established more than a decade ago (Charra et al., 1992). According to Scribner (1990) adequate control of extracellular volume is the key to treating hypertension in patients on dialysis.

Equally challenging, intravascular hypovolemia can cause intradialytic morbidities; ischemia of tissues resulting in injury to vital organs (such as the brain and heart, and loss of residual kidney function) compromises the adequacy of the dialysis treatment and increases the mortality rate (Shoji, Tsubakihara, Fujii, & Imai, 2004). The mortality rate was studied by Schreiber (2003), who found that two or more hypotensive episodes per week increase the death rate by 70%.

Occurrence of Intradialytic Morbidities

Adverse events requiring intervention are estimated to occur in 20% to 30% of HD treatments (Hlebovy & King,

2008). Specific intradialytic morbidities (ischemic events) during the HD treatment occur up to the following percentage rates (Hlebovy & King, 2008):

- Hypotension – 50%.
- Hypoxemia – 50%.
- Cramping – 20%.
- Nausea/vomiting – 15%.
- Seizures – Up to 10%.
- Angina pectoris – 5%.
- Myocardial ischemia – 22%.
- Dysrhythmias – 50%.
- Cardiac arrest – 7/100,000 treatments.
- Sudden death accounts for 25% of all deaths in the HD population.

2008 CMS *Conditions for Coverage and Interpretive Guidelines* as They Relate to Fluid Management

The CMS *Conditions for Coverage* stipulate that patients must be assessed for the appropriateness of the dialysis prescription, including blood pressure and fluid management (CMS, 2008a). This encompasses evaluating each patient's individualized fluid management needs, tracking, trending, and preventing intradialytic morbidities along with an analysis for potential root causes (CMS, 2008a). The *Interpretive Guidelines* hold facilities accountable for improving fluid management outcomes. Section §494.90, Tag V543, *Dose of Dialysis,* states that "the interdisciplinary team must provide the necessary care and services to manage the patient's volume status" (CMS, 2008a, p. 205).

The *Interpretive Guidelines* define estimated dry weight and the inter/intradialytic measures that will be used to evaluate the outcomes as follows: "A patient at [his or her] estimated dry weight should be asymptomatic and normotensive on minimum blood pressure medications, while preserving organ perfusion and maintaining existing residual renal function" (CMS, 2008a, p. 205). Target measurements for management of volume status listed on the Measurement Assessment Tool at Tag V543, *Dose of Dialysis,* also include:

- Euvolemic and normotensive: (adult) BP 130/80; (pediatric) lower of 90% of normal for age/height/weight or 130/80 (CMS, 2008b, p.1).

The *Interpretive Guidelines* require that the patient's target weight is identified and reached. The individual patient's plan of care must include treatment records that reflect the success in reaching the target weight for each treatment. If it is not attained, an assessment is needed to determine the underlying barriers interfering with this goal and a documented plan to address it (CMS, 2008a). Blood volume monitoring is mentioned as a tool to "evaluate body weight changes for gains in muscle weight vs. fluid overload" (CMS, 2008a, V504, p.189). Accountability of the team to meet individual patient goals is highlighted. "If the expected outcome is not achieved, the interdisciplinary team must adjust the patient's plan of care to achieve the specified goals" (CMS, 2008a, V559, p. 219). The patient cannot be solely responsible for not achieving goals. If patient non-adherence to the prescribed regime is identified, this is not acceptable as the only reason for not

achieving patient goals (CMS, 2008a). The plan of care must include frequent assessment of the target weight. This is addressed as follows:

- Target changes as indicated.
- Reassessment of medications.
- Root cause analysis of intradialytic morbidities.
- Scheduling an extra treatment if needed.
- Educating staff regarding fluid management strategies, machine settings, and monitoring.
- Counseling the patient regarding fluid allowances.
- Identifying causes for noncompliance, such as fear of intradialytic morbidity, prolonged recovery time, and scheduling conflicts (CMS, 2008a).

The *Interpretive Guidelines* mandate that unstable patients will require reassessment and plan of care changes monthly until stable (CMS 2008a). Examples cited for "unstable" include patients who have experienced:

- Intradialytic morbidities (any adverse event, such as cramping, hypotension, chest pain, seizures, syncope).
- Restlessness.
- Symptoms severe enough to prevent completion of the majority of dialysis treatments.
- Sudden onset of recurrent cardiac arrhythmias.
- Volume overload or depletion.
- Hypertension.
- Chronic congestive heart failure.
- Sudden onset of recurrent cardiac arrhythmia.
- Need for extra treatments for fluid removal.
- Inadequate dialysis.

The quality assessment and performance improvement (QAPI) condition (CMS, 2008a) requires facility-based assessment and improvement of care to maximize the number of patients who achieve both adequacy goals. These include successful fluid volume management and clearance of toxins (CMS, 2008a).

The interdisciplinary team must identify opportunities for improvement and track progress in adequacy of dialysis for the HD population. According to the *Conditions for Coverage* (CMS 2008a), this is done by:

- Reviewing aggregate patient data.
- Identifying commonalities among patients who do not reach minimum expected targets.
- Developing each individual patient's plan of care to address root causes.
- Implementing the plan of care.
- Monitoring the effectiveness of the plan of care.
- Adjusting portions of the plan of care that are not successful.
- Identification and prevention of intradialytic morbidities are also discussed in QAPI under medical injuries, and root cause analysis, tracking, and trending are mandated (CMS, 2008a).

Staff education and competency demonstration are now mandated in the CMS *Conditions for Coverage.* This must include the identification and treatment of intradialytic morbidities and monitoring of patients to prevent adverse events while attaining adequacy (CMS, 2008a).

The CMS *Conditions for Coverage* suggest that fluid management can be categorized as a high-risk, high-volume, problem-prone, high-cost aspect of care, and as such, is required in the facility's QAPI process (CMS, 2008a). Furthermore, the CMS *Conditions for Coverage* (2008a) indicate that optimal fluid management strategies implemented provide the right care for *every* person, *every* treatment, *every* time. Fluid management strategies need to be:

- Safe.
- Effective.
- Efficient.
- Appropriate.
- Patient-centered.
- Timely.
- Equitable.
- Providing continuity.
- Accessibile.

Team Approach for Fluid Management

Fluid management is an interdisciplinary team function. Facility managers, nephrologists, nephrology nurses, technicians, dietitians, social workers, and patients/family must all be participants of the team. The facility management team is responsible to ensure education and training programs are provided for all staff. This may include information and measures specific for optimal fluid management to achieve and maintain ideal dry weight of patients, achieve normotension, prevent intradialytic morbidities, and preserve residual kidney function. Education and training may include topics such as:

- Sodium and fluid restrictions that are individualized for the patient.
- Adequate and safe UF for the patient during the HD procedure.
- Use of diuretics for patients with residual renal function.
- Improving communication skills for all dialysis staff to promote effective patient education.
- The use of fluid management protocols, processes, equipment, and technologies that provide effective and safe methods to promote optimal fluid management during the HD treatment.
- Designating a facility fluid manager (registered nurse) for ensuring fluid management strategies are implemented and monitored for each patient.

Members of the interdisciplinary team provide and review education on fluid management with the patient to ensure continuity of information and enhanced positive patient outcomes, and encourages the patient to become a partner in his or her fluid management goals. The following provides descriptions for the fluid management roles of interdisciplinary team members.

Roles of Team Members

The nephrologist's role: To oversee and communicate their patients' medical and medication history to the interdisciplinary team to ensure thorough patient assessment and appropriate interventions. Nephrologists collaborate with other members of the patient's medical team to promote understanding of the nephrology patient's individualized medical needs.

The nephrology nurse's practice arena: Encompasses assessing and implementing fluid management strategies for the patient during HD and delegating monitoring where appropriate. The nephrology nurse is responsible for developing, implementing, and evaluating the nursing plan of care. Consistent and thorough assessment of the patient's pre/post-blood pressures trends, interdialytic weight gains, and achievement of ideal dry weight without intradialytic morbidities is necessary at every dialysis session. The effectiveness of the patient's plan of care in goal achievement is evaluated through reassessment of patient outcomes.

Dialysis technicians: Receive comprehensive education and training to accurately observe, report, and record patient changes proactively to the nephrology nurse. The nurse uses the information to determine an appropriate course of action.

The renal dietitian: Assesses body mass, analyzes dietary histories, and develops and instructs the patient through an individualized nutritional plan. The renal dietitian is expected to assist patients in achieving their nutritional goals by providing education, counseling, encouragement, and support.

The social worker: Are instrumental in assessment of patient satisfaction, motivation, and self-management with adherence to the plan of care. On-going assessment of the patient's psychosocial, financial, support of family/significant others, and other variables assist the interdisciplinary team in working with the patient to achieve improved outcomes.

The patient: At the core of the interdisciplinary team, the patient is the focus of care. A consideration for the interdisciplinary team is the patient's need for ongoing education about fluid management strategies. Encouraging the patient in self-management skills may support his or her participation as a partner in individualized fluid management goals and may foster adherence to regimes. As indicated in the *Conditions for Coverage* (CMS, 2008a), it is the responsibility of the interdisciplinary team that patients and/or designees receive information in a way they can understand. The *Conditions for Coverage* (CMS, 2008a) instructs the interdisciplinary team that patients must be informed of any changes to their dialysis prescription, adjustment in estimated dry weight being part of that prescription, and the reasons for changes.

Improvement Process in Individualized Fluid Management

The interdisciplinary team reviews fluid management for each individual patient. The team is responsible for a comprehensive patient assessment and a plan of care that addresses the needs of the patient for information and addresses ways to remove any barriers. The *Conditions for Coverage* directs the facility to encourage patient participation in care planning (for example, by offering the patient the option to participate in the interdisciplinary team care planning or to attend a planning meeting either in-person or by teleconference) (CMS, 2008a). Any changes in the plan of care, as well as rationale for changes, must be discussed with patients to the extent they desire.

The continuous quality improvement process can be applied to the individual patient's plan of care for improved outcomes. Several tools can be used for tracking, trending and analysis of fluid management outcomes. These include:

- Individual patient data collection tools:
  - Dialysis treatment log summarizing relevant patient information:
    - ➤ Pre and post-dialysis weights.
    - ➤ Pre/post/intra/interdialytic blood pressure measurements.
    - ➤ UF goal.
    - ➤ Total fluid removed.
    - ➤ Intradialytic morbidities.
  - Flow charts containing the patient's:
    - ➤ Pertinent laboratory data.
    - ➤ Test results, including diagnostic studies.
    - ➤ Residual urine output amount.
- Medical record:
  - Co-morbidities.
  - Medical history.
  - Medication review list.
  - Blood volume profiles and analysis tool (if applicable).
  - Treatment records.
  - Multidisciplinary assessments.
  - Progress notes and plan of care record.
  - Patient fluid and dietary log.
- Continuous quality improvement tools:
  - Cause-effect diagram (fish bone root cause analysis).
  - Variance (incident) reports tracking intradialytic morbidities: type, rate, time.
  - Run charts of individual patient hospitalization.
  - Patient satisfaction survey.
  - Flow charts.

Exploration of Root Causes

Exploration of potential causes of not achieving fluid management outcomes can be grouped into the six categories described by Taylor (1995). These are 1) the patient's medical history and medical condition status factors, 2) the patient's laboratory and radiologic results, 3) other patient variables, 4) medication factors, 5) hemodialysis and facility factors, and 6) interdisciplinary team factors.

Patient Medical History and Medical Condition Status Factors

- Co-morbidity factors.
- Cardiac history (CAD, atherosclerosis, MI, LVH, pericardial effusion, valve disease, pacemaker, internal defibrillator, poor ejection fraction, myopathy).
- Arrhythmias (such as bradycardia, tachycardia, atrial fibrillation).
- Hypertension.
- Respiratory disease.
- Diabetes mellitus.
- GI disturbances (nausea/vomiting/diarrhea/constipation/gastroparesis).
- Autonomic neuropathy.
- Amputations.
- Autoimmune disease.
- Skeletal muscle structural changes.
- Motor system disease.
- Polyneuropathy.
- Restless leg syndrome.

- Post transplant.
- Length of time with ESRD.
- Residual kidney function/residual urine output.
- Length of time on HD.
- Continued menses.
- Pregnancy.
- Sleep disorder.
- Septicemia.
- Temperature.
- Allergies/sensitivities/anaphylaxis.
- Type/flow/condition of access.
- High output cardiac failure related to high access blood flow.

Patient Laboratory and Radiologic Results

- Anemia.
- Hypoxemia.
- Hyper/hypokalemia.
- Hypo/hypercalcemia.
- Other electrolyte imbalances (such as sodium, magnesium).
- Parathyroid hormone (PTH)/CA x phosphorus product.
- Vitamin D levels.
- Albumin/plasma proteins.
- BUN/ANP/middle molecules.
- Serum glucose.
- Serum CO_2 and pH.
- Postdialytic alkalemia.
- Carnitine deficiency.
- Chest X-ray.
- ECHO.

Other Patient Variables

- Change in/incorrect dry weight.
- Nonadherence history.
- Skipped treatments.
- Sodium intake.
- Internal motivation.
- Lack of coordination/involvement in care planning.
- Satisfaction with HD treatments.
- Average weight gains.
- Ethnic/cultural influences.
- Appetite changes/habits.
- Posture during treatment.
- Eating during treatment.
- Size.
- Age.
- Sex.
- Self care involvement (such as home blood pressure, daily weight).
- Transportation issues.
- Social/family/peer support and pressures.
- Financial issues.
- Educational session opportunities/knowledge base.
- Beliefs.
- Amount of exercise.
- Loss of hope/negative mental attitude.
- Loss of external control.
- Invincibility belief.
- Ability to see own accountability and role.

Medication Factors

- Number/amount taken daily.
- Adherence.
- Financial resources/insurance.
- Blood pressure medications.
- Beta/calcium channel blockers.
- Diuretics.
- Digoxin.
- Phosphate binders-type/amount.
- Pain medications.
- Any vasodilator/vasoconstrictor.
- Hypertonic/normal saline administration.
- Past or present steroid therapy.
- Medication dosage.
- Time medication taken in relationship to HD treatment (pre, intra, or post-dialysis).
- Rapid administration of certain medications.
- Medication error.
- Medication side effects.
- Medication interactions.
- Drug dialyzability.

Hemodialysis/Facility Factors

- Goal.
- UF rate.
- Time into treatment.
- Inaccurate dry weight.
- Treatment time/frequency/days of week.
- Dialysate pH.
- Dialysate temperature.
- Dialysate conductivity range.
- Dialysate calcium.
- Dialysate glucose level.
- Facility protocols.
- Administration of hypertonic solutions.
- Hemolysis.
- Air embolism.
- Pyrogenic reaction.
- Dialyzer type.
- Dialyzer reaction.
- Machine calibration.
- Number of oxygen tanks/concentrators.
- Individual vs. standard plan of care/dialysis orders.
- UF controlled machine.
- Availability of blood volume monitoring (BVM).

Interdisciplinary Team Factors

- Facility management/leadership/supervision.
- Proactive vs. reactive culture.
- Quality of training programs.
- Lack of knowledge of principles/strategies/technologies available.
- Expertise of staff.
- Staff turnover rate.
- Staffing ratios.
- QAPI team plan involvement.
- Monitoring tools available and used.
- Consistency in approach and delivery.

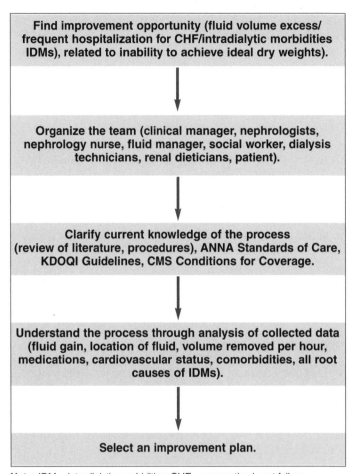

Figure 9-1
The FOCUS PDCA Approach

Find improvement opportunity (fluid volume excess/ frequent hospitalization for CHF/intradialytic morbidities IDMs), related to inability to achieve ideal dry weights).

Organize the team (clinical manager, nephrologists, nephrology nurse, fluid manager, social worker, dialysis technicians, renal dieticians, patient).

Clarify current knowledge of the process (review of literature, procedures), ANNA Standards of Care, KDOQI Guidelines, CMS Conditions for Coverage.

Understand the process through analysis of collected data (fluid gain, location of fluid, volume removed per hour, medications, cardiovascular status, comorbidities, all root causes of IDMs).

Select an improvement plan.

Note: IDM = intradialytic morbidities; CHF = congestive heart failure
Source: Used with permission from Diana Hlebovy.

- Lack of coordination in care planning.
- Belief system.
- Communication skill level.
- Attitude or frustration level related to patient non-adherence.
- Amount of support offered to patient.
- Ability to see own accountability and role.

Patient Case Study: Developing a Plan of Care Using The Plan-Do-Check-Action Cycle (see Figure 9-1)

JJ is a 46-year-old male who was admitted to the hospital 9 months ago with sudden onset of congestive heart failure and advanced kidney failure caused by primary amyloidosis. Other sequealae of his amyloidosis include autonomic neuropathy and swelling of his ankles and calves. JJ has been on chronic HD for the 3 months using a central vein catheter as access. His blood pressure has been averaging 90/60 pre-treatment. Currently, no plans have been finalized for a permanent access due to his persistently low blood pressure and the concerns that raises for adequate access perfusion to maintain its patency.

Opportunity for Improvement

While reviewing the facility monthly variance data report for episodes of intradialytic morbidities, the fluid manager noticed that JJ has had repeated occurrences of both symptomatic hypotension (80% of treatments) and cramping (60% of treatments). Hospitalization log reveals JJ has been hospitalized twice for congestive heart failure. These have occurred despite the increase in dialysis sessions from 4 hours/3 times/week, to 4 hours/5 times/week.

Measurable Goal/Patient Outcomes

- JJ will not experience symptoms of fluid volume deficit (symptomatic hypotension, cramping) related to the HD treatment.
- JJ will be free of signs and symptoms of fluid volume excess and congestive heart failure with no hospital admissions related to congestive heart failure.
- JJ will achieve an ideal dry weight (optimal volume status).
- JJ will be able to verbalize the importance of and strategies to maintain an ideal dry weight.

Meeting JJ's needs can be linked to the 2008 CMS *Conditions for Coverage* (2008a) discussed earlier in this chapter, which indicate that implementing optimal fluid management strategies must provide the right care for *every person, every treatment, every time.* Fluid management strategies need to be:

- Safe – Absence of intradialytic morbidity.
- Effective – Achieve desired goal/outcome (ideal dry weight).
- Efficient – Obtain desired effect with minimal effort, delay.
- Appropriate – Right intervention for the right problem.
- Patient-centered – Individualized plan of care; participation in plan of care and HD treatment; increased patient comfort and satisfaction with treatment.
- Timely – Proactive prevention of problems.
- Equitable – Use the fewest medication(s) or supplies as possible for interventions.
- Providing continuity – Patient care staff provide continuity from treatment to treatment.
- Accessibile – Patient has access to resources, education, technologies, and tools to achieve the desired outcomes.

Teamwork for Improved Patient Outcomes

JJ's status is unstable as defined in the *Interpretive Guidelines* under V520 related to recurrent intradialytic morbidities, hospitalizations, and inability to attain dry weight (CMS, 2008a). In order to analyze and develop action steps to resolve the problem, JJ's current patient assessment was reviewed for the development of a plan of care. The interdisciplinary team included JJ's nephrologist, primary nephrology nurse, social worker, renal dietitian, and fluid manager. To develop the most accurate, individualized plan of care, the team prepared for their meeting by reviewing JJ's medical history, recent laboratory reports, current home and dialysis treatment medication lists, and treatment flow sheets. Labs related to fluid management included:

- Albumin 4.3 (up from 3.3 upon admission).
- Pre-dialysis BUN 88.
- Glucose 98 mg/dL.
- Potassium 6.7 meq/L.

- HCT 29.1%; Hgb 9.7 gm/dL.
- Serum CO_2 23.
- Calcium/phosphorus/PTH levels, transferrin saturation, and ferritin levels were within target ranges.

Chest X-ray and ECHO showed left ventricular hypertrophy; pulmonary infiltrates were noted.

Home medications include sevelamer hydrochloride (Renagel®) 800 mg with meals, thalidomide (Thalomid®) 200 mg for the treatment of primary amyloidosis (Falk, 2006), midodrine (ProAmatine®) 5 mg on dialysis days taken 2 hours before treatment, and lorazepam (Atvan®) 1 mg as needed at bedtime.

During dialysis, JJ receives 15,000 units of erythropoietin alfa (Epoetin Alfa®) IV 3 times a week, iron sucrose for repletion 100 mg IV 3 times a week for 10 consecutive doses, and paricalcitol (Zemplar®) 8 mcg IV 3 times a week. JJ has been diagnosed with sleep apnea, and has a concentrator and CPAP machine at home.

Team Review

The renal dietitian reported that JJ's residual urine output is less than 100 ml/day. Fluid and dietary logs and his dietary prescription (2 g sodium, 1000 ml daily fluid allowance, 60 mEq potassium, 1.4 g/kg protein) and an overview of educational sessions that JJ had received provided additional information about his current status.

The social worker confirmed the patient's ability to afford prescribed medications and high-quality foods within his dietary restrictions. JJ reports his spouse as being supportive and eager to learn how to assist in preparing meals that comply with the diet prescription.

The fluid manager and primary nurse presented a brief review of the literature regarding the most current recommendations concerning fluid management:

- Relevant Literature:
  - *Core Curriculum for Nephrology Nursing,* 5th edition (Hlebovy, 2008a, 2008b; Hlebovy & King, 2008).
  - 2006 NKF KDOQI Guidelines (NKF, 2006).
  - October 2008 CMS *Conditions for Coverage* (CMS, 2008a).
- Technology and tools to assist with fluid management available include:
  - Volumetrically controlled dialysis machine with UF and sodium modeling capabilities.
  - High flux biocompatible dialyzer membrane.
  - Pulse oximeter and oxygen concentrators.
  - Hct-based BVM (monitoring blood volume and oxygen saturation).
  - Facility "no eating policy" during HD treatment.

The direct care dialysis staff were consulted for current treatment practices and insights they could provide about JJ and his treatments.

Review of JJ's treatment flow sheets shows that his intradialytic morbidities were occurring at different times in the treatment, ranging from the first hour to the last.

Interventions have included use of UF profiles that did not prevent intradialytic morbidities from developing. Currently,

JJ's UF goal is set to remove a consistent amount of fluid over the entire dialysis time.

Despite his order for treatments 5 days a week, JJ has not been able to reach his estimated dry weight of 80 kg that was established on admission.

Fluid weight has been slowly increasing; JJ is now approximately 10.5 kilograms (kg.) over the prescribed estimated dry weight. His average weight gains are 6 to 6.5 kg. Despite attempts to remove only his interdialytic fluid gain, plus the normal saline prime administered with treatment initiation, normal saline administered with treatment termination, and JJ's oral intake of a sport drink during treatment (up to 1 liter), he develops intradialytic symptoms after a 5 kg loss.

Dialysate temperature is set at 37.5 degrees Celsius. Dialysate prescription is potassium 2 mEq/L, calcium 2.5 mEq/L. Sodium modeling is prescribed from 150 meq/L to the base of 140 meq/L, the facility standard for sodium modeling.

JJ routinely receives a total of 3 doses of hypertonic saline until the last half hour of HD for prevention and/or treatment of cramping. An average 400 to 500 ml of normal saline fluid replacement is given for symptomatic hypotension each treatment. JJ insists on eating what he brings to the clinic while he is on dialysis. After the treatment has ended, JJ generally remains in the unit for 30 to 40 minutes due to orthostatic hypotension and associated dizziness. He is typically given a 12-ounce cup of chicken broth to drink post-treatment as he waits for his blood pressure to reach an acceptable level for discharge.

Staff members indicate the patient has become less communicative during the treatment; JJ listens to his music and sleeps. Because of his frequent cramping and neuropathy, JJ insists on sitting up with his feet on the floor for the majority of his treatment. JJ recently began to skip one of his weekly treatments, stating that he does not feel well during the treatment and "needs a break" during the interdialytic period. Staff members express their frustration at his perceived "non-compliant" behavior.

Root Cause Analysis

A fishbone diagram (see Figure 9-2) was used to identify and analyze potential causes of the identified problem. Several factors, including patient-related, treatment-related, medication-related, and interdisciplinary team factors, were identified as having contributed to the root causes of the problem.

Patient-Related Factors

- Underlying disease process of primary amyloidosis and its potential effect on:
  - The heart and cardiac output.
  - Autonomic neuropathy, resulting in orthostatic hypotension.
- Anemia and related hypoxemia.
- Posture (feet on floor during treatment).
- Eating during the HD treatment.
- Hyperkalemia.
- Dietary/fluid non-compliance.
- Sleep apena.

Treatment-Related Factors

- Dialysate temperature (37.5 degrees Celsius) and conductivity (sodium modeling ranging from 150 to 140 mcg/L).
- High UF rate due to interdialytic fluid weight gain.
- Administration of hypertonic saline, sodium modeling, extra normal saline.
- Difficult to assess actual dry weight due to swelling in legs (accentuated from primary disease process).
- Practice of giving 12 ounces of high-sodium chicken broth post-dialysis.

Medication-Related Factors

- Potential for medication side effects from thalidomide, such as autonomic neuropathy, orthostatic hypotension, shortness of breath, dizziness, swelling, and rash (Celgene, 1998).
- Dosage and timing of midodrine 2 hours before HD.
- Administration and long-term effects of hypertonic saline/extra saline/chicken broth.

Interdisciplinary Team Factors

- Lack of knowledge or application of principles/strategies/technologies available.
- Monitoring tools available and used.
- Consistency in approach and delivery.
- Lack of coordination in care planning.
- Negative attitude towards/frustration level related to patient non-adherence.
- Belief that intradialytic morbidities are an expected part of HD.

The PDCA Cycle

Plan

After specifying objectives, plan a change (see Figure 9-3).

Immediate action steps planned for JJ's next treatment:
- The primary nurse will assess the need for oxygen supplementation for hypoxemia through the use of pulse oximetry for pO_2 reading; BVM provides SvO_2 reading.
- Nephrologist orders:
  - Eliminate variable sodium; set and maintain the sodium base at 138 meq/L.
  - Maintain dialysate temperature between 35 degrees to 36 degrees Celsius.
  - Oxygen administration for pO_2 less than 90% or SvO_2 less than 60%.
  - Collaborate with the physician treating JJ's amyloidosis concerning thalidomide dosage.
- The primary nurse will use the available HCT-based BVM to guide fluid removal to prevent hypovolemia/hypoxemia, assess dry weight, and delegate monitoring to the dialysis technician.
- The renal dietitian will re-discuss the effects of eating on dialysis with JJ and review dietary/fluid allowances vs. choices.
- Fluid manager/primary nurse will assist the direct care staff in setting the patient's target goal. This will be based on weight gain and the lowest recent post-weight, plus the normal saline used for treatment initiation and termination. The patient's potential oral fluid intake will not be automatically added in to the goal. Adjustments will be made based on assessment of patient response as observed on BVM (Hlebovy, 2008b).

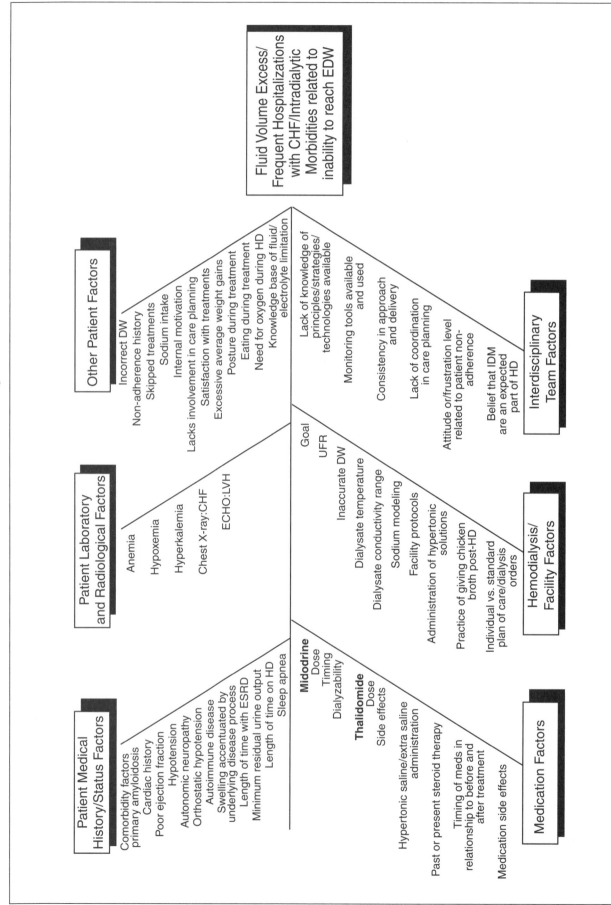

Figure 9-2
Fishbone – Cause and Effect Diagram for JJ

Fluid Volume Excess/ Frequent Hospitalizations with CHF/Intradialytic Morbidities related to inability to reach EDW

Other Patient Factors

Incorrect DW
Non-adherence history
Skipped treatments
Sodium intake
Internal motivation
Lacks involvement in care planning
Satisfaction with treatments
Excessive average weight gains
Posture during treatment
Eating during treatment
Need for oxygen during HD
Knowledge base of fluid/ electrolyte limitation

Patient Laboratory and Radiological Factors

Anemia
Hypoxemia
Hyperkalemia
Chest X-ray:CHF
ECHO:LVH

Patient Medical History/Status Factors

Comorbidity factors primary amyloidosis
Cardiac history
Poor ejection fraction
Hypotension
Autonomic neuropathy
Orthostatic hypotension
Autoimmune disease
Swelling accentuated by underlying disease process
Length of time with ESRD
Minimum residual urine output
Length of time on HD
Sleep apnea

Midodrine
Dose
Timing
Dialyzability

Thalidomide
Dose
Side effects

Hypertonic saline/extra saline administration
Past or present steroid therapy
Timing of meds in relationship to before and after treatment
Medication side effects

Medication Factors

Lack of knowledge of principles/strategies/ technologies available
Monitoring tools available and used
Consistency in approach and delivery
Lack of coordination in care planning
Attitude or/frustration level related to patient non-adherence
Belief that IDM are an expected part of HD

Interdisciplinary Team Factors

Goal
UFR
Inaccurate DW
Dialysate temperature
Dialysate conductivity range
Sodium modeling
Facility protocols
Administration of hypertonic solutions
Practice of giving chicken broth post-HD
Individual vs. standard plan of care/dialysis orders

Hemodialysis/ Facility Factors

Source: Used with permission from Diana Hlebovy.

Figure 9-3
The PDCA Cycle

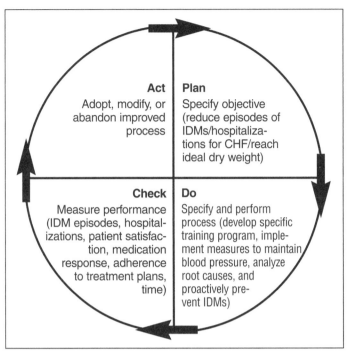

Source: Used with permission from Diana Hlebovy.

- Fluid manager/primary nurse will educate the clinic staff on strategies for fluid removal. These include:
  - Setting the UF rate to remove more fluid during the first hour of treatment.
  - Striving for a UF goal of up to 2 liters during the first hour, if tolerated.
  - Adjusting the UF goal and rate so the BVM does not demonstrate a blood volume decrease of more than minus 8% in the first hour of treatment.
  - Adjust the remaining goal over the last 3 hours of treatment, not to exceed an overall minus 15% BVM change or SvO_2 below 60%.
- The primary nurse will educate the direct care staff in JJ's plan of care. Actions include increasing the frequency of blood pressure monitoring in the last hour of treatment to every 15 minutes and planning a reduction of the UF goal based on data from BVM, SvO_2 readings, and vital signs.
- The interdisciplinary team is to engage the patient in his plan of care. Planned interventions include:
  - Asking JJ open-ended questions.
  - Discuss what is important to him (assessing his internal motivation).
  - Evaluate the patient's knowledge level concerning the importance of fluid management.
  - Identify areas of educational deficit(s) and re-educate him in those areas.
  - Discuss undesirable effects of eating during HD.
  - Review the untoward effects of the "feet down position" during HD.
  - Present strategies for fluid management that he thinks he can accomplish.

Facility plans included:
  - Provide additional educational opportunities with staff on the relationship of hypoxemia to intradialytic morbidities and safe and effective fluid management strategies.

Do
Revised plan of care was agreed upon with the patient and initiated.

The patient fluid volume assessment is outlined in Figure 9-4, resulting in the following findings:
- Complains of shortness of breath with activity, restless during sleep.
- Pre-blood pressure 88/50; pulse 60; oral temperature 35 degrees Celsius.
- Crackles audible in bilateral bases; 3+ pitting edema in ankles, thigh swelling.
- Red blistering areas noted in lower extremities.
- Neck vein distention noted.
- Pre-weight of 92 kg; gain of 6 kg from previous treatment.
- Initial SvO_2 reading of 50% (O_2 initiated).

Check
Check the effects or results of the changes.

At the end of 1 hour of HD treatment with 2 kg/2 liters of ultrafiltration removed:
- JJ's oxygenation level had improved (SvO_2 of 61%) as had his blood pressure – up to 119/78, pulse 72.
- The UF goal was adjusted to remove the remainder of his fluid weight gain and increased upward based on his BVM profile. Fluid removal is guided by changes in the SvO_2 and blood volume changes when BVM technology is used (Steuer, Harris, & Conis, 1995). The UF goal is reduced when the SvO_2 drops. Oxygen administration was initiated at 2 L/minute and increased to 3 L/minute based upon the facility's protocols.
- A dry weight check done at the end of the treatment through the BVM showed significant refill, suggesting the patient has not achieved his dry weight (Rodriguez, Domenici, Diroll, & Goykhman, 2005).
- A total of 7 L was removed without intradialytic morbidities/fluid or hypertonic solution replacement.
- At the end of the treatment, JJ rated the treatment as a 10+ (on a scale of 0 to 10).
- Post-blood pressure standing was 120/74; pulse 72; temperature 35.5 degrees Celsius.

Act
Act on what was learned in order to continue the change or modify the plan.
- The basic fluid removal plan as described above remained in effect over the next month. Dry weight checks were conducted each treatment, and no refill was noted after the eighth treatment using the BVM. This suggested the patient was at his new ideal dry weight of 82.5 kg.
- A knowledge deficit was identified about the relationship between salt and fluid gains, the difference between phosphorus and potassium, and an ongoing need for oxygen.
- An individualized education plan was subsequently designed by

Figure 9-4
Fluid Volume Assessment

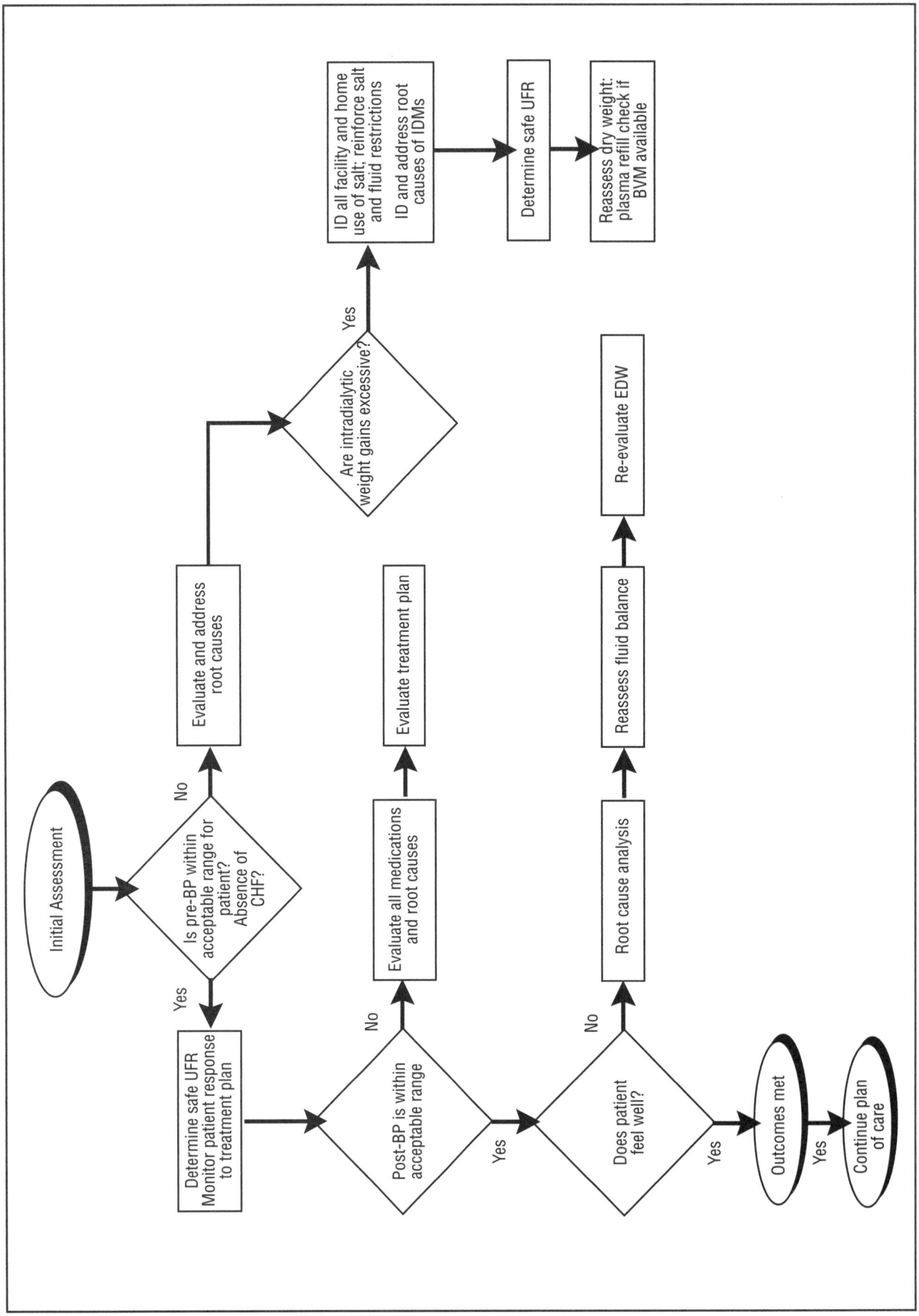

Initial Assessment

Is pre-BP within acceptable range for patient? Absence of CHF?

No → Evaluate and address root causes

Yes → Determine safe UFR Monitor patient response to treatment plan

Are intradialytic weight gains excessive?

Yes → ID all facility and home use of salt; reinforce salt and fluid restrictions / ID and address root causes of IDMs → Determine safe UFR → Reassess dry weight: plasma refill check if BVM available

Post-BP is within acceptable range

No → Evaluate all medications and root causes → Evaluate treatment plan

Yes → Does patient feel well?

No → Root cause analysis → Reassess fluid balance → Re-evaluate EDW

Yes → Outcomes met

Yes → Continue plan of care

Note: UFR = ultrafiltration rate; EDW = estimated dry weight; IDM = intradialytic morbidities; BP = blood pressure; BVM = blood volume monitoring.
Source: Used with permission from Diana Hlebovy.

the interdisciplinary team for the patient and his spouse. Meal preparation with approved alternative herbal additives was included. The thalidomide dose was reduced to 50 mg twice daily.

JJ was instructed to take his midodrine no earlier than a half hour prior to his HD treatment, and an extra dose was ordered mid-way through the treatment.

Closing the Loop

Individual patient outcomes:
- After 1 month, JJ's interdialytic fluid gains averaged 1 to 2 kg during the week, 3 kg over the weekend.
- JJ passed a verbal post re-education quiz with a score of 90%, and he was able to verbalize the importance of and strategies to maintain optimal volume status.
- There were no hospital admissions for congestive heart failure and evidence of fluid volume excess after 1 month. Following these alterations in his care, JJ's HD treatments were decreased to 4 each week. One month later, the number of treatments was reduced to 3 treatments per week.
- JJ restarted using his CPAP machine at night, and verbalized increased energy during the day and fewer episodes of shortness of breath.
- With the continued use of BVM and oxygen therapy during dialysis, JJ did not experience symptoms of fluid volume deficit during HD (such as symptomatic hypotension or cramping). He stated he does not "feel as worn out after treatments and can actually do some yard work in the evening."
- JJ is currently being referred to an access surgeon for possible arteriovenous fistula placement.
- JJ planted a garden (of flowers, not tomatoes) in the spring.

When looking at the changes made in JJ's HD management, the QAPI team adapted some of those changes into practice throughout the unit. Changes incorporated in the facility's practices included:
- Sodium modeling and hypertonic saline were eliminated from routine practices.
- Chicken broth was eliminated.
- Thermal control (maintaining the dialysate temperature between 35 to 36 degrees Celcius) was ordered for all patients by a physician.
- Re-education and reinforcement on the facility "no eating" policy and the reasons for the policy were provided for all patients.
- Proactively identifying and treating hypoxemia.

Facility-Wide Improvement Process in Fluid Management

What clinical performance measures could be explored at the facility level to indicate improvement in fluid management? Clinical performance measures include (CMS, 2008b):
- Decrease in fluid-related hospitalizations.
- Decrease in number and type of intradialytic morbidities, cardiac arrest, sudden death.
- Decrease in pre-treatment hypertension (Measurement Assessment Tool [MAT]: blood pressure 130/80 [adult]) (CMS, 2008a). (See pages 193-194 for the MAT.)
- Decrease in the number of blood pressure medications.

- Decrease in post-dialysis recovery time.
- Increase in patient satisfaction with HD treatments.
- Decrease in access failure related to hypovolemia.
- Preservation of residual kidney function/residual urine output.
- Improvement in anemia management/hemoglobin variability.
- Lower average treatment cost (results of decreased hospitalizations, and reduced use of medications/solutions and supplies to treat intradialytic morbidities).

The interdisciplinary team's review of the facility outcome data for fluid management, variance reports, analysis of individual case studies, and trending reports by facility staff for the QAPI committee meetings provide data for this continuous quality improvement process.

Tools for facility data collection for the QAPI committee include:
- Variance (incident) reports of intradialytic morbidities tracking type, rate of occurrences, and specifics (such as time, day, shift on which they occurred, UF rate).
- Hospitalization trending and analysis report.
- Network tracking reports.
- Patient satisfaction survey question results related to treatment.
- Individual data collection logs.
- Clinical performance measures of fluid management (CMS, 2008b):
  ○ Blood pressure trends.
  ○ Number of blood pressure medications/reductions.
  ○ Hospitalization rates.
  ○ Access failure rates.
  ○ Intradialytic symptom type, frequency, root causes.
  ○ Run charts to provide a picture of frequency of specific events.
  ○ Control charts to illustrate the variations that may exist.
  ○ Flow charts to visually illustrate the steps of a specific process and sequence to evaluate for complexity of the process or for missing steps.
  ○ Cause-effect diagrams (fishbone analysis).

Increased emphasis on including fluid-related patient outcomes in the adequacy assessment has increased since the Hemo Study reported that mortality rates of patients on hemodialysis have not improved with higher Kt/V and more permeable membranes (Eknoyan et al., 2002). Numerous references are now available to enable dialysis staff to keep their practices updated and current. Updates include methods to improve patient outcomes, fluid management, and reduce patient complications, which have been included in the 2006 NKF/KDOQI Clinical Practice Guidelines (NKF, 2006) and the Core Curriculum for Nephrology Nursing, 5th edition (Counts, 2008). These published reviews of technologies and strategies that have shown positive benefits in improving patient outcomes include:
- Volumetric or ultrafiltration-controlled dialysis.
- Thermal control to support blood pressure (cooler dialysate).
- HCT-based BVM: Monitoring of blood volume and oxygen saturation.
- Supplemental oxygen to prevent and treat hypoxemia.

These references showed uncertain benefit of sodium profiling and the use of hypertonic solutions. Both strategies are associated with the potential to lead to a cycle of increased thirst, increased interdialytic weight gains, hypertension, and the need for excessive UF. This increases the risk for hypotension and/or muscle cramping. The 2006 *NKF-KDOQI Clinical Practice Guidelines* state that increasing positive sodium balance by sodium profiling or using a high dialysate sodium concentration should be avoided to decrease thirst, fluid gains, and hypertension (NKF, 2006). When using UF profiling, dialysis staff need to be aware there are many variables that are not constant for any individual patient. "An individual profile may seem to emerge, but caution must be used, as this may need to vary from one HD to the next" (Hlebovy, 2008a, p. 703).

The 2008 CMS *Conditions for Coverage* and their accompanying *Interpretive Guidelines* clearly elevate the importance of fluid management as an indicator for adequacy of dialysis. The *Conditions for Coverage* emphasize fluid management's effect on hospitalizations, cardiac mortality, intradialytic morbidities, anemia, nutritional status, and access patency (CMS, 2008a). They highlight that the "ultrafiltration component of the hemodialysis prescription should be optimized with a goal to render the patient euvolemic and normotensive" (CMS, 2008a, p. 205).

The new guidelines are also more specific on the indicators to be assessed and reassessed. These indicators are to be used with root cause analysis to identify why goals are not met and why patients experience intradialytic symptoms. "The comprehensive assessment should include evaluation of the patient's pre/intra/post and interdialytic blood pressures, interdialytic weight gains, target weight, and related intradialytic symptoms (such as hypertension, hypotension, muscular cramping) along with an analysis for potential root causes" (CMS, 2008a, p. 189).

Conclusion

Principles, strategies, and technologies exist today to permit assessment and assignment of "ideal" dry weight to improve well being and survival rates for patients on HD. The nephrology nurse is able to use assessment and critical thinking skills to address individual patient needs and treatment variables. This enables the nurse to incorporate safe, effective, and proactive nursing interventions and treatment options into the HD treatment. The nephrology nurse, as part of the QAPI team, must be the champion in fluid management to enhance and improve patient outcomes. The entire dialysis team, which most importantly includes the patient, must be part of the fluid management care planning in order to achieve and maintain successful improvements in outcomes.

References

Counts, C.S. (Ed.) (2008). *Core curriculum for nephrology nursing* (5th ed.). Pitman, NJ: American Nephrology Nurses' Association.

Bleyer, A. (2008). Prevention of sudden cardiac death in dialysis patients: A nephrologist's perspective. *Dialysis & Transplantation, 77*(4),124-129.

Celgene. (1998). *Thalidomide package insert*. Retrieved February 22, 2009, from http://www.thalomid.com/pdf/Thalomid_Pl.pdf

Centers for Medicare and Medicaid Services (CMS). (2008a). *Final rule*. Retrieved February 22, 2009, from http://www.cms.hhs.gov/CFCsAndCoPs/downloads/ESRDfinalrule0415.pdf

Centers for Medicare and Medicaid Services (CMS). (2008b). *Clinical performance measures (CPM) project: Overview*. Retrieved February 22, 2009, from http://www.cms.hhs.gov/CPMProject/01_Overview.asp

Charra, B., Calemard, E., Ruffet, M., Chazot, C., Terrat, J. C., Vanel, T., et al. (1992). Survival as an index of adequacy of dialysis. *Kidney International 41*(5), 1286-1291.

Eknoyan, C., Beck, C.J., Cheung, A.K., Daugirdas, J.T., Green,T., Kusek, J.W., et al. (2002). Effect of dialysis dose and membrane flux in maintenance hemodialysis. *New England Journal of Medicine, 347*, 2010- 2019.

Falk, R.H. (2006). *The physician's guide to amyloidosis*. Danbury, CT: The National Organization for Rare Disorders.

Henning, M. (2007). Affecting Kt/V: An analysis of staff interventions. *Dialysis & Transplantation, 36*(11), 584-600.

Hlebovy, D., & King, B. (2008). Hemodialysis: Complications of hemodialysis – Prevention and management. In C.S. Counts (Ed.), *Core curriculum for nephrology nursing* (5th ed., pp. 704-716). Pitman, NJ: American Nephrology Nurses' Association.

Hlebovy, D. (2008a). Hemodialysis: Fluid removal – Obtaining estimated dry weight during hemodialysis. In C.S. Counts (Ed.), *Core curriculum for nephrology nursing* (5th ed., pp. 692-704). Pitman, NJ: American Nephrology Nurses' Association.

Hlebovy, D. (2008b). Hemodialysis: Obtaining ideal dry weight through hematocrit-based blood volume monitoring. In C.S. Counts (Ed.), *Core curriculum for nephrology nursing* (5th ed., pp. 717-724). Pitman, NJ: American Nephrology Nurses' Association.

Mees, E. (2004). Adequacy of dialysis: An inadequately applied concept. *Dialysis & Transplant, 33*(22), 738-748.

National Kidney Foundation (NKF). (2006). K/DOQI clinical practice guidelines for hemodialysis adequacy: Update 2006. *American Journal of Kidney Diseases, 48*(1, Suppl. 1), S2-S75.

Rodriguez, H.J., Domenici, R., Diroll, A., & Goykhman, I. (2005) Assessment of dry weight by monitoring changes in blood volume using Crit-Line. *Kidney International, 68*, 854-861.

Schreiber, M.J. (2003). *Intradialytic complications*. Paper presented May 2003 at the RCG Sixth Annual Medical Conference, Tucson, AZ.

Scribner, B.H. (1990). A personalized history of chronic hemodialysis. *American Journal of Kidney Disease, 16*, 511-519.

Shoji, T., Tsubakihara, Y., Fujii, M., & Imai, E. (2004). Hemodialysis-associated hypotension as an independent factor for two-year mortality in hemodialysis patients. *Kidney International, 66*: 1212-1220.

Spiegal, P., Michelis, M., Panagopoulos, G., DeVita, M.V., & Schwimmer, J.A., (2005). Reducing hospital utilization by hemodialysis patients. *Dialysis and Transplantation, 34*:3, 131-136.

Steuer, R.R., Harris, D.H., & Conis, J.M. (1995). Continuous, in-line monitoring of oxygen saturation in hemodialysis. *Dialysis & Transplantation, 24*(11), 615-620, 658.

Taylor, J. (1995). Continuous quality improvement in action: A pediatric hemodialysis case study. In G.S. Wick & E. Peacock (Eds.), *Continuous quality improvement: From concept to reality* (pp. 1-4). Pitman, NJ: American Nephrology Nurses' Association

United States Renal Data System (USRDS). (2008). *Annual data report: Atlas of chronic kidney disease and end-stage renal disease in the United States*. Bethesda, MD: National Institutes of Health, National Institute of Diabetes and Digestive and Kidney Diseases. Retrieved February 14, 2009, from http://www.usrds.org/adr.htm

Additional Readings

Charra, B., Bergstrom, J., & Scribner, B.H. (1998). Blood pressure control in dialysis patients: The importance of the lag phenomenon. *American Journal of Kidney Diseases, 32*, 720-724.

Charra, B. (1998). Dry weight in dialysis: The history of a concept. *Nephrology Dialysis Transplantation, 77*(13), 1882-1885.

Daugirdas, J.T., Blake, P.G., & Ing, T.S. (2007). *Handbook of dialysis* (4th ed.). Philadelphia: Lippincott, Williams & Wilkins.

Diroll, A., & Hlebovy, D. (2003). Inverse relationship between blood volume and blood pressure. *Nephrology Nursing Journal, 30*(4), 460-461.

Goldstein, S.L., Michael, M., & Bewer, E. (2004). Blood volume monitoring to achieve target weight in pediatric hemodialysis patients. *Pediatric Nephrology, 19*, 432-437.

Harbert, G., & Wick, G.S. (1995). Concepts and principles of quality management. In G.S. Wick, & E. Peacock (Eds.), *Continuous quality improvement: From concept to reality.* Pitman, NJ: American Nephrology Nurses' Association.

Hardnett, J., Foley, R., Kent, G., Barre, P., Murray, D., & Parfrey, P. (1995). Congestive heart failure in dialysis patients: Prevalence, incidence, prognosis and risk factors. *International Society of Nephrology, 47*, 884-890.

Harmon, E. (2003). Blood volume monitoring: Taking the guesswork out of fluid removal for the dialysis nurse. *Contemporary Dialysis & Nephrology, 24*(4), 32-34.

Hlebovy, D. (2006) Fluid management: Moving and removing fluid during hemodialysis. *Nephrology Nursing Journal, 33*(4), 441-446.

Hlebovy, D. (2006) Fluid management: Understanding its impact on morbidity and mortality. *Nephrology News and Issues, 20*(12), 75.

Hossli, S.M. (2005). Clinical management of intradialytic hypotension: Survey results. *Nephrology Nursing Journal, 32*(3), 287-292.

Jaeger, J.Q., & Mehta, R.L. (1999) Assessment of dry weight in hemodialysis: An overview. *Journal of the American Society of Nephrology, 10*, 392-403.

Johnson, D., & Sasak, C. (1995). The process of establishing a continuous quality improvement environment. In G.S. Wick & E. Peacock (Eds.), *Continuous quality improvement: From concept to reality.* Pitman, NJ: American Nephrology Nurses' Association.

Levin, N.W., & Ronco, C. (2002) *Common clinical problems during hemodialysis.* In A.R. Nissensen & S. Fine (Eds.), *Dialysis therapy* (3rd ed.). Philadelphia: Hanely & Belfus, Inc.

Patel, H., Goldstein, S., Mahan, J., Smith, B., Fried, C., Currier, H., et al. (2007). A standard, noninvasive monitoring of hematocrit algorithm improves blood pressure control in pediatric hemodialysis patients. *Clinical Journal of the American Society of Nephrology 2*, 252-257.

Pillon, L. (2006) Blood volume improves volume optimization and cardiovascular outcomes. *Nephrology News and Issues, 20*(12), 77-78.

Purcell, W., Manias, E., Williams, A., & Walker, R. (2004). Accurate dry weight assessment: Reducing the incidence hypertension and cardiac disease in patients on hemodialysis. *Nephrology Nursing Journal, 31*(6), 631-638.

Schroeder, K.L., Sallustio, J.E., Ross, E.A. (2004). Continuous haematocrit monitoring during intradialytic hypotension: precipitous decline in plasma refill rates. *Nephrology Dialysis Transplant, 19*(3), 652-656.

| Chapter 9 | CONTINUING NURSING EDUCATION EVALUATION FORM | 1.4 Contact Hours |

Clinical Application: CQI in Fluid Management with Hemodialysis   **ANNP0909**

Applying Continuous Quality Improvement in Clinical Practice contains 22 chapters of educational content. Individual learners may apply for continuing nursing education credit by reading a chapter and completing the Continuing Nursing Education Evaluation Form for that chapter. Learners may apply for continuing nursing education credit for any or all chapters.

Please photocopy this test page, complete, and return to ANNA.
You can also download this form from www.annanurse.org (choose Education - CNE Activities - Publications)
Receive continuing nursing education credit (CNE) immediately by completing the CNE evaluation process in ANNA's Online Library. Go to www.annanurse.org, and click on the Online Library icon for more information.

Name: _____

Address: _____

City: _____State: _____Zip: _____

E-mail:_____Preferred telephone: ☐ Home ☐ Work_____

State where licensed and license number: _____

CNE application fees are based upon the number of contact hours provided by the individual section. CNE fees per contact hour for ANNA members are as follows: 1.0-1.9 – $15; 2.0-2.9 – $20; 3.0-3.9 – $25; 4.0 and higher – $30. Fees for nonmembers are $10 higher.

CNE application fee for Chapter 9: ANNA member $15   Nonmember $25

ANNA Member: ☐ Yes ☐ No   ☐ Member # (if available) _____

☐ Check or money order enclosed   ☐ American Express   ☐ Visa   ☐ MasterCard

Total amount submitted:_____

Credit card number _____ Exp. Date _____

Name as it appears on the card: _____

NOTE: Your evaluation form can be processed in 1 week for an additional rush charge of $5.00.
☐ **Yes, I would like this evaluation form rush processed. I have included an additional fee of $5.00 for rush processing.**

INSTRUCTIONS

1. To receive continuing nursing education credit for an individual study after reading the chapter, complete this evaluation form.

2. Detach, photocopy, or download (www.annanurse.org) the evaluation form and send along with a check or money order payable to **American Nephrology Nurses' Assocation** to: ANNA, East Holly Avenue Box 56, Pitman, NJ 08071-0056.

3. Test returns must be postmarked by **April 30, 2011**. Upon completion of the answer/evaluation form, a certificate will be sent to you.

This section was reviewed and formatted for contact hour credit by Sally S. Russell, MN, CMSRN, ANNA Director of Education Services.

CNE Application Fee for Chapter 9
ANNA member = $15
Nonmember = $25

1. I verify that I have read this chapter and completed this education activity. _____Date _____
                                                                                                                                   Signature
2. What would be different in your practice if you applied what you have learned from this activity? (Please use additional paper if necessary.)

_____
_____
_____
_____

			Strongly disagree				Strongly agree

3. The activity met the stated objectives.
   a. Describe the importance of incorporating fluid management into the facility Quality Assessment and Performance Improvement Plan. 1 2 3 4 5
   b. Discuss the occurrence rate of intradialytic morbidities (ischemic events) during hemodialysis. 1 2 3 4 5
   c. List potential clinical performance measures. 1 2 3 4 5
   d. Identify root causes of inaccurate fluid management. 1 2 3 4 5
   e. Complete the Plan-Do-Check-Action Cycle related to fluid management. 1 2 3 4 5
4. The content was current and relevant. 1 2 3 4 5
5. The content was presented clearly. 1 2 3 4 5
6. The content was covered adequately. 1 2 3 4 5
7. How would you rate your ability to apply your learning to practice? ☐ diminished ability ☐ no change ☐ enhanced ability

Comments _____
_____

8. Time required to read the chapter and complete this form: _____ minutes

This educational activity is provided by the American Nephrology Nurses' Association (ANNA).
ANNA is accredited as a provider of continuing nursing education (CNE) by the American Nurses Credentialing Center's Commission on Accreditation (ANCC-COA).
ANNA is a provider approved of continuing nursing education by the California Board of Registered Nursing, provider number CEP 00910.
This CNE offering meets the Nephrology Nursing Certification Commission's (NNCC's) continuing nursing education requirements for certification and recertification.

Clinical Application:
Improvement Application in Acute Dialysis

Sylvia Moe, BSN, RN, CNN
Billie Axley, MS, RN, CNN

Objectives

Study of the information presented in this chapter will enable the learner to:
1. Discuss how an improvement process can be applied to the acute dialysis setting
2. Describe two examples of improvement projects in the acute dialysis setting

Introduction

Part of the challenge and excitement of working in acute dialysis clinical practice is the opportunity for the nephrology nurse to continuously look at processes to find ways to improve a patient's outcomes. Nephrology nurses may ask how the improvement process can ensure a quality program in the acute dialysis setting beyond the familiar water/dialysate and equipment manufacturer standards. One challenge of applying the improvement process in this setting could be the lack of published benchmarks against which outcomes can be compared. Nephrology nurses can, however, gain insight by looking to published experiences in other areas of health care that show the improvement process as an effective tool. Determining elements of a program to evaluate (Plan), how those elements should be measured (Do), how to analyze the results (Check), and utilizing the information gained (Act) is the starting point.

Identifying Program-Based Quality Indicators

Acute hemodialysis, according to Palevsky (2006), is initiated for signs and symptoms of renal failure, including clinical uremia, severe hyperkalemia, and pulmonary edema (see Table 10-1). Nephrology nurses know that despite major advances in both intensive care and blood purification technology over the past four decades, mortality rates associated with acute kidney injury remain high (John & Eckhardt, 2006; Palevsky, 2006).

Utilizing the experience gained from the successful application of the improvement process in the chronic kidney disease (CKD) community, the key to the improvement process in the acute setting is the commitment to an evidence-based approach to improving processes. This approach should build upon and contribute to the creation of a system in which clinical outcome events and trends could be tracked. The program can gather evidence from other programs' outcome data for best practices as benchmarks and compare this evidence to its own historical data.

Hemodialysis therapy among patients who are critically ill can frequently result in therapy-related complications. An example with which nephrology nurses may readily identify is the impact that hypotensive events can have on patient outcomes in the acute hemodialysis setting. This can include intravascular volume depletion with resulting hypotension, inadequate fluid removal, and inadequate waste product clear-

Table 10-1
Indications for Renal Replacement Therapy In the Acute Care Setting

Uremia
Fluid imbalance
Electrolyte imbalance(s) – E.g., hyperkalemia
Acid-base balance changes – Metabolic acidosis
Intoxications – E.g., acetaminophen, propylene glycol
Toxicity – E.g., radiocontrast (studies with contrast)

Source: Adapted from Bogle et al., 2008; Palevsky, 2006; Schiffl, Lang, & Fischer, 2002; Williams, Bogle, & Davey-Tresemer, 2008. Used with permission from Sylvia Moe.

ance due to early termination of a treatment, all of which can further aggravate the underlying condition (John & Eckhard, 2006). According to Henrick (2008), intradialytic hypotension remains one of the most common and vexing adverse effects occurring in 20% to 30% of standard thrice-weekly hemodialysis session. Li (2003) cited reports of up to 50% of patients experience symptomatic reductions in blood pressure following hemodialysis. When looking for guidelines for ultrafiltration (UF) of fluid in hemodialysis, nurses can review research on patients with CKD Stage 5 on dialysis that indicates UF is a component of the hemodialysis prescription and should be optimized with a goal of euvolemic and nomotensive patients in effort to improve patient outcomes (National Kidney Foundation [NKF], 2006). Fluid removal is determined clinically by the evaluation of the level of blood pressure and/or evidence of fluid overload or intravascular fluid depletion, recognizing that actual tolerance of UF varies among patients. Intradialytic hypotension is significant in critically ill patients treated in the acute care setting, and an acute dialysis program may choose to develop an improvement project addressing the occurrence of hypotensive episodes in its practice.

What data should be collected for the selected indicator? When calculating the rate of hypotensive episodes, data elements could include comparing the number of patients treated in a month to the number of patients with episodes of clinical hypotension. Additional data to consider may include an evaluation of the individual patient's treatments, including weights, blood pressures, and other intradialytic incidents. This would provide a longitudinal dynamic view of extracellular fluid volume and blood pressure changes (Hlebovy & King, 2008). Medical record audits and hemodialysis treatment flowsheets may be the source of needed data. Planning should include the development of a timeline to collect measurable data, with time allowed to provide education to team members for effective data tracking. This team member education should include several facets to facilitate trending and analysis of multiple data points. Obtaining data through a medical record chart and hemodialysis treatment flowsheet audits, as well as monitoring the indicated elements for a specified period of time will provide data needed for this analysis. The NKF Kidney Disease Outcomes Quality Initiative™ (KDOQI) guidelines suggest using a dialysis log to track and summarize relevant patient information and intradialytic events for trending (see Figure 10-1) (NKF, 2006).

Uremia and the need for renal replacement therapy among critically ill patients frequently results in therapy-related complications. Acute kidney injury is characterized by the instability of the patient's hemodynamic parameters and increased permeability of the vasculature complicating the removal of fluid, control of BUN concentrations, and compensation for metabolic acidosis (John & Eckhardt, 2006). An improvement project focus for the acute dialysis setting could be decreasing hypotensive episodes to successfully complete hemodialysis therapy in a patient with the complication of sepsis.

Goal: Decrease the Rate of Hypotensive Episodes By 25% in 6 Months

Gather baseline data (see Figure 10-2) and identify root causes:
- Episodes of hypotension:
  - Hemodialysis can be complicated by hypotension associated with aggressive fluid removal; however, autonomic dysfunction and decreased cardiac reserve are contributing factors (Cronin & Mathers, 2008). Unstable cardiovascular status, arrhythmia, pericardial tamponade, myocardial infarction, and stiff hypertrophied heart compromise the heart's ability to maintain or increased cardiac output in response to volume depletion (Hlebovy & King, 2008).
- Electrolyte imbalance:
  - Arrhythmias may develop with changes in electrolyte levels and the rate at which the electrolyte change is occurring, affecting cardiac contractility and heart rate (Helbovy & King, 2008).
- Change(s) in the patient's condition since the nephrologist examined the patient and the orders for dialysis therapy were written.

Plan: Develop an Algorithm to Optimize The Dialysis Therapy

Ultrafiltration Profiling

Dialysis equipment with UF profiling capabilities can be used to remove fluid in variable patterns as opposed to using the same UF rate throughout treatment. Alternating higher UF rates for short periods of time with lower rates may assist with capillary refill of fluid from interstitial tissues (Hlebovy & King, 2008). UF profiling can also be performed manually in the

Figure 10-1
Use of a Dialysis Log to Summarize Relevant Information of Extracellular Fluid Volume

Patient Fluid Balance
Daily weight/trends
Accurate intake and output
Blood pressure trends
Vasopressor dose(s)
Hemodynamic monitoring recordings
Intradialytic Hypotensive Events on Dialysis
Blood pressure and heart rate trends
Ultrafiltration goal
Adjustment of ultrafiltration rates in response to blood pressure trends
Ultrafiltration volume achieved
Volume support; administration of osmotic agents
Vasoactive/vasopressor rate changes
Hemodynamic monitoring changes
Blood volume monitoring

Source: Adapted from Hlebovy & King, 2008; NKF, 2006; Williams et al., 2008. Used with permission from Sylvia Moe.

acute hemodialysis practice setting by varying the rate of fluid removal based upon continuous monitoring of the patient's hemodynamic status.

Dialysate Prescription

Serum electrolytes may need to be drawn just prior to dialysis if changes in the patient's status are suspected based upon patient assessment. An increase in ectopy during the treatment may result from the rate of electrolyte changes in the patient's blood and may be resolved by utilizing dialysate with a higher level of potassium or calcium. Collaborate with the nephrologist for adjustments to the dialysate solution (Bogle et al., 2008).

Dialysate Temperature Prescription

Collaborate with the nephrologist in evaluating the advantages of a decrease in dialysate temperature. Dialysate temperatures decreased to 34 to 36 degrees Celsius may improve hemodynamic stability in patients needing a higher UF rate (Hlebovy & King, 2008).

Extending Dialysis Time Prescription

Various treatment time and blood flow combinations can be calculated to meet the selected prescription goal (NKF, 2006). Restoring electrolyte balance and maintaining normal physiologic function may need to be accomplished with slower, daily dialysis to sustain solute and fluid removal (Palevsky, 2006). Outcomes are shown to be better in patients who receive a higher delivered dose of dialysis (Luyckx & Bonventre, 2004).

Figure 10-2
Data Tracking Log Items

Patient #	Weight	24-Hour Intake Total	24-Hour Output Total	BP/HR	CVP	PAWP	Cardiac Index	Vasopressor Dose	UF Volume Achieved	Volume Support/ Osmotics	Blood Volume Monitoring	Arrythmia
Date/Time												
Date/Time												
Date/Time												
Date/Time												
Date/Time												
Date/Time												
Date/Time												
Date/Time												

Note: PAWP = pulmonary artery wedge pressure; CVP = central venous pressure; UF = ultrafiltration.
Source: Used with permission from Sylvia Moe.

Hematocrit-Based Blood Volume Monitoring As Available

Blood volume monitoring is a non-invasive measure in numerical values of hematocrit and oxygen saturation, and is a means of assessment of blood volume changes and hypoxemia. Monitoring provides an objective method to proactively prevent intravascular volume depletion (Hlebovy, 2008).

Vasopressor Prescription

The type and dose of vasopressors should be based on the patient's previous response to UF (Bogle et al., 2008).

Sodium Modeling Prescription

Collaborate with the nephrologist in evaluating the use of osmotic support via sodium modeling when available and the patient's response to the sodium modeling prescription. It is important to note, however, that the sodium modeling option will need consideration because the NKF KDOQI does not support sodium profiling based upon reported incidence of increased thirst and interdialytic weight gains (Hlebovy, 2008; NKF, 2006).

Maintain and Sustain Improved Outcomes

In the *Act* step of the improvement process, successful strategies are incorporated into the acute program's processes, in this case, to minimize hypotensive events during hemodialysis. These strategies include:
- Monitoring vital signs and responding to changes with adjustment in the UF rate.
- Using UF profiling as available or altering UF rates manually based upon the patient's response to therapy.
- Reducing the dialysate temperature as prescribed.
- Monitoring hematocrit-based blood volume, as available.
- Utilizing hemodynamic monitoring information.
- Titrating vasopressors as prescribed in the acute care setting.
- Using dialysate sodium modeling only if and as prescribed by the nephrologist.
- Considering use of daily dialysis treatments.

Avoiding hypotension helps to ensure the delivery of adequate dialysis therapy by preventing early termination of the treatment. Low blood pressure can compromise dialysis adequacy by impairing tissue perfusion (Hlebovy & King, 2008). Advantages may be found in daily dialysis as well as with the use of volumetric control of UF (Schiffl, Lang, & Fischer, 2002). Using algorithm steps (see Figure 10-3) and gathering relevant patient data, the continuous quality improvement team may identify which steps produce successful outcomes (such as a reduction in the rate of hypotensive episodes from the baseline rate), which could be considered for incorporation into a best practice guideline for providing adequate hemodialysis in the acute care setting.

Use of Personal Protective Equipment for Infection Control Measures – Improvement Project

Another example of a clinical practice indicator in which an inpatient program's staff could apply the improvement process is staff use and observation of infection control practices. This can include the use of personal protective equip-

Figure 10-3
Algorithm Diagram

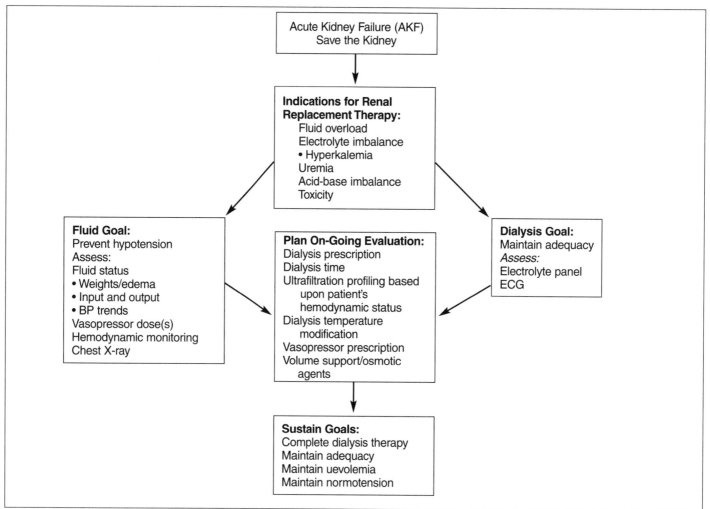

Acute Kidney Failure (AKF)
Save the Kidney

Indications for Renal Replacement Therapy:
Fluid overload
Electrolyte imbalance
• Hyperkalemia
Uremia
Acid-base imbalance
Toxicity

Fluid Goal:
Prevent hypotension
Assess:
Fluid status
• Weights/edema
• Input and output
• BP trends
Vasopressor dose(s)
Hemodynamic monitoring
Chest X-ray

Plan On-Going Evaluation:
Dialysis prescription
Dialysis time
Ultrafiltration profiling based
    upon patient's
    hemodynamic status
Dialysis temperature
    modification
Vasopressor prescription
Volume support/osmotic
    agents

Dialysis Goal:
Maintain adequacy
Assess:
Electrolyte panel
ECG

Sustain Goals:
Complete dialysis therapy
Maintain adequacy
Maintain uevolemia
Maintain normotension

Source: Used with permission from Sylvia Moe.

ment and consistent application of infection control practices to protect patients from cross-contamination. The state of uremia results in impaired immune function. This enhances susceptibility to infection and puts the patient at risk for bacteremia and potentially sepsis (Arduino et al., 2008). These complications further impact the patient's hemodynamic stability. Using the improvement process, nurses would start the project by gathering data. The question at baseline would be, "What is the current compliance rate among the HD staff members?" Obtaining a baseline compliance rate in this case could require data from observational assessment.

An example of baseline observational assessment could include:
• Wearing gloves when at risk of contamination by body fluids.
• Washing hands or using a gel before and after glove use.

• Wearing a barrier gown and face protection when at risk of blood exposure.
• Cleaning of patient station according to policy and procedure; such as the bed and rails, side table, and the hemodialysis equipment, including the blood pressure cuff.
• No eating, drinking, or applying lipstick in the patient care area.

The observational assessment can be followed by staff interviews to identify root causes of non-compliance:
• Identified barriers/key causes.
• Staff were not aware of all details in the personal protective equipment policy.
• Staff did not always think about wearing personal protective equipment in the busy patient care area.
• Correct sizes of personal protective equipment is not always readily available to staff.

Next Steps in the Improvement Process

Plan/Do

- Review the personal protective equipment audit findings with all staff during a staff meeting.
- Review personal protective equipment policies and procedures with all staff; post policies and procedures in the break room.
- Assign staff members to ensure all hemodialysis sites are stocked with needed sizes and personal protective equipment is easy for dialysis staff to locate.

Check

Repeated observational assessment/audit after a specified period of time:
- Percent compliant.
- Percent breaks in compliance.

Act

- Institute quarterly infection control/personal protective equipment assessments, rotating team members who perform the audits.
- Staff members not meeting 100% compliance assigned to attend an infection control/personal protective equipment inservice.

Access Plan Activated for Patients with Catheters Improvement Project

Acute nephrology nurses also care for many patients on chronic hemodialysis who enter the acute care setting. Nephrology nurses are concerned about what they can do for these patients that could influence their mortality and morbidity outcomes. This third example of an improvement process in the acute dialysis setting involves an interdisciplinary team. Which processes could be improved to increase the rate of permanent access for patients with CKD who initiate hemodialysis treatments in the acute setting?

- **Problem statement:** Patients new to dialysis admitted for initiation of dialytic therapy in the inpatient setting may be discharged with neither a permanent access nor a consult with a vascular surgeon for placement of a permanent access.
- **Analyze:** Audit 10% of the medical records for past 3 months for baseline of patients who began chronic hemodialysis. Audit revealed less than 30% of patients initiating treatment had a permanent access or plans in place for placement of permanent access prior to discharge.
- **Goal:** Select a timeframe (6 months) and target goal percentage (50%) of patients initiating chronic hemodialysis who will receive permanent access placement or vascular surgeon consult made prior to discharge to the outpatient facility.

Key Causes

- Lack of a patient education plan in place for vascular accesses.
- No process in place for inpatient staff to follow up with nephrologists for the order on vein mapping and/or vascular surgeon consult.

Plan/Do

- The interdisciplinary team met with nephrologists. They asked how they could help in the process for patients new to hemodialysis to undergo vein mapping and/or a vascular access consult while the patient is in the hospital or has an appointment scheduled prior to discharge.
- Staff checked the patient orders at the first hemodialysis treatment for vein mapping/vascular surgeon's consult, and if not present, notified the rounding nephrologist.
  - A tracking tool was developed to monitor vein mapping and vascular surgeon consult status of for patients new to chronic hemodialysis.
- A patient education plan developed for staff using the "Fistula First" (CMS, 2008) resources to educate patients on vascular access.

Check

After 6 months, data showed 62% of all new patients on chronic hemodialysis initiated in the inpatient program had placement of (or a consult for placement of) a permanent access before discharge to their chronic hemodialysis facility. *Goal met!*

Act

- Incorporate successful processes into program policy.
- Add a quarterly report of outcomes to hospital improvement committee and nephrologists.
- Select a new goal of 70% of patients new to chronic hemodialysis with vascular access placed, vascular surgeon consult, or scheduled appointment with a vascular surgeon prior to discharge to the outpatient program.
- Add education for all new patients on access site protection during hospitalization and education for hospital staff on vein preservation.

Conclusion

We return to the original question, "How can the improvement process ensure a quality program in the inpatient acute dialysis setting?" A key to the improvement process is in the commitment to an evidence-based approach. It should build upon and contribute to the creation of a system in which clinical outcome trends, such as hypotensive events, could be tracked and analyzed to gather evidence for best practices. This evidence-based approach can be found in following the principles of the improvement process. The process always begins with gathering data to identify an opportunity for improvement, identifying root causes of the problem, addressing the root causes with realistic action steps, and then gathering data again to determine if the plan provided the desired outcomes. Incorporating successful action steps into the daily routine ensures that the achieved outcomes will continue. Using continuous quality improvement for any improvement process can be a fun team problem-solving experience, with challenges and opportunities for improvement following a time proven method.

References

Arduino, M.J., Arnold, E., Axley, B., Butera, E., Curry, G., & Peacock, E.J. (2008). Infection control. In C.S. Counts (Ed.), *Core curriculum for nephrology nursing* (5th ed., pp. 969-1006). Pitman, NJ: American Nephrology Nurses Association.

Bogle, J.L., Craig, M., Williams, H.F., Garrigan, P.L., Davey-Tresemer, J., & Dalton, T.L. (2008). Acute care: Hemodialysis in the acute care setting. In C.S. Counts (Ed.), *Core curriculum for nephrology nursing* (5th ed., pp. 176-214). Pitman, NJ: American Nephrology Nurses' Association.

Cronin, S.C., & Mathers, T.R. (2008). Care of the older adult with chronic kidney disease: Opportunities to improve health and quality of life for the older adult. In C.S. Counts (Ed.), *Core curriculum for nephrology nursing* (5th ed., pp. 931-966). Pitman, NJ: American Nephrology Nurses' Association.

Henrick, W. (2008). Intradialytic hypotension: A new insight to an old problem. *American Journal of Kidney Disease, 52*(2), 209-210.

Hlebovy, D. (2008). Fluid removal: Obtaining estimated dry weight during hemodialysis. In C.S. Counts (Ed.), *Core curriculum for nephrology nursing* (5th ed., pp. 692-704). Pitman, NJ: American Nephrology Nurses Association.

Hlebovy, D., & King, B. (2008). Hemodialysis: Complications of hemodialysis – Prevention and management. In C.S. Counts (Ed.), *Core curriculum for nephrology nursing* (5th ed., pp. 704-716). Pitman, NJ: American Nephrology Nurses' Association.

John, S., & Eckardt, K. (2006). Renal replacement therapy in the treatment of acute renal failure – Intermittent and continuous. *Seminars in Dialysis, 19*, 455-464.

Li, J. (2003). Medication for hemodialysis-induced hypotension. *Medscape Internal Medicine 5*(2). Retrieved July 24, 2008, from http://www.medscate.com/viewarticle/463204

Luyckx, V.A., & Bonventre, J.V. (2004). Dose of dialysis in acute renal failure. *Seminars in Dialysis, 17*(1), 30-36.

National Kidney Foundation (NKF). (2006). *Kidney Disease Outcomes Quality Initiative: Clinical practice guidelines and clinical practice recommendations; Guideline 5. Control of volume and blood pressure.* Retrieved February 3, 2009, from http://www.kidney.org/professionals/kdoqi/guideline_upHD_PD_VA/hd_guide5.htm

Palevsky, P.M. (2006). Dialysis modality and dosing strategy in acute renal failure. *Seminars in Dialysis, 19*(2), 165-170.

Schiffl, H., Lang S., & Fischer, R. (2002). Daily hemodialysis and the outcome of acute renal failure. *New England Journal of Medicine, 346*(5), 305-310.

Williams, H.F., Bogle, J.L., & Davey-Tresemer, J. (2008). Acute kidney injury and acute renal failure. In C.S. Counts (Ed.), *Core curriculum for nephrology nursing* (5th ed., pp. 144-175). Pitman, NJ: American Nephrology Nurses' Association.

Additional Readings

Burrows-Hudson, S., & Prowant, B. (2005). *ANNA nephrology nursing standards of practice and guidelines for care.* Pitman, NJ: American Nephrology Nurses' Association.

Center for Medicare and Medicaid Services (CMS). (2008). *Fistula First.* Retrieved February 3, 2009, from http://www.fistulafirst.org

Chapter 10 — CONTINUING NURSING EDUCATION EVALUATION FORM — 1.4 Contact Hours

Clinical Application: Improvement Application in Acute Dialysis

ANNP0910

Applying Continuous Quality Improvement in Clinical Practice contains 22 chapters of educational content. Individual learners may apply for continuing nursing education credit by reading a chapter and completing the Continuing Nursing Education Evaluation Form for that chapter. Learners may apply for continuing nursing education credit for any or all chapters.

Please photocopy this test page, complete, and return to ANNA.
You can also download this form from www.annanurse.org (choose Education - CNE Activities - Publications)
Receive continuing nursing education credit (CNE) immediately by completing the CNE evaluation process in ANNA's Online Library. Go to www.annanurse.org, and click on the Online Library icon for more information.

Name: _____

Address: _____

City: _____ State: _____ Zip: _____

E-mail: _____ Preferred telephone: ☐ Home ☐ Work _____

State where licensed and license number: _____

CNE application fees are based upon the number of contact hours provided by the individual section. CNE fees per contact hour for ANNA members are as follows: 1.0-1.9 – $15; 2.0-2.9 – $20; 3.0-3.9 – $25; 4.0 and higher – $30. Fees for nonmembers are $10 higher.

CNE application fee for Chapter 10: ANNA member $15   Nonmember $25

ANNA Member: ☐ Yes ☐ No   ☐ Member # (if available) _____

☐ Check or money order enclosed   ☐ American Express   ☐ Visa   ☐ MasterCard

Total amount submitted: _____

Credit card number _____ Exp. Date _____

Name as it appears on the card: _____

NOTE: Your evaluation form can be processed in 1 week for an additional rush charge of $5.00.

☐ **Yes, I would like this evaluation form rush processed. I have included an additional fee of $5.00 for rush processing.**

INSTRUCTIONS

1. To receive continuing nursing education credit for an individual study after reading the chapter, complete this evaluation form.

2. Detach, photocopy, or download (www.annanurse.org) the evaluation form and send along with a check or money order payable to **American Nephrology Nurses' Assocation** to: ANNA, East Holly Avenue Box 56, Pitman, NJ 08071-0056.

3. Test returns must be postmarked by **April 30, 2011**. Upon completion of the answer/evaluation form, a certificate will be sent to you.

This section was reviewed and formatted for contact hour credit by Sally S. Russell, MN, CMSRN, ANNA Director of Education Services.

CNE Application Fee for Chapter 10
ANNA member = $15
Nonmember = $25

1. I verify that I have read this chapter and completed this education activity. _____ Date _____
   Signature

2. What would be different in your practice if you applied what you have learned from this activity? (Please use additional paper if necessary.)
   _____
   _____
   _____
   _____

	Strongly disagree				Strongly agree
3. The activity met the stated objectives.					
a. Discuss how an improvement process can be applied to the acute dialysis setting.	1	2	3	4	5
b. Describe two examples of improvement projects in the acute dialysis setting.	1	2	3	4	5
4. The content was current and relevant.	1	2	3	4	5
5. The content was presented clearly.	1	2	3	4	5
6. The content was covered adequately.	1	2	3	4	5

7. How would you rate your ability to apply your learning to practice?   ☐ diminished ability   ☐ no change   ☐ enhanced ability

Comments _____
_____

8. Time required to read the chapter and complete this form: _____ minutes

This educational activity is provided by the American Nephrology Nurses' Association (ANNA).
ANNA is accredited as a provider of continuing nursing education (CNE) by the American Nurses Credentialing Center's Commission on Accreditation (ANCC-COA).
ANNA is a provider approved of continuing nursing education by the California Board of Registered Nursing, provider number CEP 00910.
This CNE offering meets the Nephrology Nursing Certification Commission's (NNCC's) continuing nursing education requirements for certification and recertification.

Clinical Application: CQI in Solid Organ Transplant

Pat Weiskittel, MSN, RN, CNN, ACNP,BC

Objectives

Study of the information presented in this chapter will enable the learner to:
1. Discuss two quality indicators for solid organ transplantation and the continuous quality improvement method for each.
2. Identify immunosuppressive medications commonly used post-transplant.

Overview
1. Graft survival is the primary outcome for all recipients of solid organ transplants.
2. There is an increased focus on controlling co-morbidities that affect patient and graft survival.
3. There is an evolution of shared care with primary care providers and community-based nephrologists.
4. The value of health maintenance processes is appreciated.
5. There is heightened interest in decreasing drug toxicity and side effects and their relation to quality of life.

Introduction

The field of solid organ transplantation spans slightly more than half a century. Outcomes of the early decades (from the 1950s to the 1970s) stressed technical success, graft survival, biologic measures (such as laboratory values), and acute care issues. Only the healthiest patients were considered for transplantation. As the science of transplantation has evolved, it has become the preferred treatment option for individuals with end stage organ failure (Smith, 2003). The achievement of technical (surgical) success shifted priorities to an increased understanding of the immune response and the efficacy of pharmacologic therapies. The development of more sophisticated and expensive immunosuppressive agents since the 1980s broadened the focus of outcomes to include efficient and effective resource utilization. During this period, short-term graft survival increased, and the occurrence of acute rejection decreased markedly (Smith, 2003). Strategies for outcome improvement transitioned from a single patient to a group of patients with a specific disease entity, such as patients with diabetes. As graft survival increased, the eligibility criteria became less restrictive. The immune response continues to be a major factor guiding clinical research and the development of therapeutic agents (Smith, 2003). However, as mastery of the learning curve by clinicians has occurred, the emphasis has changed from individual, immediate care of the patient to the continuum of care for the life of the patient and the transplanted organ. Health-related quality-of-life and economic measures have been added to biologic measures utilized to determine continuous quality improvement (CQI) in solid organ transplantation.

Outcome Measures

The primary outcome measure for recipients of solid organ transplants continues to be graft survival (Danovitch, 2005). However, CQI must be assessed in all phases of the transplant process. Some outcome measures reflect the quality of the transplant program, and others are specific to patient care issues. The phases of the transplant process include the pre-transplant period, the immediate peri-transplant period, and the post-transplant period (Danovitch, 2005)

Quality Indicator: Overall Patient Outcome

The United Network for Organ Sharing (UNOS) (2008a, 2008b) transplant program reports outcome measures, two of which are kidney – 1-year graft survival and 1-year patient survival:
• Kidney Single – Organ Transplantation Only: 1-year graft survival, U.S. 92% (UNOS, 2008a).
• Kidney Single – Organ Transplantation Only: 1-year patient survival, U.S. 96% (UNOS, 2008b).

Plan

Designate one team member to monitor graft and patient survival at 3 month intervals:
• Document reason for graft loss.
• Document cause of patient death and status of graft function at time of death.
• Compare results of outcomes with previous year data.
• Compare outcome results with national transplant data outcomes.

Do

Team review of outcome measures every 3 months:
• Team discussion and review of all incidents of graft loss.
• Team review of causes of all patient deaths.

Check

Evaluation of findings compared to overall standard measure. If the desired outcome is not achieved:
• Review causes of graft loss.
• Review immunosuppressive protocols utilized.
• Review acceptance criteria utilized for the donor (deceased or living) and recipient.
• Identify factors that have an impact on the patient and graft survival at 1 year.
• Compare center results with national data for graft and patient survival.

Act

- Make appropriate changes in immunosuppressive protocols, and target drug levels and criteria for selection of donor and recipient.
- Continue tracking the results of patient and graft survival every 3 months.

Pre-Transplant Period

Success during this period is dependent upon the infrastructure and processes in place to expedite movement of the potential recipient from evaluation to listing (Danovitch, 2005). This may be from a deceased donor transplant or recipients of a scheduled kidney or possibly liver live donor transplant. The following measures may be used to evaluate program effectiveness and identify organization, system, and patient problems. The infrastructure and processes may be efficient but not effective if the patient fails to complete the work up in an appropriate time frame.

Program quality improvement measures for this period would include:

- Time from referral to completion of patient evaluation.
- Time from completion of the evaluation to listing on the deceased donor waitlist or the scheduling of a live donor transplant.
- Evaluation of the donor advocate program.
- Maintenance of the deceased donor waitlist:
  - Patient morbidity.
  - Patient mortality.
  - Length of waiting time.
  - Utilization of paired exchange programs.

Data can be used to compare results from other transplant programs and to identify possible resources needed to improve these outcomes.

Quality Indicator: Program-Specific Indicator For the Pre-Transplant Period

Efficiency and effectiveness of the pre-transplant process is defined by the total time from Initial Assessment to Listing on the deceased donor list or scheduled for living donor transplant surgery.

Plan

Assess the current time from Initial Assessment to Listing on the deceased donor list or scheduled for transplant surgery:

- Set a target of 8 weeks for a patient to complete the pre-transplant process.
- Outline the current process used by the transplant program to assess patients for consideration for transplantation.
- Identify the current method of communication with the referring provider/facility.
- Identify an individual to track the progress of each patient through the pre-transplant process.
- Use a flow sheet to track the progress of each patient in the program.

Do

Educate all members of the pre-transplant team concerning the plan:

- Educate patients about their responsibilities in progressing through the pre-transplant process.
- Track the patient flow though the pre-transplant process for 3 months.

Check

At 3 months, the length of time to complete the pre-transplant process averaged 12 weeks. The team identified several challenges to the process:

- Evaluation of procuring dental clearance during the evaluation period found half of the patients did not obtain clearance.
- Getting patients scheduled for colonoscopy, and scheduling patients for cardiac workup and clearance.
- Communication with the referring provider/facility revealed that letters mailed requesting the needed work up added at least 5 to 7 days to the time frame for scheduling.
- Provider office personnel or facility transplant designees not familiar with the immediacy of the requests and the need to send results of testing to the transplant center as soon as available.

Act

- Provide a list of dental clinics to patients who do not have a dentist.
- Identify patient groups that require the most intensive work up, and devise the most efficient and effective method of completing the work up.
- Discuss with the referring provider/facility to identify a contact in the office/facility to fax or send secure electronic mail to the request for work up.
- Establishing a contact in the office/facility also provides a contact for those designated to communicate delays in the workup to the transplant center

Quality Indicator: A Program-Specific Indicator

The Centers for Medicare and Medicaid Services (CMS) – *Conditions for Coverage* require transplant centers to keep their waitlist up to date (CMS, 2007).

Plan

Waitlist management includes:

- Updating the patient's clinical information.
- Remove patients from the list if transplanted, expired, or other clinical condition requires removal from the waitlist.
- Notify the Organ Procurement and Transplantation Network (OPTN) within 24 hours of removal from the transplant program waitlist.

Do

- Review the duties of all transplant team members.
- Identify specific team member as the waitlist manager.
- Identify a back-up person for the waitlist manager.
- Based upon the waitlist volume, determine the appropriate interval needed to maintain current patient information.

Table 11-1
Surgical Complications

Kidney	Urine leak	Wound infection	Wound dehiscence	Lymphocele	Arterial or venous thrombosis
Liver	Bile leak	Hepatic artery thrombosis or stenosis	Caval or bile duct stenosis	Portal vein complication	Primary non-function
Heart	Allograft dysfunction	Hemorrhage	Fluid imbalance	MI or dysrhythmia	Right or left ventricular failure
Lung	Volume depletion	Pleural bleeding	Low SVR High cardiac output	Hypoxia	Vascular anastamosis problems
Pancreas	Pancreatic edema	Anastamotic leak	Wound complications	Blood glucose control	

Sources: Freeman et al., 2008; McLean & Barr, 2008.
Adapted and used with permission from Pat Weiskittel.

○ Example: one-third of waitlist is reviewed quarterly.
• Establish contacts at each provider/facility to obtain/update information.

Check
• Evaluate results of team members' review of duties, training of backup waitlist manager, and the interval determined for maintaining current patient information.

Act
• Develop a tracking package to monitor/update information.
• Develop a letter to the patient and provider/facility to be issued if the patient is placed on hold or removed from the waitlist.
• Send a letter to providers and patients explaining the need for updated information and the waitlist manager's contact information.
• Evaluate the process quarterly; make changes as needed.

Peri-Transplant Period

Program outcomes include:
• Length of stay of the recipient.
• Length of stay of the live donor (kidney or liver).
• Percentage of recipients with delayed graft function.
• Acute rejection episodes.
• Infections:
  ○ IV line infection.
  ○ Urinary tract infection.
  ○ Pneumonia.
  ○ Wound infections.

Issues of concern in the 3 to 6 months immediately post-transplant are related to technical complications, graft function, rejection episodes, attainment of therapeutic drug levels, identification and treatment of toxicity related to immunosuppression, and monitoring for infectious process-es. Bacterial infections are most common during this period (for example, placement of ureteral stents intraoperatively in the recipient of a transplanted kidney) (see Table 11-1) (Danovitch, 2005).

Plan
• Monitor urinary tract infection (UTI) occurrences.

Do
• If incidence of UTIs increases, initiate review of adherence to policy for stent placement and time until removal.

Check
• If policy adherence is in place, review policy for best practice based upon current published literature and research.

Act
• Institute policy changes to address the increase incidence of UTIs in this population based upon implementation of best practice with resulting decrease in infections.

Intense immunosuppression with multiple agents is used during the first 3 to 6 months post-transplant for all recipients of solid organs to prevent rejection of the graft. The result of this immunomodulation is an increased risk for bacterial, viral, and fungal infections (Danovitch, 2005). Along with common bacterial infections, uncommon pathogens, such as *legionella, nocardia, mycobacteria, listeria,* and *pneumocystis carinii,* may be acquired. Fungal infections include *candida, aspergillus, toxoplasmosis, cryptococcus,* and *histoplasmosis* (Danorvitch, 2005). Viral pathogens include the herpes viruses (simplex, Epstein Barr, cytomegalovirus, varicella zoster, human herpes 6 and 7), hepatitis B and C, and polyomavirus (BK nephropathy) only in recipients of kidneys. Utilizing prophylaxis against oral candida, the herpes viruses and pneumocystis have decreased their frequency in the immediate post-transplant period (Danovitch, 2005). Tracking the incidence of these pathogens and an increase in the incidence would trigger an evaluation of the immunosuppressive protocols and re-examination of prophylaxis therapy.

Assessment of graft function and issues related to immunosuppression guide treatment decisions during the first 3 to 6 months (Danovitch, 2005). A decrease in graft function may be caused by rejection, infection (such as polyomavirus in kidney transplant), or drug toxicity. The gold standard for determining the cause of alterations in organ function is a biopsy (Danovitch, 2005). The diagnosis of rejection, infection, or toxicity will guide changes in immunosuppressive therapy.

Quality Indicator: Immediate Post-Transplant Period

CMS *Conditions for Coverage* (CMS, 2007) require a multidisciplinary discharge planning for post-transplant care.

Plan
- The transplant team will identify the components of the discharge plan.
- The discharge planning team to include patient and family, transplant physician, nurse-coordinator, pharmacist, social worker, dietitian, and financial counselor.

Do
- Begin discharge planning with the patient and family at the time of admission.
- The planning team develops a schedule of interviews with the patient and family.
- At the time of admission, meet with the patient and family to review the process the patient will experience, the critical care stay, and/or transfer to the transplant unit.
- Schedule daily contact by the discharge team to review the plans for discharge.
- The pharmacist reviews medications with patient and family on a daily basis. Table 11-2 lists immunosuppressive medications commonly used.
- Determination of pharmacy to be used for obtaining discharge medications; review written list of medications and provide upon discharge.
- The social worker identifies any problems with family support and transportation to follow-up visits to the transplant clinic.
- The financial counselor reviews medication coverage and out-of-pocket expenses with the patient and family.
- The physician determines discharge date and plan for follow-up visits.
- The nurse-coordinator meets with the patient and family to reinforce discharge plan and provide written instructions for follow-up.

Check
- At first follow-up visit, review the discharge plan, and determine effectiveness of the process.

Act
- Make changes as necessary based upon results of the review.

Quality Indicator: Removal of Ureteral Stents after Transplantation

Plan
- Determine the use of ureteral stents by the transplant surgeons.
- Determine the appropriate time frame for stent removal.

Do
- Educate the patient and family on the stent in place and the time frame for removal.
- The patient record must reflect the placement of the stent.
- Identify the process for tracking stent placement and removal.
- Identify a specific team member to track stent placement and removal.
- Consult with urology department for outpatient stent removal.

Check
- Evaluate: At first follow-up visit, review the stent removal process for effectiveness and patient understanding.

Act
- At the time of discharge, remind the patient and family that a stent is in place and will require removal at a determined number of weeks post-transplant.
- Contact urology department to schedule a date for stent removal.
- Follow up to ensure stent removal and place note in chart with the date of stent removal.
- Monitor patient at subsequent follow-up visits for any adverse events following stent removal.

Post-Transplant Period

As immunosuppressive therapy has improved and acute rejection markedly decreased, patients are surviving longer with a functioning graft (Danovitch, 2005). The paradigm has shifted from acute care to the continuum of care focus extending to the management of co-morbidities, health maintenance, and long-term quality of life. The centralization of care no longer takes place at the transplant center but is shared with primary care providers and community-based nephrologists, hepatologists, cardiologists, endocrinologists, and pulmonologists (current practice, no reference, date). The importance of controlling diabetes, minimizing cardiovascular risk factors, and controlling hypertension and hyperlipidemia are recognized as factors that have an impact on long-term graft and patient survival (Danovitch, 2005). Sharing care responsibilities with primary care providers will open the avenue for patients to preserve health maintenance. These include yearly flu vaccine, assessment of skin for the presence of precancerous or cancerous lesions, colonoscopy screening at appropriate intervals, mammo-

Table 11-2
Immunosuppressive Medications Commonly Utilized

Agent	Action	Major Side Effects
Mycophenolate mofetil Mycophenolic acid	An antimetabolite selectively inhibiting proliferation of T and B lymphocytes.	Bone marrow suppression, GI distress, malignancies.
Azathioprine	6 mercaptopurine (MP) antimetabolite interfering with DNA/RNA synthesis reducing proliferation of lymphocytes.	Bone marrow suppression, hair loss, hepatic dysfunction, pancreatitis.
Corticosteroids	Inhibits production of IL-1 and IL-2 reducing the ability of lymphocytes to mount an immune response.	Hyperglycemia, Cushingoid features, increased appetite, salt and water retention, GI distress, hyperlipidemia, osteoporosis, easy bruising.
Cyclosporine (calcineurin inhibitor)	Interferes with the production of IL1 and IL2 affecting T lymphocyte activation factor and growth factor preventing an immune response.	Nephrotoxicity, hepatotoxicity, neurotoxicity, hypertrichosis, gingival hyperplasia, GI distress, hirsuitism, hypertension, hyperkalemia, hyperlipidemia, hyperesthesia, malignancy, hyperglycemia.
Tacrolimus (calcineurin inhibitor)	Inhibits T cell activation by impairing the activation for IL-2, IL-3, IL-4, tumor necrosis factor, and gamma interferon.	Nephrotoxicity, hypertension, neurotoxicity, parethesias, insomnia, headache, sleep disturbances, diabetes mellitus, malignancies.
Sirolimus (TOR inhibitor)	Inhibits T cell activation and proliferation in response to antigenic and cytokine stimulation. Inhibits antibody production.	Hyperlipidemia, diarrhea, anemia, arthralgia, acne, thrombocytopenia, hypokalemia, delayed wound healing, rash, mouth sores.
Polyclonal preparations Antilymphocyte globulin Thymoglobulin	Decreases the number and activity of T lymphocytes.	Hypersensitivity response, hypotension, rash, arthralgias and myalgias, leukopenia and thrombocytopenia, opportunistic infections.
Monoclonal antibody Preparations Muromonab CD3	Combines with the T3 complex on the surface of T lymphocytes inhibiting proliferation and lysis of transplanted cells.	First dose: flu-like symptoms, chest pain and tightness, GI distress, viral infections and lymphoma long-term, flash pulmonary edema.
Interleukin-2 receptor antagonists, Basiliximab, daclizumab	Chimeric and humanized monoclonal antibody preparations that bind to the CD 25 or Tac subunit of the IL-2 receptor on activated T lymphocytes inhibiting IL-2 mediated activation and proliferation.	No major side effects have been noted when compared to placebo.

Source: Ekberg et al., 2007.
Adapted and used with permission from Pat Weiskittel.

grams and pap smears for females, and PSA and digital rectal examinations for males. These quality indicators are now recognized as important for the transplant population as well as the general population (Danovitch, 2005).

Although short-term graft survival statistics have peaked, long-term survival continues to decrease over time (Ahsan, 2006). Long-term issues related to graft loss are:

- Chronic rejection in all organ types.
- Chronic allograft nephropathy.
- Coronary artery vasculopathy in recipients of heart transplants.
- Recurrent disease in recipients of both liver and kidney transplants.
- Calcineurin inhibitor toxicity in native kidneys.
- Non-adherence with immunosuppression regimens.

Examples of therapeutic indicators to be monitored in patients with renal transplant include drug levels, serum creatinine and estimated glomerular filtration rate (eGFR), urine protein and creatinine ratio, and yearly 24-hour urine for protein and creatinine (Danovitch, 2005). Other transplanted organs will have indicators specific to that organ's functions. Changes in these baseline values guide further assessment and work up.

Recent studies evaluating the efficacy and relative toxic effects of various immunosuppressive regimens will provide guidance in determining future immunosuppressive protocols that will provide the best short and long-term success. Graft loss both at the early and late stages has been associated with non-adherance to the medication regimen. Quality of life related to side effects from immunosuppression, complexity of the regimen, history of non-adherance, and relationship with the provider have all been associated with non-adherance (Chisholm & Weiskittel, 2005). According to Chisholm and Weiskittel (2005), adherence is higher among patients who have trust and confidence in their health care providers. Providers instill confidence by considering patient preferences and their economic circumstances when prescribing and taking the time to assess medication adherence on a regular basis. Economic factors, including the cost of medications and the loss or lack of long-term coverage for medications, has led to nonadherence and subsequent graft dysfunction. This can lead ultimately to graft loss if not addressed (Chisholm & Weiskittel, 2005). The monitoring of side effects, blood levels, and renal function offers clues to the diagnosis of nonadherence. These issues are of great importance in the pediatric and adolescent populations. Medication side effects have major social and psychological impact on the quality of life of these two populations (Hathaway et al., 2003). The effects on growth and development, ability to continue with peers in the education arena, and the availability of a strong social support structure affect the course for recipients of both pediatric and adolescent organ transplants (Magee, Krishnan, Benfield, Hsu, & Schneider, 2008).

The indicators employed to assess CQI in organ transplantation change with the progression from short-term to long-term survival. The primary outcome continues to be graft and patient survival. As grafts and patients survive longer, other outcomes that would benefit from a CQI program may come to the forefront. In the previous half century, the transplant community has seen focus progress from outcomes for a single patient encompass the continuum of care over the life of the organ for recipients of all transplants.

Quality Indicator: Maintenance of Therapeutic Levels of Immunosuppressive Agents Plan

Plan
- Maintain therapeutic level of calcineurin inhibitors to prevent rejection.
- Dose adjustment of agents based upon monitored drug levels.

Do
- Educate the patient and family on specifics of when and how to take medications.
- Provide written instructions on how to take immunosuppressive medications.
- Educate the patient and family concerning medications that may interact with transplant immunosuppressive agents.
- Reinforce with the patient and family to hold immunosuppressive medications prior to having blood drawn for drug levels.
- Identify the appropriate therapeutic range based on time after transplantation.

Check
- Evaluate effectiveness of the plan for patients to maintain therapeutic immunosuppressive agents.

Act
- Schedule the same team members to see the patient on each visit as possible to provide consistency and develop a level of trust and a milieu of comfort for the patient.
- Monitor drug levels with each follow-up visit.
- Confirm with the patient that medication was not taken prior to blood draw.
- Perform a medication reconciliation with each visit.
- Review medication side effects with patient and family at each visit.
- Ask the patient and family about any over-the-counter agents or medications obtained from another provider.
- If the measured drug level is not therapeutic, contact the patient and family to re-educate on factors involved in maintaining a therapeutic level, timing of dose prior to blood draw, and ingestions of any other drugs or agents that may affect the blood level of the therapeutic drug.
- Schedule redraw of blood level or adjust doses as indicated.

Quality Indicator: Health Maintenance

Plan
Patients undergoing a renal transplant need continuing health maintenance:
- Flu vaccine annually.
- Pneumococcal vaccine as recommended.
- Colonoscopy at age 50 and scheduled thereafter based on initial findings.
- PSA for males annually starting at age 50.

- Mammograms for females age 40 or earlier if assessed at risk.
- Dental follow up, particularly patients on cyclosporine who may develop gum hyperplasia.

Do
- Educate the patient and family regarding the importance of maintenance health care.
- Emphasize that recipients of transplants are at high risk for infection and malignancy.
- Ensure patient has a primary care provider.

Check
- Evaluate the effectiveness of the plan for patients' successful health maintenance.

Act
- Determine on a yearly basis if the patient has had health maintenance visits.
- Maintain communication with the patient's primary care provider.
- Request documentation of health maintenance activities for the transplant record.

Conclusion

This chapter has provided an overview of transplantation in the current era. The field of transplantation has traditionally focused only on patient and graft survival as quality indicators, but the focus has now broadened to include program and patient outcomes. CQI must encompass all phases of the transplant process. Each transplant program must perform an evaluation of all three phases of the process and determine the outcomes of their services and areas for improvement.

References

Ahsan, N. (2006). Guiding kidney transplantation to successful long-term outcomes. *Nephrology Updates, 2*(5), 1-13.

Centers for Medicare and Medicaid Services (CMS). (2007). *CMS requirements in the Federal Register, 72*(61), 15204. Retrieved March 4, 2009, from www.cms.hhs.gov/CFCsAndCoPs/Downloads/trancenterreg2007.pdf

Chisholm, M.A., & Weiskittel, P. (2005). Strategies for improving adherence to post transplant immunosuppressive regimens. *Nephrology Updates, 2*(4), 1-9.

Danovitch, G.M. (2005). *Handbook of kidney transplantation.* Philadelphia: Lippincott Williams and Wilkins.

Ekberg, H., Tedesco-Sival, H., Demirbas, A., Vitko, S., Nashan, B., Gurkan, A., et al. (2007). Reduced exposure to calcineurin inhibitors in renal transplantation. *The New England Journal of Medicine, 357*(25), 2562-2575.

Freeman, R.B., Steffick, D.E., Guidinger, M.K., Farmer, D.G., Berg, C.L., & Merion, R.M. (2008). Liver and intestine transplantation in the United States, 1997-2006. *American Journal of Transplantation, 8*(Part 2), 958-976.

Hathaway, D., Barr, M.L., Ghobrial, R.M., Rodrigue,J., Bogner, S., Prendergast, M.M., et al. (2003). The PORTEL registry: Overview and selected findings. *Progress in Transplantation, 13*(Suppl), 3-13.

Magee, J.C., Krishnan, S.M., Benfield, M.R., Hsu, D.T., & Schneider, B.L. (2008). Pediatric transplantation in the United States 1997-2006. *American Journal of Transplantation, 8*(Part 2), 935-945.

Mc Lean, M.K., & Barr, M.L. (2008). Current state of heart transplantation. *Transplantation Updates, 2*(3), 3-10.

Smith, S.L. (2003). *Quality aspects of transplantation.* Retrieved December 26, 2008, from http://www.medscape.com/viewarticle/451346

United Network for Organ Sharing (UNOS). (2008a). *Kidney. 1-year graft survival, adult.* Retrieved December 24, 2008, from http://www.ustransplant.org/csr/current/csrDefault.aspx

United Network for Organ Sharing (UNOS). (2008b). *Kidney. 1-year patient survival, adult.* Retrieved December 24, 2008, from http://www.ustransplant.org/csr/current/csrDefault.aspx

Addditional Reading

Dickinson, D.M., Arrington, C.J., Fant, G., Levine, G.N., Schaubel, D.E., Pruett, T.L., et al. (2008). SRTR program-specific reports on outcomes: A guide for the new reader. *American Journal of Transplantation, 8*(Part 2), 1012-1026.

| Chapter 11 | CONTINUING NURSING EDUCATION EVALUATION FORM | 1.4 Contact Hours |

Clinical Application: CQI in Solid Organ Transplant   **ANN0911**

Applying Continuous Quality Improvement in Clinical Practice contains 22 chapters of educational content. Individual learners may apply for continuing nursing education credit by reading a chapter and completing the Continuing Nursing Education Evaluation Form for that chapter. Learners may apply for continuing nursing education credit for any or all chapters.

Please photocopy this test page, complete, and return to ANNA.
You can also download this form from www.annanurse.org (choose Education - CNE Activities - Publications)
Receive continuing nursing education credit (CNE) immediately by completing the CNE evaluation process in ANNA's Online Library. Go to www.annanurse.org, and click on the Online Library icon for more information.

Name: _____

Address: _____

City: _____ State: _____ Zip: _____

E-mail:_____ Preferred telephone: ☐ Home ☐ Work _____

State where licensed and license number: _____

CNE application fees are based upon the number of contact hours provided by the individual section. CNE fees per contact hour for ANNA members are as follows: 1.0-1.9 – $15; 2.0-2.9 – $20; 3.0-3.9 – $25; 4.0 and higher – $30. Fees for nonmembers are $10 higher.

CNE application fee for Chapter 11: ANNA member $15   Nonmember $25

ANNA Member: ☐ Yes ☐ No   ☐ Member # (if available) _____

☐ Check or money order enclosed   ☐ American Express   ☐ Visa   ☐ MasterCard

Total amount submitted:_____

Credit card number _____ Exp. Date _____

Name as it appears on the card: _____

NOTE: Your evaluation form can be processed in 1 week for an additional rush charge of $5.00.

☐ **Yes, I would like this evaluation form rush processed. I have included an additional fee of $5.00 for rush processing.**

INSTRUCTIONS

1. To receive continuing nursing education credit for an individual study after reading the chapter, complete this evaluation form.

2. Detach, photocopy, or download (www.annanurse.org) the evaluation form and send along with a check or money order payable to **American Nephrology Nurses' Association** to: ANNA, East Holly Avenue Box 56, Pitman, NJ 08071-0056.

3. Test returns must be postmarked by **April 30, 2011**. Upon completion of the answer/evaluation form, a certificate will be sent to you.

This section was reviewed and formatted for contact hour credit by Sally S. Russell, MN, CMSRN, ANNA Director of Education Services.

CNE Application Fee for Chapter 11
ANNA member = $15
Nonmember = $25

---

1. I verify that I have read this chapter and completed this education activity. _____ Date _____
   Signature

2. What would be different in your practice if you applied what you have learned from this activity? (Please use additional paper if necessary.)

   _____
   _____
   _____
   _____

	Strongly disagree				Strongly agree
3. The activity met the stated objectives.					
a. Discuss two quality indicators for solid organ transplantation and the continuous quality improvement method for each.	1	2	3	4	5
b. Identify immunosuppresive medications commonly used post-transplant.	1	2	3	4	5
4. The content was current and relevant.	1	2	3	4	5
5. The content was presented clearly.	1	2	3	4	5
6. The content was covered adequately.	1	2	3	4	5

7. How would you rate your ability to apply your learning to practice?   ☐ diminished ability   ☐ no change   ☐ enhanced ability

Comments _____
_____

8. Time required to read the chapter and complete this form: _____ minutes

This educational activity is provided by the American Nephrology Nurses' Association (ANNA).
ANNA is accredited as a provider of continuing nursing education (CNE) by the American Nurses Credentialing Center's Commission on Accreditation (ANCC-COA).
ANNA is a provider approved of continuing nursing education by the California Board of Registered Nursing, provider number CEP 00910.
This CNE offering meets the Nephrology Nursing Certification Commission's (NNCC's) continuing nursing education requirements for certification and recertification.

Clinical Application: CQI in Peritoneal Dialysis

Linda Dickenson, BSN, RN, CNN, CQHP
Billie Axley, MS, RN, CNN

Objectives

Study of the information presented in this chapter will enable the learner to:
1. Discuss how regulations and published standards of care can assist nephrology nurses in peritoneal dialysis in continuous quality improvement (CQI) activities.
2. Identify nursing involvement in quality activities for quality assessment and performance improvement (QAPI).
3. Describe a model for a CQI/QAPI program for peritoneal dialysis.
4. Provide an example of the CQI process in a peritoneal dialysis home therapy program.

Overview

There is a growing focus on nurses' involvement in quality activities in the healthcare environment. Nephrology nurses can combine their knowledge and skills to deliver safe and effective patient-centered care using the principles and concepts of continuous quality improvement (CQI). This chapter will explore quality as a core competency for nephrology nurses and provide a description of how nurses working in peritoneal dialysis contribute to quality improvement for improved patient outcomes.

Introduction

Quality assessment and performance improvement (QAPI) for care at home is addressed in the *Conditions for Coverage*, published by the U.S. Department of Health and Human Services, Centers for Medicare and Medicaid Services (CMS) (2008c). The QAPI condition regarding care at home provides the requirements and interpretative guidelines for the focus on aggregate outcomes for patients on peritoneal dialysis (PD) (CMS, 2008c). Dialysis facilities that are certified to provide home dialysis services and stand alone PD programs must ensure, through the interdisciplinary team, that home dialysis services are at least equivalent to the services offered to patients receiving care with in-center programs (CMS, 2008c). The QAPI program continually assesses and monitors the effectiveness of the processes and systems within the home therapies program. The QAPI program uses a CQI process to focus daily attention on improvement. This planned and systematic process provides ongoing evaluation of patient outcomes by defined indicators to assure patients' quality of care.

QAPI in a PD Program

The QAPI program must achieve measurable improvement in health outcomes and reduction in medical errors (CMS, 2008c). The focus of the PD QAPI program is on aggregate patient outcomes through tracking and analysis of identified quality indicators, and the interdisciplinary team's goal of improving outcomes. The QAPI focus differs from the patient plan of care, which focuses on the individual patient's plan of care and outcomes. Quality indicators, as identified by the *Conditions for Coverage*, include monitoring and addressing treatment adequacy, anemia management, mineral bone disease management, infection control, patient satisfaction, medication errors, and medical injuries (CMS, 2008c). The *Conditions for Coverage* stipulate that the PD program's medical director must actively participate in the QAPI program (CMS, 2008c). Utilizing the standards described in the regulations and the CQI process, the PD nurse can identify opportunities for improvement in the PD program. Methods for the tracking and trending of data may include:

- Reviewing laboratory reports listing aggregate patient data.
- Using dialysis product manufacturer software programs for tracking and trending infections.
- Reviewing internal or corporate survey results.
- Trending patient and staff complaints or grievances, medical injuries, and medical errors (clinical variances, occurrences, and adverse events).

An opportunity for improvement can be identified when collected data elements cross a predetermined threshold (Pozgar & Santucci, 2007).

CMS (2008b) provided a tool, the Measures Assessment Tool (MAT), to assist the nephrology community in reviewing the required quality indicators to be addressed in a QAPI program. The indicators required by CMS for the PD QAPI program are outlined in the Federal Register, *Conditions for Coverage in End Stage Renal Disease Facilities* under paragraph 494.110 (CMS, 2008c). (Editor's Note: Please see Chapter 19, Table 19-1, pp. 193-194, for the complete MAT.)

The MAT (CMS, 2008b) includes the following items to be monitored by the PD programs QAPI team:

- PD adequacy.
- Nutritional status (albumin).
- Mineral bone metabolism (calcium, phosphorus, and parathyroid hormone [PTH]).
- Anemia (mean hemoglobin, mean hematocrit, serum ferritin, transferritin saturation, or reticulocyte hemoglobin content [CHr]).
- Patient satisfaction and grievances.
- Peritonitis rate, exit site, and tunnel infection rate.
- Medical injuries and medical errors identification.
- Vaccinations (hepatitis B, influenza, and pneumococcal).
- Health outcomes – Physical and mental functioning as surveyed annually with the Kidney Disease Quality of Life (KDQOL) tool (Life Options, 2009; The Renal Network, 2008).
- Health outcomes – Patient survival (standard mortality ratio [SMR]).

KDQOL

KDQOL is included in the oversight and management of patients on PD as a result of a recommendation from the Institute of Medicine (IOM) in 1993. Functional and health-related quality-of-life outcomes should be included in the overall management of patients with end stage renal disease (ESRD), and KDQOL provides this assessment (Thomas-Hawkins & Mapes, 2005).

A CQI Model

A model for improvement using the Plan-Do-Study-Act (PDSA) cycle, a systematic method for action, is a powerful and proven tool for improvement (Langley, Nolan, Nolan, Norman, & Provost, 1996). The "Plan" is developed around what the team is trying to accomplish – determining the goal and what is being measured to know that improvement is occurring, and deciding upon the changes or action steps to be made to accomplish the goal. The "Do" is the implementation of the changes or action steps that can be a combination of evidence-based interventions and those specifically applicable to the culture of the program. "Study" is the improvement model step in which the results of the changes are evaluated to see if the plan is on track to produce the desired effect. "Act" is the adoption or rejection of the changes or action steps. If the action step has resulted in improvement, it can be adopted into routine practice. Action steps that have not resulted in improvement are rejected or modified, and the cycle of the PDSA begins again (Jain, 2005).

Using the PDSA model, the CQI team:
- Reviews the aggregate patient data.
- Analyzes aggregate data for commonalities among patients who do not reach the expected outcomes.
- Brainstorms for root causes; uses tools of CQI to assist in organizing root causes.
- Develops action steps (Plan) to address 1 or 2 root causes.
- Implements the plan (Do).
- Monitors (Study) the effectiveness of the plan.
- Acts by adjusting portions of the plan that are not successful and incorporates successful actions into the PD program's policy and procedures.

Once an opportunity for improvement has been identified, a written action plan can be developed by a CQI team. A CQI action plan is basically a "to do" list, indicating the "Plan" or steps that will be taken to address the identified opportunity for improvement. One difference between an action plan and a "to do" list is that the action plan includes the name of the responsible person to ensure each action step is accomplished. An effective action plan contains a target date for completion of each step and a section for follow up of the outcome of each action step. A written action plan assists the QAPI CQI team to keep track of the information gathered for the project and serves as a tool to update the status of the plan. The written action plan should include (see Figure 12-1):
- Identified opportunity for improvement:
  - An opportunity for improvement exists when there is a gap between where an outcome is and where the outcome should be.
  - The team uses data to make an objective statement of the current outcome status. Example: "50% of the patients on PD have albumin greater than 4.0 mg/dL."

- Identified root cause to be addressed in the action plan:
  - Brainstorming is one of the CQI tools the team can use to identify possible root causes of an opportunity for improvement. The team may use other CQI tools to assist in organizing the brainstorming activity.
  - The team then selects 1 or 2 root causes to be addressed by the action plan.
- Improvement goal:
  - A target or goal is written in objective terms.
  - Example: "85% of patients on PD will have albumin equal to or greater than 4.0 mg/dL.
- Timeline for the plan:
  - The CQI action plan includes the targeted date for reaching the stated goal.
  - Example: "85% of patients on PD will have a serum albumin equal to or greater than 4.0 mg/dL within six (6) months."
- Team members identified:
  - The members of the interdisciplinary team to be involved in the improvement project are listed on the action plan, such as RN, renal dietitian, and social worker.
- Action steps:
  - The CQI team documents their "to do" list under action steps.
  - Each action step is assigned to a team member to ensure completion.
- Target date:
  - A target date for each action step provides the team with a reminder of a point at which a check is performed.
  - If the step is not completed by the target date, the team may ask, "Why not?" The team can select a new date for completion or determine if the timeline was realistic.
  - If the step is completed, the team member responsible for the action step gathers data to check if the action step is becoming a successful part of the plan for improvement.
  - If the action step does not result in goal accomplishment, the team can stop the step or modify it based upon what has been learned during the study.
- Follow up:
  - Reviewing the written action plan, team members can identify the results of the action steps completed and action steps modified.
  - At the end of the project timeline, outcomes can be identified and documented in the follow-up column.
  - If successful, then the "Act" part of the PDSA cycle incorporates the steps taken into the routine facility procedure.
  - If the plan is not successful, another key cause is identified and/or the plan is revised, and other action steps are documented and instituted.

Resources for QAPI

The NKF Kidney Disease Outcomes Quality Initiative™ (KDOQI) *Clinical Practice Guidelines* serve as a resource to the QAPI team when developing action plans to improve outcomes for patients using PD as their renal replacement therapy (NKF, 2001). Resources for the CQI action plan can be found in additional published guidelines for care, such as the

Figure 12-1
Action Plan Form

Project: Example – Reducing Peritonitis Rates			
Opportunity Statement: Reduce peritonitis rates by increasing months between cases from current rate of 14.9 months.			
Goal: Achieve a rate of 30 months between new peritonitis cases within 1 year.			
Key Cause: Break in connection technique by patients.			
Team Members: PD nurses, renal dietitian, renal social worker, and medical director for PD program.			
Action Step	**Person Responsible**	**Target Date**	**Follow Up/Date Completed (Status, etc.)**
1. Review peritonitis cases for the last 3 years and identify any common causes for peritonitis by compiling data for criteria decided upon in previous quality improvement meetings.	Registered nurses	03/31	Completed 03/25. Reported results at March QAPI meeting on 03/28. Most common cause(s) identified. Root cause(s) brainstormed – Selected patient break in connecting technique for improvement project.
2. Review all patients' connecting technique either at patient's next clinic visit or during a home visit.	PD nurses	04/30	Completed 04/30. All patients' connecting technique was observed. Patients not following connection technique as trained were re-educated.
3. Make a home visit to check on patient's technique in the home setting at the end of new patient training.	PD nurses	06/30 and ongoing. Check results every 3 months.	06/30. All new patients had a home visit after completing training, connection technique observed. 09/30. All new patients had a home visit after completing training, connection technique observed. 12/31. All new patients had a home visit after completing training, connection technique observed.
4. Recheck all new patients in 90 days for connecting technique either at a clinic visit or a home visit.	PD nurses	06/30 and ongoing. Check results every 3 months.	06/30. All patients trained in last 90 days were observed for connecting technique. 09/30. Four (4) of the six (6) patients in this group were observed for connecting technique at 90 days. 12/31 Five (5) of eight (8) patients in this group were observed for connection technique at 90 days.
5. Make a home visit if patient changes modality (CAPD to cycler).	PD nurses	06/30 and ongoing. Check results every 3 months.	06/30. All patients who changed modality received a home visit; connection technique observed. 09/30. All patients who changed modality received a home visit; connection technique observed. 12/31. All patients who changed modality received a home visit; connection technique observed.
Added action step 04/04 6. All current patients using a cycler will be provided with and trained to use an assist device to spike dialysate bags. All future new cycler patients will be trained to use assist device to spike bags.	PD nurses	05/31 and ongoing	05/31. Target date not met. New target date 06/30. 06/30. Completed training all current patients to use assist device. 09/30. All new cycler patients provided with and trained to use assist device to spike bags. 12/31. All new cycler patients provided with and trained to use assist device to spike bags.
Added action step 05/24 7. Develop and implement an ongoing re-training for all patients; developed "training sheets."	PD nurses	06/01	05/27. Completed "training sheets" and will begin using as of 06/01. 09/30. All patients have been instructed in cleanliness, exit site care, and exchange procedure using the "training sheets." 12/31. All patients have been instructed in fluid management, dialysis medications, and emergency procedures using the "training sheets."
12/31			Peritonitis rates decreased with an improvement in new peritonitis cases to 26.6 months between cases.
Added action step 01/25 8. Revised the patient training process based upon team experience and incorporated new PD training guidelines for the program.	PD nurses	02/08	Goal of 30 months between new peritonitis cases in one year achieved. Incorporated successful action steps into program's policy and procedures.
			CQI team determined to select a new goal and develop new action plan. Will incorporate successful action steps from this action plan into new plan.

Source: Used with permission from Linda Dickenson and Billie Axley.

CMS *Clinical Performance Measures* (CPMs) (CMS, 2008a) and the American Nephrology Nurses' Association's *Nephrology Nursing Standards of Practice and Guidelines for Care* (Burrows-Hudson & Prowant, 2005). These guidelines can be very useful in determining a goal, identifying root causes, and developing the steps for an action plan. Guidelines for anemia management, mineral bone disease, nutrition, adequacy of dialysis, cardiovascular disease management, management of hypertension, and management of diabetes for patients with CKD have been published. Insight on how guidelines are developed is provided by the American Diabetes Association (ADA) *Clinical Practice Guidelines,* as well as the NKF KDOQI *Clinical Practice Guidelines.* According to the ADA, clinical practice guidelines are based on the review of relevant literature by highly trained clinicians. The reviewing clinicians, after weighing the quality of evidence that ranges from rigorous double-blind clinical trials to expert opinion, draft recommendations that are further reviewed by workgroups. Finally, they are submitted for approval to an executive committee (ADA, 2007). Clinical practice guidelines are revised on a regular basis and subsequently published, as is done with the NKF KDOQI updates.

The NKF's Dialysis Outcomes Quality Initiative (DOQI) guidelines were released in 1997, and subsequently, the KDOQI guidelines have expanded the clinical areas addressed, having a significant positive impact on improving patient outcomes (NKF, 2009). They have provided the nephrology community with 22 guidelines on topics ranging from vascular access for patients on dialysis, hemodialysis, and peritoneal dialysis to chronic kidney disease itself. All published guidelines followed the rigorous KDOQI process and were developed by independent volunteer work groups (NKF, 2009). A current update is the Kidney Disease: Improving Global Outcomes (KDIGO), with the first clinic practice guidelines published in April 2008 entitled, *Prevention, Diagnosis, Evaluation, and Treatment of Hepatitis C in Chronic Kidney Disease.* Two additional clinical practice guidelines are being published in 2009, with two more slated for 2010 (KDIGO, 2009). The KDIGO guideline development process is evidence-based. Evidence will be graded and the recommendations guided through an interdisciplinary approach. Proposed guidelines will be subjected to a professional organizational and peer review process, inviting comments from international groups and professionals whose practice the guidelines will affect (KDIGO, 2009).

Example of CQI in a PD Program

Figure 12-1 is an example of a PD program's CQI team's action plan evaluating the effectiveness of their processes to ensure results meet or exceed the targeted goal. A CQI team was formed to address improving peritonitis rates in their PD population:

- With the program's peritonitis rate of 14.9 months between new cases, the CQI team was formed to address the opportunity for improvement.
- The team gathered data of peritonitis rates from the previous three years and analyzed the results for commonalities. The team used brainstorming for the CQI tool to identify possible root causes for the problem. The CQI tool, a fishbone diagram (see Figure 12-2), was developed to help the team in categorizing the possible causes of peritonitis.

- The root cause identified by the CQI team to address was patient technique with the connection procedure. Action steps were developed, and all steps were documented on an action plan form with team members' assignments and target dates for follow up by the interdisciplinary team.
- Documentation on the action plan form provided the team the ability to track completion dates of action steps, follow up on action steps, and results of action step in an organized and efficient manner.
- The improvement project produced positive results as evidenced by a decrease in peritonitis rates within the first 9 months of the project. Holding true to the concept of CQI, the PD CQI team did not stop with improved rates. The plan continued with the goal of reaching the facility target within the specified time frame of 1 year and succeeded.
- The team then selected a new goal and new action steps, striving for even better outcomes. The new plan incorporated the previously successful action steps plus additional steps.

Continuous quality improvement means the process continues as team members strive to continually improve care provided to patients on PD. Utilizing the principles of CQI, the facility was able to decrease their peritonitis rate from 1:14.9 months to 1:26.6 months within a 9-month time frame. They achieved their target goal of 1:30 months between new cases within one year.

In order to maintain communication during the project with the program's QAPI committee, the CQI team provided an update on the action plan's status at each QAPI meeting. The QAPI team can also be an excellent resource to the CQI team if they find themselves facing challenges or barriers in their improvement project. The CQI team kept the PD program's staff members informed of the project and its status by reporting on the updated action plan at each staff meeting. An informed staff can be an excellent resource to the CQI team and can be crucial to the data collection process for the project.

Conclusion

Nephrology nurses can actively participate in improvement activities that will benefit all patients by using the concepts and principles of the CQI process for PD home therapy. These principles provide a method for problem solving that nurses often find resemble the nursing process. The PD nurse can lead the process to identify opportunities for improvement, identify root causes, develop action plans, and monitor or check the results of an action plan's implementation. Using CQI in the PD program, nurses can work with the interdisciplinary team and patients to improve outcomes, resulting in an enhanced quality of life for patients and their families.

References

American Diabetes Association (ADA). (2007). *Clinical practice recommendations.* Retrieved Feb 28, 2009, from http://www.diabetes.org/for-health-professionals-and-scientists/cpr.jsp

Burrows-Hudson, S., & Prowant, B.F. (2005). *Nephrology nursing standards of practice and guidelines for care.* Pitman, NJ; American Nephrology Nurses' Association.

Centers for Medicare and Medicaid Services (CMS). (2008a). *Clinical performance measures.* Retrieved March 11, 2009, from http://www.cms.hhs.gov/CPMProject/

Centers for Medicare and Medicaid Services (CMS). (2008b). *Measures assessment tool.* Retrieved March 11, 2009, from http://www.

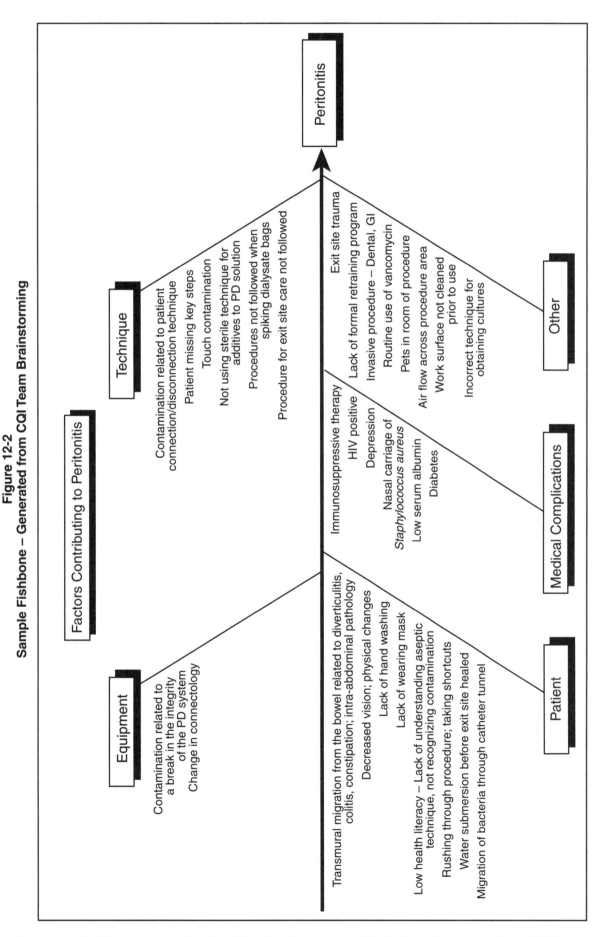

Figure 12-2
Sample Fishbone – Generated from CQI Team Brainstorming

Factors Contributing to Peritonitis

Peritonitis

Technique
Contamination related to patient connection/disconnection technique
Patient missing key steps
Touch contamination
Not using sterile technique for additives to PD solution
Procedures not followed when spiking dialysate bags
Procedure for exit site care not followed

Other
Exit site trauma
Lack of formal retraining program
Invasive procedure – Dental, GI
Routine use of vancomycin
Pets in room of procedure
Air flow across procedure area
Work surface not cleaned prior to use
Incorrect technique for obtaining cultures

Equipment
Contamination related to a break in the integrity of the PD system
Change in connectology

Medical Complications
Immunosuppressive therapy
HIV positive
Depression
Nasal carriage of *Staphylococcus aureus*
Low serum albumin
Diabetes

Patient
Transmural migration from the bowel related to diverticulitis, colitis, constipation; intra-abdominal pathology
Decreased vision; physical changes
Lack of hand washing
Lack of wearing mask
Low health literacy – Lack of understanding aseptic technique, not recognizing contamination
Rushing through procedure; taking shortcuts
Water submersion before exit site healed
Migration of bacteria through catheter tunnel

Source: Satalowich & Prowant, 2008. Used with permission from Linda Dickenson and Billie Axley.

cms.hhs.gov/SurveyCertificationGenInfo/downloads/SCletter 09-01.pdf

Centers for Medicare and Medicaid Services (CMS). (2008c). *Medicare program: Conditions for coverage for end-stage renal disease facilities*. Washington, DC: Federal register.

Jain, M. (2005). *Road map for quality improvement.* Retrieved March 11, 2009, from http://quality.mjain.net

Kidney Disease: Improving Global Outcomes (KDIGO). (2009). *Clinical practice guidelines.* Retrieved March 11, 2009, from http://www.kdigo.org/clinical_practice_guidelines/index.php

Langley, G.L., Nolan, K.M., Nolan, T.W., Norman, C.L., & Provost, L.P. (1996). *The improvement guide: A practical approach to enhancing organizational performance.* San Francisco: Jossey-Bass Publishers.

Life Options. (2009). *KDQOL-36™ online.* Retrieved April 5, 2009, from http://www.lifeoptions.org

National Kidney Foundation (NKF). (2001). K/DOQI Clinical practice guidelines for peritoneal dialysis adequacy, 2000. *American Journal of Kidney Diseases, 37*(Suppl 1), S65-S136.

National Kidney Foundation (NKF). (2009). *NKF-KDOQI guidelines.* Retrieved March 11, 2009, from http://www.kidney.org/PROFESSIONALS/kdoqi/guidelines.cfm

Pozgar, G., & Santucci, N. (2007). *Legal aspects of health care administration* (pp. 455-460). Sudberry, MA: Jones & Bartlett Publishers.

Satalowich, R.J., & Prowant, B.F. (2005). Peritoneal dialysis complications. In C.S. Counts (Ed.), *Core curriculum for nephrology nursing* (pp. 825-847). Pitman, NJ: American Nephrology Nurses' Association.

The Renal Network. (2008). *KDQOL resources.* Retrieved April 5, 2009, from http://www.therenalnetwork.org/services/kdqol.php

Thomas-Hawkins, C., & Mapes, D. (2005). The dialysis outcomes and practice patterns study (DOOPS). In C.S. Counts (Ed.), *Core curriculum for nephrology nursing* (pp. 473-494). Pitman, NJ: American Nephrology Nurses' Association.

Additional Reading

National Kidney Foundation (NKF). *K/DOQI Clinical practice guidelines.* Retrieved March 11, 2009, from http://www.kidney.org/Professionals/kdoqi/

| Chapter 12 | CONTINUING NURSING EDUCATION EVALUATION FORM | 1.3 Contact Hours |

Clinical Application: CQI in Peritoneal Dialysis　　　　　　　　　　**ANNP0912**

Applying Continuous Quality Improvement in Clinical Practice contains 22 chapters of educational content. Individual learners may apply for continuing nursing education credit by reading a chapter and completing the Continuing Nursing Education Evaluation Form for that chapter. Learners may apply for continuing nursing education credit for any or all chapters.

Please photocopy this test page, complete, and return to ANNA.
You can also download this form from www.annanurse.org (choose Education - CNE Activities - Publications)
Receive continuing nursing education credit (CNE) immediately by completing the CNE evaluation process in ANNA's Online Library. Go to www.annanurse.org, and click on the Online Library icon for more information.

Name: _____

Address: _____

City: _____State: _____Zip: _____

E-mail:_____Preferred telephone: ☐ Home ☐ Work_____

State where licensed and license number: _____

CNE application fees are based upon the number of contact hours provided by the individual section. CNE fees per contact hour for ANNA members are as follows: 1.0-1.9 – $15; 2.0-2.9 – $20; 3.0-3.9 – $25; 4.0 and higher – $30. Fees for nonmembers are $10 higher.

CNE application fee for Chapter 12: ANNA member $15   Nonmember $25

ANNA Member: ☐ Yes ☐ No   ☐ Member # (if available) _____

☐ Check or money order enclosed   ☐ American Express   ☐ Visa   ☐ MasterCard

Total amount submitted:_____

Credit card number _____ Exp. Date _____

Name as it appears on the card: _____

NOTE: Your evaluation form can be processed in 1 week for an additional rush charge of $5.00.
☐ **Yes, I would like this evaluation form rush processed. I have included an additional fee of $5.00 for rush processing.**

INSTRUCTIONS

1. To receive continuing nursing education credit for an individual study after reading the chapter, complete this evaluation form.

2. Detach, photocopy, or download (www.annanurse.org) the evaluation form and send along with a check or money order payable to **American Nephrology Nurses' Assocation** to: ANNA, East Holly Avenue Box 56, Pitman, NJ 08071-0056.

3. Test returns must be postmarked by **April 30, 2011**. Upon completion of the answer/evaluation form, a certificate will be sent to you.

This chapter was reviewed and formatted for contact hour credit by Sally S. Russell, MN, CMSRN, ANNA Director of Education Services.

CNE Application Fee for Chapter 12
ANNA member = $15
Nonmember = $25

1. I verify that I have read this chapter and completed this education activity. _____Date _____
　　　　　　　　　　　　　　　　　　　　Signature

2. What would be different in your practice if you applied what you have learned from this activity? (Please use additional paper if necessary.)
_____
_____
_____
_____

	Strongly disagree				Strongly agree
3. The activity met the stated objectives.					
a. Discuss how regulations and published standards of care can assist nephrology nurses in peritoneal dialysis in continuous quality improvement (CQI) activities.	1	2	3	4	5
b. Identify nursing involvement in quality activities for quality assessment and performance improvement (QAPI).	1	2	3	4	5
c. Describe a model for a CQI/QAPI program for peritoneal dialysis.	1	2	3	4	5
d. Provide an example of the CQI process in a peritoneal dialysis home therapy program.	1	2	3	4	5
4. The content was current and relevant.	1	2	3	4	5
5. The content was presented clearly.	1	2	3	4	5
6. The content was covered adequately.	1	2	3	4	5

7. How would you rate your ability to apply your learning to practice?　☐ diminished ability　☐ no change　☐ enhanced ability

Comments _____
_____

8. Time required to read the chapter and complete this form: _____ minutes

This educational activity is provided by the American Nephrology Nurses' Association (ANNA).
ANNA is accredited as a provider of continuing nursing education (CNE) by the American Nurses Credentialing Center's Commission on Accreditation (ANCC-COA).
ANNA is a provider approved of continuing nursing education by the California Board of Registered Nursing, provider number CEP 00910.
This CNE offering meets the Nephrology Nursing Certification Commission's (NNCC's) continuing nursing education requirements for certification and recertification.

Clinical Application: CQI Aspects of the Therapeutic Apheresis Program

Judy Kauffman, BSN, RN, CNN
Linda Myers, BSN, RN, CNN
Regina M. Rohe, BS, RN, HP(ASCP)
Billie Axley, MS, RN, CNN

Objectives

Study of the information presented in this chapter will enable the learner to:
1. Describe the use of continuous quality improvement for improving processes in the therapeutic apheresis program.
2. Identify potential outcome indicators for application in a therapeutic apheresis program.

Introduction

Therapeutic apheresis is a group of blood separation procedures used in the management of a wide variety of diseases encompassing neurology, hematology, oncology, nephrology, and rheumatology (Rohe, Smith, & Wilson, 2008). The physician overseeing the apheresis program evaluates the appropriateness of the therapy when it is requested. This assessment includes a detailed patient history and diagnosis, the patient's clinical assessment, and the application of available clinical practice guidelines. Guidelines for therapeutic apheresis have been developed by professional organizations, including the American Medical Association (AMA), the American Society for Apheresis (ASFA), and the American Association of Blood Banks (AABB) (Rohe et al., 2008). A therapeutic apheresis clinical team may consist of the attending specialty physician, the physician overseeing the apheresis program, and the staff performing the procedure. The apheresis clinical team works collaboratively with the patient, the patient's family, direct patient care providers, and the facility's pharmacy and blood bank staff members. This is to ensure that the patient receives appropriate, safe, and effective therapy.

The application of continuous quality improvement (CQI) in therapeutic apheresis programs evolves from working with standards of practice and guidelines for care developed by professional organizations, such as the ASFA, AABB, and the American Nephrology Nurses' Association (ANNA). Apheresis programs rely upon these professional organizations when developing policies and procedures for clinical practice and when choosing outcomes indicators to include in the facility's CQI program. Application of CQI in a therapeutic apheresis program, as in any clinical setting, is virtually unlimited and can be tailored to the specific type of therapeutic procedure provided.

Using Failure Mode and Effect Analysis In an Apheresis Program

When used as a CQI tool, *failure mode and effect analysis* (FMEA) allows for an assessment of risk or of identifying ways in which a "product, process, or service might fail" (Brassard, Finn, Ginn, & Ritter, 2002, p. 111). The FMEA tool can guide a team in the development of actions to minimize that risk, and a form can be created to serve as the documentation tool for the process improvement activities (see Figure 13-1) (Brassard et al., 2002). David Krugh addressed risk reduction using an example from his experience. He described FMEA as providing a method of identifying and preventing process/system issues. The goal, as explained by Krugh, is to prospectively identify improvements that will reduce risk, such as following the steps of a process and identifying a risk of an "unintended" adverse effect (Krugh, n.d.). The FEMA tool assists the team in identifying the opportunity for improvement, can lead the team in determining what data to collect, and helps define the opportunity for improvement (Brassard et al., 2002). Krugh's example used the tool to address an improvement opportunity of reducing the chance of an adverse effect (Krugh, n.d.).

Assessment of the critical processes involved in providing apheresis treatments were obtained through:
- Tracking results of the program's identified quality indicators.
- Audits.
- Adverse event reports.
- Regulatory requirements.
- Literature review.
- Questions posed by the interdisciplinary team and brainstorming.

Additional elements in the use of risk identification for unintended adverse events may include:
- An interdisciplinary team.
- Focusing is on process/system issues.
- Developing the flow chart of the process.
- Using a cause and effect diagram for analysis of what is causing the problem.

Using the FMEA method, a team can begin by utilizing the identified process to create a flowchart, providing a visual map of the process. By examining the steps in the flowchart, the team can identify potential ways in which the process could fail ("failure mode") and the potential outcomes for the patient. This exercise helps the team identify where the opportunities are for improving the process (Krugh, n.d.).

Using the FMEA model, the team can assign a risk identification score to an "opportunity for improvement" process. This is a numerical score of 1 to 10, with 1 being low and 10 being high, using:

Figure 13-1
Failure Mode and Effects Analysis (FEMA) Tool

Process:										
Process Step	Inputs	Failure Mode	Failure Effects/ Severity	1-2 Key Causes/ Occurrence	Controls/ Dectection	RPN	Action Steps	Person Responsible	Target Date	Follow-Up/ Outcomes

Note: RPN = risk priority number.
Source: Adapted from Brassard, Finn, Ginn, and Ritter, 2002. Used with permission from Billie Axley.

- Severity – "[The] rate the severity of the failure effect the customer experiences" (Brassard et al., 2002, p. 213).
- Occurrence – "Determine how often the cause of the failure mode occurs" (Brassard et al., 2002, p. 213).
- Detection - "Determine how effective the current controls can detect the cause of the failure mode" (Brassard et al., 2002, p. 213). An example of detection scoring would be
  - "If a good detection system (such as an automated feedback system) is in place, assign a 1 or 2..."
  - "If no controls are in place, assign a 10..." (Brassard et al., 2002, p. 213).

The team then applies a mathematical product of the "severity, frequency, and detection ratings" for each identified failure mode. This product provides a *"risk priority number"* that can then be used to prioritize the identified failure modes to be addressed. A risk priority number score ranges from 1 to 1000, 1 being the lowest and 1000 being the highest (Brassard et al., 2002). Krugh (n.d.) provides a risk priority number "rank priority" range as follows:
- "Equal to or greater than 250 is significant."
- "100 to 249 is less important."
- "Less than 100 is not important" (p. 8).

Krugh (n.d.) provides an additional mathematical product that can be used to determine a "criticality rating." This rating is used to identify a process that has poor patient outcome (severity rating high) but may not be easily detected, resulting in a lower risk priority number score. In this calculation, the failure mode is numerically scored (1 to 4) for frequency and severity.
- Frequency:
  - "Frequent (4), occasional (3), uncommon (2), remote (1)."
- Severity:
  - "Catastrophic (4), major (3), moderate (2), minor (1)" (Krugh, n.d., p. 8).

The mathematical product of this frequency and severity provides a "hazard score 1 to 16," 1 being the lowest and 16 being the highest (Krugh, n.d., p. 8). The team can use a risk priority number and criticality ratings to evaluate an identified opportunity for improvement. The team can then use a CQI tool, such as the cause and effect (or "fishbone") diagram to brainstorm what is causing the problem or opportunity for improvement. The CQI team can select 1 to 2 of the problem's causes or sources to address from the cause and effect diagram with an action plan for improvement.

Use of Checklists as a Tool in CQI

Another CQI tool that is useful in the improvement process is the checklist. The use of checklists to ensure that critical steps are performed with each apheresis procedure can provide the framework for patient care staff to avoid errors and missed steps. Monitoring the completion of procedural checklists can assist the apheresis program in building clinical variance tracking tools and employing CQI techniques to reduce errors while increasing patient safety (Riley, Justison, Povrzenic, & Zabetakis, 2002). The use of clinical practice guidelines to establishment safety standards is recognized by the Joint Commission as a means to develop evidence-based procedures and protocols. This provides clinicians with "...instructions on how to conduct specific therapeutic procedures within the scope of services offered..." (Riley et al., 2002, p. 285).

Therapeutic Apheresis

Many clinical decisions are required for the safe and efficient delivery of therapeutic apheresis and are based upon the type of therapeutic apheresis procedure needed to treat the patient's disease.

Plasmapheresis or Therapeutic Plasma Exchange

When therapeutic plasma exchange is used as a treatment for a specific disease, one of the first clinical considerations is the volume of plasma to exchange. Therapeutic plasma exchange is a treatment prescribed by volume and not by time (Rohe et al., 2008). Calculation of the individual patient's plasma volume is necessary to determine the end point of each treatment session and to establish the volume of replacement fluid required for each procedure.

The exchange of plasma volumes requires consideration of several patient safety factors:

- Anticoagulation:
  - The larger the volume of plasma exchanged leads to greater exposure of the patient to an anticoagulant (such as citrate, heparin).
- Blood products:
  - The larger the volume of plasma exchanged, the longer the patient's exposure to blood products used for volume replacement will be.
- Time:
  - The larger the volume of plasma exchanged, the longer the procedure will take. This increases the potential for the patient to experience potential side effects and adverse events (Rohe et al., 2008).
- Pediatrics:
  - Specific formulas should be used to calculate the total blood volume for children. Additional resources for apheresis therapy in pediatrics are listed in the suggested readings at the end of this chapter.
- Fluid management in therapeutic plasmapheresis:
  - Replacement volume:
    - ➤ A desired patient outcome in a therapeutic plasma exchange is to maintain an isovolemic fluid status, avoiding both hypovolemia and fluid overload (Burrows-Hudson & Prowant, 2005). The patient's calculated plasma volume is used to determine the volume of replacement fluid needed when performing a therapeutic plasma exchange procedure.
  - Fluid type:
    - ➤ A process must be in place to ensure fluid replacement is appropriate for the disease process and the patient's medical treatment plan.
    - ➤ 5% albumin:
      - ✓ If the pharmacy determines a need to create the 5% albumin solution from a more concentrated solution of albumin, a safety check process must be put in place to ensure the concentrated albumin volume is diluted with the appropriate amount of 0.9% sodium chloride solution. Dilution with other IV solutions (such as sterile water) creates a hypo-osmolar solution and results in hemolysis of red blood cells (Rohe et al., 2008). The CQI safety check process must be in place to support these courses of action.
- A process must be in place to ensure fluid replacement is available in an efficient time frame to satisfy the patient's medical treatment plan.
  - Using CQI, the apheresis team and facility pharmacy staff can work together to establish and maintain an efficient communication and delivery process:
    - ➤ The CQI team looks at cycle time – The time between when an order is placed by the physician to the time the calculated replacement fluid volume is at the patient's bedside or apheresis location (*Plan*).
    - ➤ The CQI team identifies the steps in the cycle time. Steps can be selected for improvement, and action steps are developed and implemented (*Do*).
    - ➤ After a specified time frame, the team reviews the cycle time and evaluates whether the action steps resulted in improvement (*Check*).

- ➤ Action steps resulting in improvement are incorporated into a protocol to maximize efficient cycle time (*Act*).
- ➤ A quality indicator of cycle time can be included in the apheresis program's quality assessment and performance improvement (QAPI) program to ensure improvement is maintained over time. (Note: QAPI is nomenclature from the ESRD *Conditions for Coverage*, not the CRRT community [Centers for Medicare and Medicaid [CMS], 2008].) Once an improvement has become part of the program's standard operating procedure, the indicator can be moved progressively from monthly monitoring to quarterly, to bi-annually, and then ultimately, to an annual frequency.
- ➤ When the replacement fluid is fresh frozen plasma or cryoprecipitate-depleted plasma, an established protocol is necessary to ensure an efficient process for obtaining the required volume of blood products just prior to the plasma exchange procedure.
- Monitor the patient's extracorporeal red cell volume due to the cardiac and oxygenation implications.
  - No patient treated with therapeutic apheresis should have an extracorporeal red cell volume percentage greater than 15% for adults (McLeod et al., 2005); 10% is the suggested maximum safe extracorporeal volume for pediatric patients (Burrows-Hudson & Prowant, 2005).
  - If a patient with a small total blood volume or low red cell volume needs apheresis, donor red blood cells (RBCs) may be used to prime the extracorporeal circuit to avoid exceeding a safe extracorporeal volume.
    - ➤ If the circuit has been primed with blood, reinfusion of RBCs remaining in the circuit at the end of the procedure is usually not necessary.

Cytapheresis

A cell depletion procedure, or cytapheresis, is not an exchange, but rather a separation and removal of a particular cell type. In leukapheresis, for example, the cells targeted for removal are white blood cells (leukocytes). During thrombocytapheresis or plateletapheresis, the cells targeted for removal are platelets (Rohe et al., 2008). All components of the patient's blood are returned to the patient except for the targeted cells and any volume of plasma removed in conjunction with the targeted cells. Issues identified for particular scrutiny in cytapheresis procedures can include:

- Monitoring citrate infusion and appropriate calcium infusion.
  - Process and safeguards are in place for therapy that requires the infusion of a high volume of citrate during cytapheresis.
- Verifying the quality of the collection.
  - A process is in place to verify that the collection of the specific targeted cell population is occurring.

Erythrocytapheresis

Erythrocytapheresis, or red blood cell exchange, can be used in treatment of several urgent situations, including sickle cell anemia crisis. The CQI program must monitor the calculation of the red cell volume needed for a safe and effective RBC exchange.

To ensure the patient receives a safe, effective, and timely treatment, it is prudent to monitor that the cycle time is efficient for RBC exchange procedures, as is done with a therapeutic plasma exchange. The cycle time for an RBC exchange is defined as the time from when the order for the treatment and blood products is placed to the time when the RBCs are available for use with the apheresis procedure. A sickle cell crisis warrants an efficient cycle time to enhance treatment efficacy. The cycle time includes steps that ensure that the appropriate units of RBCs are found, matched, prepared, and available for the procedure. The challenges involved in the process of obtaining multiple units of RBCs include:

- Locating packed RBC units that are ABO compatible and hemoglobin S negative.
- Crossmatching and screening for antibodies.
- Washing all units to reduce potential allergens.
  ○ This procedure can take up to 30 minutes.
- Ensuring that all units of RBCs are available for transfusion at the same time.

Plan

- Using the flowchart tool, the CQI team can gather data by charting the steps in their process. This begins with the physician's written order and ends with the RBC units available at the apheresis treatment location.
- By flowcharting each step occurring in the actual process from beginning to end, the team can assess their current process for missing or unnecessary steps, or complex steps that might be simplified.
- Comparing the flowchart of what is actually happening to the facility's written procedure or protocol can be revealing. This can help the team identify if there are steps that are not being done efficiently, or if extra steps that do not contribute to the efficiency of the process have been added over time.

Do

- Performing a time study (actually timing each step in the flow chart) can help the CQI team identify which steps may be streamlined to reduce the complexity and completion time.
- Team members involved in the process work together to determine more efficient methods to complete the identified steps. This creates an opportunity for improvement and to develop action steps with specified time frames.

Check

- The team's action plan articulates when to evaluate the results of the action steps.
- The team can learn which action steps are producing successful outcomes and which are not resulting in improvement. Action steps that are not demonstrating improvement can be removed from the plan by periodically checking for results at specified intervals.
- At each checkpoint, the team may learn new information about the process and add additional action steps into the improvement plan.

Act

- Action steps that resulted in improvement are incorporated into the apheresis program's policy, procedure, or protocol.
- Once an improved process is in place, the QAPI committee monitors the process to ensure continuation of the improvement.

Potential CQI opportunities exist for all types of apheresis procedures. These include monitoring of:

- Laboratory studies:
  ○ A goal for patients undergoing apheresis therapy is to maintain their electrolyte balance within safe parameters. Review patients' laboratory results and nursing assessment for signs and symptoms of electrolyte(s) depletion. Follow established guidelines for care that include monitoring sodium, potassium, magnesium, phosphorous, calcium, and bicarbonate (Burrows-Hudson & Prowant, 2005).
  ○ Laboratory studies are ordered by the physician.
    ➤ Monitor the patient's pre-treatment calcium and potassium for low levels that might require replacement.
      ✓ Observe the patient for clinical signs and symptoms of hypocalcemia and/or hypokalemia. Serially monitor blood levels during therapy based upon the nurses' assessment, as ordered.
      ✓ Laboratory tests for electrolytes may be ordered 2 to 4 hours post-treatment to assess the need for additional replacement.
    ➤ Patients are monitored for signs and symptoms of low ionized calcium levels. Ionized calcium levels decrease in the plasma of patients undergoing therapeutic apheresis. This is a result of citrate anticoagulation, removal of calcium in the patient's plasma, and the intrinsic calcium-binding properties of albumin used as a replacement fluid during a therapeutic plasma exchange (McLeod et al., 2005).
    ➤ The complete blood count (CBC) is monitored pre and post-RBC exchange.
    ➤ The CBC is assessed pre and post-leukapheresis or plateletpheresis procedures. A mid-procedure CBC may be ordered to monitor both treatment progress and the amount of blood cells removed other than the targeted cell type.
    ➤ Patients receiving plasmapheresis for hyperviscosity syndromes generally have a daily order for serum viscosity to assess the reduction of the identified protein.
    ➤ Other laboratory studies that are known indicators for underlying disease may be ordered at the discretion of the physician.
- Patient medications.

Patient Medications

Another important aspect of providing safe and effective apheresis procedures includes pre-treatment evaluation of the patient's medications. Important categories of medications to note can include:

- *Angiotensin-converting enzyme inhibitors (ACE-I).* ACE-I inhibitors must be stopped 24 to 48 hours prior to some apheresis procedures (or longer in cases of renal failure). This is to prevent increased risk of allergic/anaphylactoid reactions "that may decrease a patient's ability to inactivate bradykinin" (McLeod et al., 2005, p. 22). These reactions have been primarily associated with selective depletion columns for low-density lipoprotein (LDL) and protein A immunoadsorption (McLeod et al., 2005). "Beta blockers may prevent an increase in heart rate in response to hypotension" (McLeod et al., 2005, p. 27).

- "Calcium channel blockers and nitroglycerin paste may prevent vasoconstriction in response to fluid volume shifts" (McLeod et al., 2005, p. 27).
- Drugs that bind to plasma proteins may be removed during therapeutic plasma exchange (Burrows-Hudson & Prowant, 2005).
- "Immunoglobulins may be removed during a therapeutic plasma exchange" (McLeod et al., 2005, p. 12).
- Plasma cholinesterase is removed during a therapeutic plasma exchange, "which would increase a subsequent anesthesia risk if urgent surgery were required" (McLeod et al., 2005. p. 28).
- The medical team evaluates the need to hold medications prior to procedure.
- Evaluate patients on vasopressors, pain medications, and continuous IV drips for dose adjustments due to removal during therapeutic apheresis, especially during plasma exchange.

Track and Trend Outcome Indicators

Using published standards of practice and guidelines for patient care, the apheresis program can select quality indicators to track and trend for CQI. Audun Fredriksen defined a quality indicator as being based on "...a consensus of scientific judgment, which can be objectively measured and thereby express indirectly the level of quality" (Fredriksen, 2005, p. 11). Fredriksen goes on to say that chosen indicators must be:

- Valid – Indicators must measure what they were intended to measure.
- Reliable – Indicators must yield data that are reproducible over time.
- Sensitive – Be able to detect changes.
- Relevant and useful – Indicators are not measurements made just for the sake of measuring something.
- Not "fixed" or static – Indicators represent choices and decisions made by health care professionals; they are dynamic, not static, in order to meet the changing needs of a program.
- Improving – Indicators selected by the healthcare team meet the needs of monitoring and improving their own program's performance (Fredriksen, 2005).

Healthcare professionals can help the team identify opportunities for improvement by tracking and trending selected outcome indicators in the therapeutic apheresis program. These indicators may include those that reflect the safety and efficacy of individual patient treatments.

- No signs/symptoms of air embolism.
- No hemolysis of red blood cells.
- No events of volume deficit due to volume removal and no events of volume overload due to infusion of fluids during the procedure.

Assessment Elements

- Stable weight.

- No blood pressure alterations.
- No change in apical heart rate, peripheral pulses (radial, pedal).
- Heart sounds, regular with S1 and S2, absence of S3, no evidence of jugular vein distention.
- No alterations in respiratory rate and/or breath sounds.
- Stable hemodynamic parameters (such as central venous pressure or pulmonary artery wedge pressure elements).
- No alterations in level of consciousness (Burrows-Hudson & Prowant, 2005).

Allergic Reactions Are Minimized

- Pre-medications are recommended before infusing large quantities of fresh frozen plasma or cryoprecipitate-reduced plasma (CRP) (Rohe et al., 2008).
- Plan for pre-treatment medications to prevent allergic reaction if the patient evaluation reveals a history of allergic reactions to blood products, such as hives or urticaria.
- Plan for a response to allergic reactions during apheresis procedure.
  - Consider establishing a physician-approved protocol to assist in the immediate treatment of an emergency situation.
  - Establish a patient-specific pre-treatment protocol for patients with predictable or unusual allergic reactions.
  - Monitor platelet loss during apheresis procedures other than thrombocytapheresis.
    - ➤ Platelet removal may occur during apheresis and may be significant in leukapheresis.

Monitor Coagulation Factor Reduction

- Transient coagulopathy routinely occurs post-apheresis.
  - Patients scheduled for surgery within 24 hours post-procedure should have a prothrombin time (PT) and partial thromboplastin time (PTT) measured and corrected as necessary.
  - Fresh frozen plasma may be included instead of, or in addition to, colloids as replacement solution for correction purposes.
  - If colloid replacement plasmapheresis procedures are done daily, a pre-procedure PT, PTT, and fibrinogen should be done prior to each procedure to determine if fresh frozen plasma needs to be included in the replacement solution.
  - Consider checking coagulation factors prior to removal of a central venous line catheter. The physician overseeing the apheresis therapy may order fresh frozen plasma administered at the end of a therapeutic plasma exchange in preparation for the removal of a central line catheter.
  - Adequate extracorporeal blood circuit anticoagulation is maintained without the patient experiencing citrate toxicity.
  - Citrate is added to the blood circuit as blood is drawn from the patient.
  - Selection of correct anticoagulant citrate dextrose (ACD) formula for centrifugal apheresis machines with microprocessors is essential (Rohe et al., 2008).

○ Selection of the ACD to whole blood ratio is adequate to anticoagulate the extracorporeal circuit.

○ Consider process for calcium replacement:

➤ Critically ill patients and patients sensitive to citrate may have an order for continuous calcium infusion to prevent symptoms of hypocalcemia (Rohe et al., 2008).

• CQI indicators may reflect the outcome of aggregate procedures. For example:

○ Targeted laboratory parameters were achieved.

○ Clinical disease manifestations improve.

○ All adverse events are avoided.

Venous Access for Apheresis Procedures

The function of vascular access devices is included in the desired outcome to deliver a safe and effective apheresis treatment. The vascular access must provide adequate and consistent blood flow rates (Burrows-Hudson & Prowant, 2005).

• Peripheral access can be used when the planned number of procedures is low and intermittent.

• Central venous catheters (CVCs):

○ Provide two ports of venous access.

○ Minimize opportunities for infection:

➤ Monitor exit site for signs, symptoms.

➤ Follow procedure for dressing changes.

➤ Use checklist during insertion.

✓ A CQI project was implemented and reported by Johns Hopkins Medical Center to reduce the CVC infection rate. A checklist was constructed from guidelines, and conditional statements were reworded into a checklist of simple steps. These include washing hands and putting a sterile dressing over the catheter site after the line is inserted. Consistent use of the checklist was associated with a reduction in CVC infection rates (Wylie, 2009).

CQI Consideration in Additional Types Of Therapeutic Apheresis

As a fascinating, newer technology, cascade (or secondary filtration) is a technology that can be used for the treatment of a number of disease states. An example is cascade apheresis for homozygous familial hypercholesterolemia. Whole blood is first separated, and the plasma is passed through a filter specific for the targeted plasma component (low-density lipoprotein). This secondary filtration of the plasma allows all blood components to be returned to the patient except for the absorbed component (Rohe et al., 2008). Secondary filtration procedures can also be applied to immunoadsorption therapies. Many of the guidelines for care of the patient undergoing apheresis already discussed in this chapter can be applied to these therapies. Current literature and the equipment manufacturer's operator manual can assist the team in developing initial guidelines to monitor quality indicators specific to the procedure.

Conclusion

Opportunities will always exist for providers to identify areas upon which improvement can be explored and implemented. The work to develop and implement operational and procedural changes to help prevent and reduce errors belongs to everyone. Therapeutic apheresis programs rely upon the unique missions and perspectives of professional organizations, federal and state government agencies, and accreditation groups to develop program standards and provide a platform for CQI initiatives (Riley et al., 2002). Therapeutic apheresis is yet another arena in which a CQI program provides structure to identify opportunities for improvement, implement change, measure outcomes, and provide solutions to challenges.

References

Brassard, M., Finn, L., Ginn, D., & Ritter, D. (2002). *The Six Sigma memory jogger II.* Salem, NH; GOAL/QPC.

Burrows-Hudson, S., & Prowant, B.F., (Eds.). (2005). *Nephrology nurse standards of practice and guidelines for care.* Pitman, NJ; American Nephrology Nurses' Association.

Centers for Medicare and Medicaid Services (CMS). (2008). *Conditions for coverage for end stage renal disease facilities.* Washington, D.C.: Federal Register.

Fredriksen, A. (2005). Quality indicators – Why and how. *Transfusion and Apheresis Science, 32*(1), 11-12.

Krugh, D. (n.d.). *Risk reduction strategies.* Retrieved February 14, 2009, from http://www.apheresis.org/~DOCUMENTS/Fri_230_Krugh_Galleon_II_&_III.pdf

McLeod, B.C., Crookston, K., Eder, A., King, K., Kiss, J., Sarode, R., et al. (Eds.). (2005). *Therapeutic apheresis: A physician's handbook* (1st ed., p. 9). Bethesda, MD: American Association of Blood Bank Press.

Riley, J.B., Justison, G.A., Povrzenic, D., & Zabetakis, P.A. (2002). Designing an integrated extracorporeal therapy service quality service. *Therapeutic Apheresis, 6*(4), 282-287.

Rohe, R.M., Smith, S.J., & Wilson, J. (2008). Therapeutic plasma exchange. In C.S. Counts (Ed.) *Core curriculum for nephrology nursing* (5th ed., pp. 279-297). Pitman, NJ: American Nephrology Nurses' Association.

Wylie, I. (2009). *Checklists offer a cure for many ills.* Retrieved March 25, 2009, from http://www.ft.com/cms/s/0/abfaa628-f6c8-11dd-8a1f-0000779fd2ac.html

Additional Readings

American Society for Apheresis Standards and Education Committee. (1996). Organizational guidelines for therapeutic apheresis facilities. *Journal Clinical Apheresis, 11*(1), 42-45.

Mokrzycki, M.H., & Kaplan, A.A. (1994). Therapeutic plasma exchange: Complications and management. *American Journal of Kidney Disease, 23*(6), 817-827.

Centers for Medicare and Medicaid Services (CMS). (1992). *NCD for apheresis (therapeutic pheresis) (110.14).* Retrieved March 25, 2009, from http://www.cms.hhs.gov/mcd/viewncd.asp?ncd_id=110.14&ncd_version=1&basket=ncd%3A110%2E14%3A1%3A Apheresis+%28Therapeutic+Pheresis%29

Cobe Spectra Operator's Manual. (2007). *Essentials guide.* Gambro BCT, Inc.

Kim, H.C. (2000). Therapeutic pediatric apheresis. *Journal of Clinical Apheresis, 15*, 129-157.

McLeod, B.C., Price, T.H., & Weinstien, R. (Eds.). (2003). *Apheresis: Principles and practice* (2nd ed.). Bethesda, MD: AABB Press.

National Marrow Donor Program. (2006). *Apheresis center participation criteria.* Retrieved March 25, 2009, from http://www.marrow.org/ABOUT/About_Us/NMDP_Network/Maintaining_NMDP_Standards/AC_Participation_Criteria_PDF/criteria_ac.pdf

Palepu, R., Murfaugh, A., Barnett, E., Smith, M., Pamintuan, M.L., & Linenberger, M. (n.d.). *Effects of central venous catheter (CVC) size on the performance and cost of extracorporeal photophersis (ECP) for graft-versus-host disease (GVHD).* Retrieved March 25, 2009, from http://www.apheresis.org/~DOCUMENTS/Thurs_230_Palepu_Grand_Ballroom_AB.pdf

| Chapter 13 | CONTINUING NURSING EDUCATION EVALUATION FORM | 1.5 Contact Hours |

Clinical Application: CQI Aspects of the Therapeutic Apheresis Program **ANNP0913**

Applying Continuous Quality Improvement in Clinical Practice contains 22 chapters of educational content. Individual learners may apply for continuing nursing education credit by reading a chapter and completing the Continuing Nursing Education Evaluation Form for that chapter. Learners may apply for continuing nursing education credit for any or all chapters.

Please photocopy this test page, complete, and return to ANNA.
You can also download this form from www.annanurse.org (choose Education - CNE Activities - Publications)
Receive continuing nursing education credit (CNE) immediately by completing the CNE evaluation process in ANNA's Online Library. Go to www.annanurse.org, and click on the Online Library icon for more information.

Name: _____
Address: _____
City: _____ State: _____ Zip: _____
E-mail:_____ Preferred telephone: ☐ Home ☐ Work_____
State where licensed and license number: _____

CNE application fees are based upon the number of contact hours provided by the individual section. CNE fees per contact hour for ANNA members are as follows: 1.0-1.9 – $15; 2.0-2.9 – $20; 3.0-3.9 – $25; 4.0 and higher – $30. Fees for nonmembers are $10 higher.

CNE application fee for Chapter 13: ANNA member $15   Nonmember $25

ANNA Member: ☐ Yes ☐ No   ☐ Member # (if available) _____
☐ Check or money order enclosed   ☐ American Express   ☐ Visa   ☐ MasterCard
Total amount submitted:_____
Credit card number _____ Exp. Date _____
Name as it appears on the card: _____
NOTE: Your evaluation form can be processed in 1 week for an additional rush charge of $5.00.
☐ **Yes, I would like this evaluation form rush processed. I have included an additional fee of $5.00 for rush processing.**

INSTRUCTIONS

1. To receive continuing nursing education credit for an individual study after reading the chapter, complete this evaluation form.

2. Detach, photocopy, or download (www.annanurse.org) the evaluation form and send along with a check or money order payable to **American Nephrology Nurses' Assocation** to: ANNA, East Holly Avenue Box 56, Pitman, NJ 08071-0056.

3. Test returns must be postmarked by **April 30, 2011**. Upon completion of the answer/evaluation form, a certificate will be sent to you.

This chapter was reviewed and formatted for contact hour credit by Sally S. Russell, MN, CMSRN, ANNA Director of Education Services.

> **CNE Application Fee for Chapter 13**
> **ANNA member = $15**
> **Nonmember = $25**

1. I verify that I have read this chapter and completed this education activity. _____ Date _____
   Signature

2. What would be different in your practice if you applied what you have learned from this activity? (Please use additional paper if necessary.)
   _____
   _____
   _____
   _____

	Strongly disagree				Strongly agree
3. The activity met the stated objectives.					
a. Describe the use of continuous quality improvement for improving processes in the therapeutic apheresis program.	1	2	3	4	5
b. Identify potential outcome indicators for application in a therapeutic apheresis program.	1	2	3	4	5
4. The content was current and relevant.	1	2	3	4	5
5. The content was presented clearly.	1	2	3	4	5
6. The content was covered adequately.	1	2	3	4	5

7. How would you rate your ability to apply your learning to practice? ☐ diminished ability ☐ no change ☐ enhanced ability

Comments _____
_____

8. Time required to read the chapter and complete this form: _____ minutes

This educational activity is provided by the American Nephrology Nurses' Association (ANNA).
ANNA is accredited as a provider of continuing nursing education (CNE) by the American Nurses Credentialing Center's Commission on Accreditation (ANCC-COA).
ANNA is a provider approved of continuing nursing education by the California Board of Registered Nursing, provider number CEP 00910.
This CNE offering meets the Nephrology Nursing Certification Commission's (NNCC's) continuing nursing education requirements for certification and recertification.

Clinical Application:
CQI in Continuous Renal Replacement Therapy

Helen F. Williams, MSN, RN, CNN
Tana Waack, BSN, RN
Billie Axley, MS, RN, CNN

Objectives

Study of the information presented in this chapter will enable the learner to:
1. Explore quality indicators that could be applied to a continuous renal replacement therapy program.
2. Describe an interdisciplinary improvement project conducted in an acute care setting.

Overview

In this chapter, the reader will find the focus is on using principles and concepts of continuous quality improvement (CQI) to ensure every patient receives safe and effective continuous renal replacement therapy (CRRT). Suggestions are presented for the use of quality indicators in monitoring patient outcomes to identify opportunities for improvement.

Introduction

In continuous renal replacement therapy (CRRT), a small volume of the patient's blood is continuously pumped from a central venous access to flow though a filter and then back to the patient. As the blood passes through the filter, toxins and excess electrolytes move from the patient's blood through the filter's semipermeable membrane by diffusion and/or convective transport. Fluid removal from the patient's blood in the filter is accomplished by the process of ultrafiltration, the transport of water across a membrane. Both processes occur on a controlled and continuous basis over an extended period of time (Chrysochoou, Marcus, Sureshkumar, McGill, & Carlin, 2008; Dirkes & Hodge, 2007).

Management of the patient with acute kidney injury has become complex in today's intensive care units (ICU), with the increased incidence of sepsis and multi-organ system failure caused by many different disease processes (DiMuzio, 2008). Hemodynamic instability of these critically ill patients can require the administration of large volumes of intravenous (IV) fluids and vasoactive drugs to support the patient's blood pressure and maintain essential organ perfusion. Patients with acute kidney injury in ICU need a therapy that temporarily provides the elements of renal function while the failing kidneys are given time to regain their function. DiMuzio (2008) cites a multi-hospital, multi-country study of nearly 30,000 ICU patients in which about 6% of the population developed acute kidney injury. Among these ICU patients, the risk factors for increased mortality included the use of vasopressors, mechanical ventilation, and medical risk factors, such as shock, sepsis, and combined liver-kidney failure (DiMuzio, 2008).

In patients with acute kidney injury, further nephron injury from repeated or continued ischemia due to hypotension should be avoided to prevent further, possibly irreversible, damage. With this added concern about the patient's hemodynamic stability, the difficulty in removing excess fluid and toxins during intermittent hemodialysis without causing hypotensive episodes is well recognized by nephrology practitioners. Therefore, utilization of CRRT, a slower, less aggressive therapy, provides an important alternative for these critically ill patients (Dirkes & Hodge, 2007). Nephrology and critical care clinicians have increasingly recognized the efficacy of this 24-hour therapy in providing renal replacement therapy while minimizing fluctuations in the patient's hemodynamic stability (DiMuzio, 2008).

Dirkes and Hodge (2007) explain the benefit of removing fluid over a longer period of time with CRRT compared to the shorter time frame of intermittent hemodialysis (HD) in the following example. To remove 3 liters of plasma water over 4 hours with intermittent HD would generate a constant net ultrafiltration rate of 12.5 mL/minute. Removing the same volume of fluid over 24 hours using CRRT would yield a net ultrafiltration rate of only 2 mL/minute. This difference makes CRRT an ideal therapy for critically ill patients.

Patients experiencing acute kidney injury also suffer from a build up of uremic toxins and waste products. The serum electrolytes become abnormal, frequently reaching life-threatening levels. Acid-base balance is also adversely affected. Patients are often catabolic, leading to further symptoms of disruption of homeostasis. Solute removal in CRRT, another of its major functions, like fluid removal, occurs slowly over time, returning the patient to a more stable physiologic state. Achieving and then maintaining that balance while the body heals and regains its own equilibrium are essentials of the CRRT process that demand the highest quality of patient care (DiMuzio, 2008).

When looking for what is meant by "quality" in the healthcare arena, the Institute of Medicine (IOM) (2001) provides one definition: "...the degree to which health services for individuals and populations increase the likelihood of desired health outcomes and are consistent with current professional knowledge" (p. 44). In the past few years, the Joint Commission has expanded its quality healthcare focus from review of policies, procedures, and facilities to include the exploration of process improvement in the organization, patient safety, and patient outcomes (Hall, Shirley, & Barnsteiner, 2008).

Monitor for Achieving Therapy Goals

Monitoring the patient and CRRT device to achieve prescribed therapy goals is a collaborative team effort between nephrology nurses and the ICU nursing staff (Craig, 2008). Individual patient treatment goals for CRRT may include correction and management of fluid balance, adequate uremic waste product removal, correction and maintenance of electrolytes levels, and facilitation of nutritional management through parenteral or enteral administration (Axley, 2005).

Documentation of patient and equipment monitoring during CRRT is done on a continuous basis. It may be performed hourly, but it can vary based upon program protocols and the individual patient's needs. By monitoring and documenting patient data and equipment parameters, the patient care team can work together to ensure the patient receives a safe and effective treatment while achieving therapy goals.

Concepts and principles of CQI can be applied to the selection of quality indicators following recommendations for nursing management and guidelines for care of the patient during CRRT (Burrows-Hudson & Prowant, 2005; DiMuzio, 2008; Dirkes & Hodge, 2007; Paton, 2007). CRRT is a complex therapy with many factors that interact and can affect the provision of quality care. Determining what indicators are important to monitor can be based on the impact they have on achieving the overall therapy goals. They may be selected based on experience and a desire to improve facility outcomes, problems that have occurred that need resolution, or implementation of evidence-based practice improvements. Suggestions for consideration related to patient assessment, monitoring, and evaluation are presented below.

Monitor Fluid Volume Balance

If too little fluid is removed, the patient's fluid overload can worsen; if too much fluid is removed, the patient can become hypovolemic (DiMuzio, 2008).
- Cardiovascular parameters:
  - Blood pressure, heart rate and rhythm, heart sounds, jugular venous distention (JVD), peripheral pulses, capillary refill.
  - Central venous pressure (CVP), pulmonary capillary wedge pressure (PCWP), cardiac output (CO), cardiac index (CI), mixed venous oxygen saturation (SvO_2)
- Respiratory parameters:
  - Respiratory rate, adventitious lungs sounds, chest X-ray, oxygen saturation, arterial blood gasses.
  - Ventilator modality and settings – peak-inspiratory pressure, FiO_2, positive end-expiratory pressure (PEEP).
- Ultrafiltration (UF) parameters:
  - Hourly intake and output monitoring:
    - ➤ Intake – IV fluids, blood products, nutritional support.
    - ➤ Output – Urine, stool, drainage (wounds, chest tube, NG).
    - ➤ Hourly calculation of UF rate to meet prescribed fluid removal goal.
- Treat hypotensive episodes:

  - Fluid volume replacement.
  - Reduction of UF rate.
- Administer vasopressors as ordered to maintain mean arterial pressure for organ perfusion.

Monitor Electrolyte Balance
- Establish patient's baseline and monitor labs as ordered.
- Evaluate electrolyte contribution from all fluid sources.
- Electrolyte replacement managed based on laboratory results and confirmed with patient assessment:
  - Abnormal electrolyte levels may require adjustment in the CRRT system solutions.
  - Treat imbalance with intermittent electrolyte replacement.

Monitor Acid/Base Balance
- Establish the patient's baseline and monitor labs as ordered:
  - Evaluate arterial blood gases for metabolic decompensation.
  - Evaluate metabolic panel for bicarbonate deficit.
  - Evaluate metabolic acidosis.
- Evaluate CRRT system solutions for adjustment:
  - Evaluate use of bicarbonate-based solutions.
  - Evaluate all other sources of bicarbonate in cases of metabolic alkalosis.

Monitor Body Temperature
- Extracorporeal blood circuit exposure to room temperature and room temperature solution:
  - Fluid/blood warmer.
  - Warming blanket.
- Monitor for infection since fever may be masked by cooling effect of extracorporeal circulation:
  - Trend white cell count for elevation.
  - Monitor increase in immature WBCs.

Monitor Vascular Access for CRRT
- Line connections are visible and secure.
- Positional flows from access – Reposition the patient, treat hypovolemia, replace catheter.

Monitor Anticoagulation
Increase CRRT circuit patency to avoid patient complications.
- Heparin:
  - Dose adjustments made based on activated partial thromboplastin time (aPTT).
  - Monitor platelet count for thrombocytopenia.
  - Monitor for development of heparin-induced thrombocytopenia (HIT).
  - Heparinization may not be indicated in patients with recent surgery, GI bleeding (melena or bloody stools, NG drainage), sepsis, hepatic failure, presence of thrombocytopenia.
  - Hct/Hgb monitored as prescribed for loss of blood.
- Trisodium citrate (TSC):
  - Citrate interrupts the clotting cascade by binding with calcium within the CRRT circuit.

○ The citrate/calcium bound molecules are partially removed from the blood by diffusion in the filter.

○ Calcium replacement is infused post-circuit or through a central venous catheter to replace the calcium losses as the blood returns to the patient (Craig, 2008).

○ Monitor ionized calcium levels of the patient and the extracorporeal circuit.

○ Dose adjustments made based on the patient's ionized calcium level.

➤ Monitor the patient for development of signs of hypocalcaemia.

➤ Monitor the patient's labs for development of alkalosis due to metabolism of citrate into bicarbonate.

➤ Monitor for hepatic inability to metabolize citrate.

• Direct thrombin inhibitors — Argatroban, lepirudin:

○ Cleared by the liver and kidneys.

○ Monitor liver function.

○ Lepirudin may not be indicated for patients with renal failure.

• Normal saline (NS) flushes:

○ Reduces stagnation of blood in the filter to minimize clotting of the fibers/membrane.

○ Volume of flushes are included when calculating the UFR to prevent fluid overload.

At the same time that patient monitoring and assessment is crucial, nurses must also monitor and manage the CRRT system's extracorporeal circuit. Concepts and principles of CQI can again be applied to the selection of quality indicators following recommendations for nursing management and guidelines for care of the patient during CRRT (Burrows-Hudson & Prowant, 2005; Craig, 2008; DiMuzio, 2008; Dirkes & Hodge, 2007; Paton, 2007).

Monitor Blood Flow Rate

• Small solute removal is dependent upon the amount of blood moving though the CRRT filter.

• May be limited by vascular access.

Monitor CRRT Solutions

Meet prescription – Dialysate and replacement fluids.

• Dialysate: Prescribed fluid infused into the outer compartment of the filter; small molecular wastes and excess electrolytes diffuse from high concentration in the patient's blood into the dialyzing fluid (continuous venovenous hemodialysis [CVVHD] and continuous venovenous hemodiafiltration [CVVHDF]).

○ Dialysate fluid prescription is based upon the patient's electrolyte status:

➤ Monitor sodium, potassium, bicarbonate, chloride, calcium, phosphorus, and magnesium laboratory results to determine the need for repletion.

➤ Monitor the development of dysrhythmias.

○ Dialysate fluid prescription can be based upon the patient's acid/base balance:

➤ Adjust to maintain metabolic control.

➤ Ensure fluids containing bicarbonate are not excessively warmed to prevent bicarbonate coming out of solution as carbon dioxide bubbles.

○ Dialysate is appropriately labeled by pharmacy.

○ Dialysate content is checked to match the prescription with verification documented by two RNs prior to use.

• Replacement fluids: Prescribed sterile (IV grade) fluid infused into the blood compartment of the filter, which increases the volume of ultrafiltrate, thereby increasing convective clearance.

○ Convective clearance:

➤ The process of carrying solutes across a semipermeable membrane along with the solution in which they are carried.

➤ Larger molecules tend to clear better with convection than with diffusion.

○ Solutions may vary by practice protocols:

➤ Normal saline alone or mixed with selected electrolytes.

➤ Prescribed physiological fluids to mimic normal plasma water content.

➤ Custom or commercially prepared solutions to meet individual patient metabolic control needs.

➤ Commercially prepared solution, including citrate for regional anticoagulation.

➤ The rate of administration may be adjusted to replace any excess ultrafiltration removed hourly during the process of CVVH or CVVHDF.

Monitor Prescribed CRRT Fluid Flow Rates To Evaluate Adequacy of Clearance

• Dialysate fluid flow is set at prescribed rate (Dirkes & Hodge, 2007). Dialysate flow rate determines the amount of small molecule waste clearance.

• Replacement fluid flow is set at prescribed rate. Replacement fluid flow rate determines the amount of middle and large molecule clearance.

• Monitor laboratory values for urea clearance.

• Calculate dialysis dose in ml/kg/hour using total effluent volume and total actual treatment time.

Monitor Machine Circuit Pressures Alarms

• Machine and alarm parameters are set to notify the nurse of changes in the CRRT circuit pressure readings: Venous (return) pressure, arterial (access) pressure, transmembrane pressure (TMP).

• System pressure changes and trends can reflect circuit issues including:

○ Clotting in the extracorporeal circuit.

○ Flow from the vascular access.

○ Disconnection of the system's bloodlines from the vascular access.

○ Issues related to dialysate and/or replacement solution flows.

Monitor Integrity of Pump Tubing Segments And/or Integrity of Transducer or Pressure Pods

• No visible shearing of pump segment material.

• No pressure variations or fluid leaks.

Figure 14-1
Example of a CRRT Quality Indicator Trending Tool

Indicator Audit 10% of Medical Records	Threshold	Jan	Feb	Mar	Apr	May	Jun	Jul	Aug	Sep	Oct	Nov	Dec
Vital signs every hour (including temperature)	100%												
Ultrafiltration parameters documented every hour	100%												
Cardiovascular assessment every 4 hours	90%												
Respiratory assessment documented every 4 hours	90%												
Electrolytes monitored every 6 hours	90%												
Acid/base monitored every 6 hours	90%												
Vascular access monitored every hour	100%												
Anticoagulation settings every hour	100%												
Blood flow rate every hour	100%												
Dialysate/replacement fluid flow rate every hour	100%												
Circuit pressure readings monitored every hour	100%												
Integrity of blood pump segment every 4 hours	90%												
Blood loss greater than 50 ml	1%												
Air embolism	0%												
Hemolysis	0%												
Clotted circuit	10%												
Incorrect dialysate/ replacement fluid used	0%												
Vascular access removed due to infection	0%												

Source: Used with permission from Billie Axley.

Monitor System to Minimize Interruption Of Therapy

- Clotting in the circuit – Routinely monitor for visible clotting in the circuit and for changes in system pressure readings; replace the circuit prior to system clotting to prevent patient blood loss.
- Air in the circuit – Secure and monitor system connections to prevent air from entering the system; ensure the venous return line is placed in air detector since micro-bubbles in blood may or may not be visible.
- Filter blood leak – Blood leak alarm may signal failed integrity of filter fiber(s); prepare for immediate system change.

- Follow the program protocol for the time CRRT system can be in recirculation mode before required discard (resources include manufacturer's guidelines, infection control, and blood bank services) due to system disconnection during patient transport to other departments, such as radiology or surgery.
- Follow program protocol and manufacturer recommendations for routine systems change.
- Evaluate actual hours of treatment per day as well as the reasons for treatment interruptions (operating room, interventional radiology, MRI or CT, nephrology staff's ability to respond to restart therapy, ICU staff skills in problem solving to prevent interruptions).

Apply CQI to Ensure Safe and Effective Delivery Of CRRT

With the mainstreaming of CRRT, it has become advantageous to have a formal CQI program in place for monitoring aggregate patient and equipment quality indicators, contributing to safe and effective care to all patients receiving this therapy. As identified previously in this chapter, concepts and principles of CQI can be applied to the selection of quality indicators. In addition to the quality indicators identified as recommendations for nursing management of the patient during CRRT, additional aggregate patient care indicators tracked could include:

- Patients will have minimal loss of blood related to the CRRT:
  - Review adverse event reports.
- Patients will have no air embolism related to the CRRT:
  - Review adverse event reports.
- Effective collaboration between nephrology and ICU nursing staff:
  - Review documentation of bedside training and communication.
  - Review staff satisfaction reports.
- Internal survey activities – Audit selected percentage of medical records for adherence to policy/protocol could include:
  - Patient assessment and monitoring performed and documented.
  - Equipment parameters monitored and documented.
  - CRRT fluid parameters monitored and documented.
  - Fluid removal calculations performed and documented.
  - CRRT pre-treatment machine alarm self-test performed and documented.
  - Treatment parameters met prescriptions.
  - Equipment preventive maintenance performed according to manufacturer's guidelines and documented.
  - CRRT program using HD equipment follows specific quality indicators related to water purification:
    - ➤ Test product water for chlorine and chloramines.
    - ➤ Test dialysate conductivity and pH.
    - ➤ Monthly test of water and dialysate for colony count and endotoxin testing.
    - ➤ Scheduled American Academy of Medical Instrumentation (AAMI) water analysis.
    - ➤ Scheduled equipment preventive maintenance.
- External survey results:
  - The Joint Commission.
  - Centers for Medicare and Medicaid Services (CMS).
  - State surveys.
  - Occupational Safety and Health Administration (OSHA) survey.

Figure 14-1 presents an example of a CRRT quality indicator trending tool.

Organization Structure to Manage Opportunities For Improvement

The CRRT program's CQI committee can stimulate nurses' involvement in quality activities by welcoming suggestions for improvement opportunities. Patients undergoing CRRT benefit from the program's use of CQI as a method for solving problems. The CQI committee reviews selected quality indicators and analyzes them for trends as well as variations from the expected outcome(s). These identified variances are ranked and prioritized for the CQI team to address with an action plan for improvement.

The CQI committee may decide to review a few selected quality indicators at each meeting. A calendar can be created to rotate various reports to ensure that all areas of concern are addressed on a regular basis. Additional activities can be added to the calendar as needed. It is important to ensure there is adequate time on the CQI committee meeting agenda to review current action plans that have been updated by CRRT team members. Attach the action plans to the meeting minutes to provide a consistent flow of information from the committee to all CRRT team members.

Example of CQI in CRRT

An inpatient dialysis program providing CRRT identified an opportunity for improvement while reviewing the quality indicator, "The CRRT system will maintain patency." According to the quality indicator-tracking tool, the circuit clotting rate had exceeded the threshold as determined by the committee as an alert to initiate a CQI project.

A CQI project team was selected for the improvement project and began its work by reviewing the adverse event reports for circuit clotting events. The review revealed an increase in clotting events that coincided with an update in equipment technology. The improvement team members interviewed CRRT nephrology nurses and ICU staff members concerning the increase in frequency of CRRT circuit clotting and their perceived competence in managing the treatment after the technology update. Interviews provided the team with several possible root causes of the problem. One factor was a low confidence level of the ICU nurses to monitor and troubleshoot the CRRT system. Another factor was the inconsistent review of equipment monitoring provided to the ICU staff by nephrology nurses with each set up and/or daily visit. The CQI team utilized a small core workgroup of nephrology nurses and ICU nurses to develop an action plan for improvement.

Goal

Decrease interruption of CRRT due to circuit clotting to level below the established threshold.

Plan

Step 1. Establish written protocols for:
- Defining responsibilities for ICU and nephrology nurses.
- Monitoring machine parameters.
- Managing machine alarms.
- Reviewing CRRT operations with the ICU nurse at each change of shift and at each set up of the circuit.

Step 2. Identify a team of nephrology nurse "superusers" to serve as resources to all staff members providing CRRT by:
- Providing education to all staff members on CRRT equipment operations, including bedside review of troubleshooting alarms.
- Ensuring each system was checked near the beginning of each shift for signs of clotting:

Figure 14-2
Example of a CQI Action Plan

Goal: Decrease interruption of CRRT due to circuit clotting to below threshold in six months.

Action Step: Plan and Do	Team Member(s)	Target Date	Follow Up: Check
1. Establish written protocols for responsibilities of ICU and dialysis nurses for: • Monitoring machine parameters and machine alarms • Reviewing CRRT operations with the ICU nurse at each change of shift and at each set-up of the circuit.	Nurse Managers and 2 staff RNs	August	CRRT theory and machine operation classes were already offered on a monthly basis to new ICU staff members. Classes added for experienced users regarding technology upgrades to system.
2. Identify a team of nephrology nurse "superusers" to serve as resources to all staff members providing CRRT. • Provide education to all staff members on CRRT equipment operations, including beside review of troubleshooting alarms. • Ensure each system is checked near the beginning of each shift for signs of clotting; if signs of clotting are present communicate plan to change circuit before clotting of system; use opportunity to provide visualization of signs of clotting with the ICU nurse • At the beginning of each work shift, review monitoring machine parameters and management of alarms with the ICU nurses.	Superusers	September	Superuser team was expanded with additional education and skill building opportunities for nephrology staff members.
3. Include CRRT competencies in the ICU nurse's skills lab and competency reviews. Superusers participate in competency skills labs and check-offs for ICU nurses.	Superusers	October and on-going	The nephrology nurses attended the competency labs to support the collaborative initiative.
			Check: Six months after initiation of the improvement project, the number of CRRT procedures being performed increased, and clotting events decreased below threshold levels. The number of clotted systems within the first 4 hours decreased by 68%. Additional improvement identified: the number of calls received by the nephrology nurse on call after midnight decreased by 87%.
Act: 1. The action steps were incorporated into the CRRT program's standard of practice with written policies and procedures. 2. The quality indicator of "The CRRT system will maintain patency" continued to be monitored on a regular basis to ensure sustained improvement.			

Source: Used with permission from Billie Axley and Tana Waack.

○ If signs of clotting were present, communicate plan to change circuit before the system clots.

○ Use opportunity to provide guidance in visualizing signs of clotting with the ICU nurse.

• Reviewing monitoring machine parameters and management of alarms with ICU nurses at the beginning of each work shift.

Step 3. Include CRRT competencies in the ICU nurses' skills lab and reviews:

• Superusers were scheduled to participate in competency skills labs and check-offs for ICU nurses.

• Nephrology nurses attended the competency labs to support the collaborative initiative.

Do
Initiate action steps.

Check Outcomes
Six months after initiation of the improvement project, the number of CRRT procedures being performed increased, and clotting events decreased below threshold levels. The number of clotted systems within the first 4 hours decreased by 68%.

The need to contact the nephrology nurse on call diminished as the number of calls received after midnight decreased by 87%.

Act

The action steps were incorporated into the CRRT program's standard of practice with written policies and procedures. The quality indicator of "The CRRT system will maintain patency" continued to be monitored on a regular basis to ensure sustained improvement. Figure 14-2 presents an example of a CQI Action Plan.

CQI Applied to Other Methods of Renal Replacement Therapy

Slow extended daily dialysis (SLEDD) is a therapy similar to CRRT, although the treatment is completed in a shorter time. SLEDD treatments are 6 to 12 hours each day instead of 24 hours of continuous treatment. Some differences will exist when selecting quality indicators for tracking and trending in SLEDD. Fluid management monitoring is more frequent due to the shorter treatment time and higher UF rate. SLEDD may not require anticoagulation because blood flow rates are faster than with longer therapies. Studies have demonstrated that SLEDD therapy provides effective waste removal and supports cardiovascular stability as efficiently as CRRT (Dirkes & Hodge, 2007).

Other non-renal applications of CRRT include the treatment of sepsis and decompensated heart failure (Dirkes & Hodge, 2007). Whatever the application of the therapy, the nurse is an integral part of assessment and monitoring patient and equipment parameters, and identification, tracking, and trending the quality indicators. These important functions serve to identify opportunities for improvement to achieve high quality, safe patient care.

Conclusion

Hall and colleagues (2008) observe that "...many nurses will find that discussions of the need for safe, patient-centered, high-quality care resonate with the values that drew them into nursing" (p. 418). The acquisition of the skills necessary for successful quality improvement initiatives can be achieved through nurses' education about their use to enhance the quality of care (Hall et al., 2008). CQI must be an integral part of CRRT programs to monitor safety and efficacy of CRRT because the use of this complex therapy is on the rise. Rebecca Patton, President of the American Nurse Association (ANA) (2008), states that "The nursing profession has done extraordinary work related to quality" (p. 14), observing that nurses make a difference in quality improvement and patient outcomes. As a collaborative nephrology and ICU team, nurses can work together to collect accurate data, make improvements at the bedside, and become involved in the CQI process to significantly enhance the care of patients with acute and chronic renal failure.

References

Axley, B. (2005). *Continuous renal replacement therapy for the critically ill patient.* Lecturer, Vanderbilt School of Nursing Critical Care Program, Nashville, TN.

Burrows-Hudson, S., & Prowant, B.F. (Eds.). (2005). *Nephrology nursing standards of practice and guidelines of care.* Pitman, NJ: American Nephrology Nurses' Association.

Chrysochoou, G., Marcus, R.J., Sureshkumar, K.K., McGill, R.L., & Carlin, B.W. (2008). Renal replacement therapy in the critical care unit. *Critical Care Nursing Quarterly, 34*(4), 282-290.

Craig, M. (2008). Slow extended daily dialysis (SLEDD) and continuous renal replacement therapies (CRRT), In C.S. Counts (Ed.), *Core curriculum for nephrology nursing* (5th ed., pp. 231-278). Pitman, NJ: American Nephrology Nurses' Association.

DiMuzio, C. (2008). CRRT spells success against acute renal failure in critically ill patients. *American Nurse Today, 3*(5), 9-11.

Dirkes, S., & Hodge, K. (2007). Continuous renal replacement therapy in the adult intensive care unit: History and current trends. *Critical Care Nurse, 27*(2), 61-66, 68-72, 74-80.

Hall, L.W., Shirley, M.M., Barnsteiner, J.H. (2008). Quality and nursing: Moving from a concept to a core competency. *Urologic Nursing, 28*(6), 417-426.

Institute of Medicine (IOM). (2001). *Crossing the quality chasm: A new health system for the 21st century.* Washington, D.C.: National Academies Press.

Paton, M. (2007). CRRT: Help for acute renal failure. *Nursing Made Incredibly Easy!, 5*(5), 28-38.

Patton, R.M. (2008). From your ANA president: PR, P4R, P4P, VBP. Connecting the dots—with all of the "P's." *American Nurse Today, 3*(5), 14.

Additional Reading

Waack, T. (2007). *Providing CRRT: A collaborative effort between ICU and dialysis.* Abstract. 12th Annual International Conference on Continuous Renal Replacement Therapy, San Diego, CA.

| Chapter 14 | CONTINUING NURSING EDUCATION EVALUATION FORM | 1.3 Contact Hours |

Clinical Application: CQI in Continuous Renal Replacement Therapy

ANNP0914

Applying Continuous Quality Improvement in Clinical Practice contains 22 chapters of educational content. Individual learners may apply for continuing nursing education credit by reading a chapter and completing the Continuing Nursing Education Evaluation Form for that chapter. Learners may apply for continuing nursing education credit for any or all chapters.

Please photocopy this test page, complete, and return to ANNA.
You can also download this form from www.annanurse.org (choose Education - CNE Activities - Publications)
Receive continuing nursing education credit (CNE) immediately by completing the CNE evaluation process in ANNA's Online Library. Go to www.annanurse.org, and click on the Online Library icon for more information.

Name: _____

Address: _____

City: _____ State: _____ Zip: _____

E-mail:_____ Preferred telephone: ☐ Home ☐ Work _____

State where licensed and license number: _____

CNE application fees are based upon the number of contact hours provided by the individual section. CNE fees per contact hour for ANNA members are as follows: 1.0-1.9 – $15; 2.0-2.9 – $20; 3.0-3.9 – $25; 4.0 and higher – $30. Fees for nonmembers are $10 higher.

CNE application fee for Chapter 14: ANNA member $15   Nonmember $25

ANNA Member: ☐ Yes ☐ No   ☐ Member # (if available) _____

☐ Check or money order enclosed   ☐ American Express   ☐ Visa   ☐ MasterCard

Total amount submitted:_____

Credit card number _____ Exp. Date _____

Name as it appears on the card: _____

NOTE: Your evaluation form can be processed in 1 week for an additional rush charge of $5.00.

☐ **Yes, I would like this evaluation form rush processed. I have included an additional fee of $5.00 for rush processing.**

Instructions

1. To receive continuing nursing education credit for an individual study after reading the chapter, complete this evaluation form.

2. Detach, photocopy, or download (www.annanurse.org) the evaluation form and send along with a check or money order payable to **American Nephrology Nurses' Association** to: ANNA, East Holly Avenue Box 56, Pitman, NJ 08071-0056.

3. Test returns must be postmarked by **April 30, 2011**. Upon completion of the answer/evaluation form, a certificate will be sent to you.

This chapter was reviewed and formatted for contact hour credit by Sally S. Russell, MN, CMSRN, ANNA Director of Education Services.

> **CNE Application Fee for Chapter 14**
> **ANNA member = $15**
> **Nonmember = $25**

---

1. I verify that I have read this chapter and completed this education activity. _____ Date _____

   Signature

2. What would be different in your practice if you applied what you have learned from this activity? (Please use additional paper if necessary.)

   _____
   _____
   _____
   _____

	Strongly disagree				Strongly agree
3. The activity met the stated objectives.					
a. Explore quality indicators that could be applied to a continuous renal replacement therapy program.	1	2	3	4	5
b. Describe an interdisciplinary improvement project conducted in an acute care setting.	1	2	3	4	5
4. The content was current and relevant.	1	2	3	4	5
5. The content was presented clearly.	1	2	3	4	5
6. The content was covered adequately.	1	2	3	4	5

7. How would you rate your ability to apply your learning to practice?   ☐ diminished ability   ☐ no change   ☐ enhanced ability

Comments _____
_____

8. Time required to read the chapter and complete this form: _____ minutes

---

Clinical Application:
Improving Quality for Children with Kidney Disease: Unique Dimensions

Helen Currier, BSN, RN, CNN
Deborah H. Miller, MSN, CNS, CNN

Objectives

Study of the information presented in this chapter will enable the learner to:
1. Explain how children differ clinically from adults.
2. Discuss benchmarking methodologies for assessing and treating chronic kidney disease and end stage renal disease in children.
3. Describe one way to build a quality culture of care in a pediatric setting.

Introduction

The Institute of Medicine defines high-quality care as care that is safe, timely, effective, efficient, equitable, and patient-centered (Agency for Healthcare Research and Quality [AHRQ], 2007). Children and adolescents comprise 25% of the United States (U.S.) population. While children consume few health care dollars relative to adults, their long life span means that the impact of investments in quality will be longer lasting (AHRQ, 2007).

Children differ from adults in several ways that are important for measuring and improving the quality and safety of their care. Children present unique healthcare problems: they are at greater risk for serious breathing difficulties, less tolerant of blood loss, more vulnerable to head injury, and require special tests and equipment for diagnosis and treatment (Children's Hospital and Research Center Oakland, 2009). Children also have a limited ability to communicate their needs. "Children often lack the communication skills to tell caregivers if something is wrong, which increases the responsibility of caregivers to carefully monitor their care to keep them safe," states Mark R. Chassin, MD, MPP, MPH, president of The Joint Commission (The Joint Commission, 2008, p. 4).

Children also present the challenge of anatomical and physiological immaturity, which changes with age. For example, obtaining and interpreting vital signs in children may present more difficulty simply because it can be challenging to obtain accurate values. Children may be uncooperative, and properly sized equipment may not be readily available. Normal values vary with age, making recognition of abnormalities more challenging (Dieckmann, Gausche-Hill, Brownstein, & the American Academy of Pediatrics [AAP], 2006). Finally, treating pediatric emergencies requires specialized knowledge and experience that can be found at a hospital that provides pediatric care.

Preventing Pediatric Medical Errors

The Joint Commission's mission is to continuously improve the safety and quality of care provided to the public through the provision of healthcare accreditation and related services that support performance improvement in healthcare organizations. The purpose of The Joint Commission's National Patient Safety Goals is to promote specific improve-ments in patient safety. These requirements highlight problem-atic areas in health care and describe evidence and expert-based solutions to these problems. The requirements focus on *system-wide* solutions. The National Patient Safety Goals have included efforts to improve the accuracy of patient identifica-tion, improve the effectiveness of communication among care-givers, and reduce the risk of healthcare-associated infections (The Joint Commission, 2008).

Children vary in weight, body surface area, and organ sys-tem maturity, which affect their ability to metabolize and excrete medications. There are few standardized dosing regi-mens for children, with most medication dosing requiring body weight or body surface area calculations. The causes of med-ication errors are multi-factorial. Therefore, medication error improvement programs must focus on system improvements and team communication (AAP, 2003).

In pediatrics, incorrect dosing is the most commonly reported medication error, including computation errors of dosage and dosing interval. To reduce the risk of pediatric medication errors, The Joint Commission (2008) suggests that healthcare organizations take a series of specific actions, including:

- Use the Joint Commission's National Patient Safety Goals and Medication Management.
- Use standards to guide safe medication practices for pedi-atric patients.
- Weigh all pediatric patients in kilograms, which then becomes the standardized weight used for prescriptions, medical records, and staff communication.
- Do not dispense or administer drugs classified as high risk until the patient has been weighed (unless in an emergency situation).
- Require prescribers to write out how they arrived at the proper dosage, such as dose per weight or body surface area, so that the calculation can be double checked by a pharmacist, nurse, or both.
- Use pediatric-specific medication formulations and concen-trations when possible.

Pediatric End Stage Renal Disease (ESRD)

Measures of the quality of health care that are meaningful for adults cannot be assumed to have the same applicability to health care for children. Children differ fundamentally from adults in their development, dependency, patterns of illness and disability, and demographic characteristics (Zadrozny, Power, Nishimi, & Kizer, 2004). For example, mortality and morbidity rates in children who are on dialysis are markedly lower than those in adult patients on dialysis, although they are substantially higher than in the general pediatric population. Thus, "...while mortality hospitalization rates are important outcome indicators for pediatric ESRD programs, they are insufficient" (Goldstein et al., 2004, p. 846). "The pediatric ESRD patient is a member of a unique sub-population of ESRD patients. The cause of ESRD in the pediatric patient differs markedly from the adult patient; treatment modality in the pediatric ESRD patient differs substantially from the adult patient; and outcomes such as growth, development, and school attendance are also unique to the pediatric ESRD patient" (Andreoli et al., 2005, p. 2263).

Benchmarking

Chronic Kidney Disease

The North American Pediatric Renal Trials and Collaborative Studies (NAPRTCS) offers excellent benchmarking opportunities for pediatric ESRD programs. NAPRTCS was organized by pediatric nephrologists in 1987 as a registry initially devoted to children who had received renal transplants. It has since been expanded to include children who receive maintenance dialysis therapy and children with chronic kidney disease (CKD). A report is generated annually to examine multiple characteristics of this population, including patient and allograft survival, immunosuppressive medication regimens, anemia status, growth, school attendance, dialysis adequacy, dialysis access types and complications, and peritonitis rates (NAPRTCS, 2008). These data can be used to generate best practice benchmarking for process improvement. Individual centers are also given reports of their patient outcomes to compare with the national outcomes (Andreoli et al., 2005).

Acute Kidney Injury

Since January 2001, the Prospective Pediatric Continuous Renal Replacement Therapy (ppCRRT) Registry Group has been collecting data from multiple U.S. pediatric centers. The purpose is to obtain demographic data regarding pediatric patients who receive continuous renal replacement therapy (CRRT), assess the effect of different CRRT prescriptions on circuit function, and evaluate the impact of clinical variables on patient outcomes. Many issues plague the pediatric acute kidney injury outcome literature. These include data only from single-center sources, a relative lack of prospective study, mixture within studies of renal replacement therapy modality without stratification, and inconsistent use of methods to control for patient illness severity in outcome analysis. The ppCRRT Registry Group reports have described prevalent methods for pediatric CRRT and offered insight as to which methods may lead to better outcomes (Goldstein et al., 2004). A CRRT example is as follows:

- Identify a problem area such as reduced CRRT circuit life. Before embarking on a comparison with another program, know the circuit data, program protocols, policies/procedures, and outcomes. For example, data will include machine brand, blood pump flow rate, catheter size and anatomical site, extracorporeal circuit volume, priming fluid,

dialysis or replacement fluid composition, and anticoagulation method. This establishes a baseline performance, providing a point against which an improvement effort can be measured.
- Identify potential partners – If one is interested in improving the circuit life in children on CRRT, it may be helpful to identify other pediatric practitioners who face similar circuit priming and anticoagulation challenges. These practitioners may reside in critical care and/or nephrology departments.
- Identify data sources – Examine the very best outcomes in the ppCRRT registry circuit data:
  ○ Filter life-span (hours).
  ○ Reason for circuit change:
    ➤ Clotting.
    ➤ Access malfunction.
    ➤ Machine malfunction.
    ➤ Unrelated patient indication (for example, needs CT scan).
    ➤ CRRT discontinued.
- Survey practitioners/programs for measures and practices. Surveys are sometimes distributed within e-mail discussion groups (for example, mailto:pedcrrt-admin@listhost.uchicago.edu). Results are typically reported by a neutral party and blinded to protect confidential data. Other professional networking opportunities exist at educational meetings addressing pediatric CRRT (CRRTOnline.com, 2009; Pediatric CRRT, 2008).
- Visit "best practice" facilities to identify leading edge practices. Programs typically agree to mutually exchange information beneficial to all parties. Another option is to invite the expert(s) to your facility – either informally or by a consulting arrangement.
- Determine gaps between identified best practices and current practices.
- Implement new and improved practices. Take leading-edge practices and develop implementation plans that include identification of specific opportunities (such as protocols, policies/procedures, and/or care delivery models), associated cost/benefits, and a plan for marketing the idea to your organization.
- Evaluate.

Quality Assurance Performance Improvement (QAPI) Priorities for Children with CKD

- Patient safety, particularly in dialysis settings.
  ○ Prime examples include minimizing extracorporeal volume and preventing exsanguination in hemodialysis (HD) and preventing dialysate overfill in automated controlled peritoneal dialysis (PD).
- Preventive care, including (but not limited to) immunization, injury prevention (for example, falls), and avoidable hospitalizations (see Figure 15-1a and 15-1b).
  - One example of injury prevention is the Falls Risk Assessment (see Figure 15-2). Assessment tools created for use in the adult dialysis population to evaluate the potential for falls are not appropriate for use with pediatric patients. Environmental factors, such as size of furniture/equipment (the examination table), develop-

Figure 15-1a

Hospitalizations 2009																								
Hemodialysis	Jan		Feb		March		April		May		June		July		Aug		Sept		Oct		Nov		Dec	
Diagnosis	Days	Pts	Days	Pts	Days	Pts	Days	Pts	Days	Pts	Days	Pts	Days	Pts	Days	Pts	Days	Pts	Days	Pts	Days	Pts	Days	Pts
Access/AVF Placement																								
Access Clotted/Declot/AVF Placed																								
Access/AVF Revision/Col/Clotted																								
Hyperphosphatemia/ Hyperkalemia																								
G-Button Placement																								
Anemia																								
Nephrectomy																								
Renal Osteodystrophy/Septic Arthritis																								
Catheter Replacement																								
Thrombectomy																								
Fever																								
Gastroenteritis																								
Hyperkalemia																								
Hypertension																								
Hypertension/ Fluid Overload																								
Initiate HD																								
Graft Rejection																								
Med/Psychosocial Issues																								
HD Tunnel Infection/ Initiate Peritoneal Dialysis																								
Sepsis/Line Sepsis																								
MRSA Sepsis																								
Malnutrition/Bilateral SCFE																								
Other Issues																								
Pain Issues/Abdominal Pain																								
Other Issues																								
Psychosocial Issues																								
Respiratory Issues																								
Seizure Issues/Hypertension																								
Pulmonary Capilliaritis																								
Total	0	0	0	0	0	0	0	0	0	0	0	0	0	0	0	0	0	0	0	0	0	0	0	0

Note: SCFE = slipped capital femoral epiphysis, G-button = gastrostomy button.
Source: Used with permission from Helen Currier, Texas Children's Hospital.

Figure 15-1b

Hospitalizations 2009																								
Peritoneal Dialysis	Jan		Feb		March		April		May		June		July		Aug		Sept		Oct		Nov		Dec	
Diagnosis	Days	Pts	Days	Pts	Days	Pts	Days	Pts	Days	Pts	Days	Pts	Days	Pts	Days	Pts	Days	Pts	Days	Pts	Days	Pts	Days	Pts
Nephrectomy																								
Catheter Malfunction/ Temp HD																								
Catheter Malfunction																								
Dehydration																								
Abdominal Pain																								
Fever/Hypertension																								
Gastroenteritis																								
Hernia/Repair																								
Surgery/Hydrocele																								
Septic																								
Hyperkalemia																								
Hyperphosphatemia/ Hyperkalemia																								
Hypertension/Fluid Overload/ Complications to HD																								
Hypertension/Fluid Overload																								
Hypertension																								
Transfusion																								
Infected PICC Line																								
Initiate CCPD Training																								
Seizure Issues																								
Non-Dialysis/Other Infections																								
PD Machine Malfunction																								
Peritoneal/Pleural Fistula/Pulmonary Effusion																								
Transplant																								
Tumor/Ocular Pressure																								
Peritonitis																								
Catheter Removal (hole)/Temp HD																								
Pre-Transplant																								
Respiratory Infection																								
Multi-Organ Failure																								
Severe Anemia/Med Issues																								
Tunnel Infection/Catheter Removed/Temp HD																								
Total	0	0	0	0	0	0	0	0	0	0	0	0	0	0	0	0	0	0	0	0	0	0	0	0

Source: Used with permission from Helen Currier, Texas Children's Hospital.

Figure 15-2
Example: Quality Indicator Tracking Tool (Pediatric)

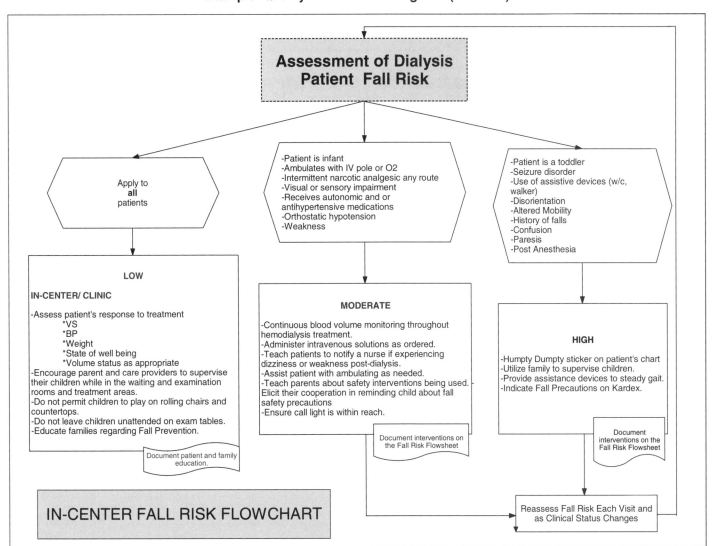

Source: Used with permission from Helen Currier, Texas Children's Hospital.

mental factors such as "learning to walk," and body weight changes with growth, drove a different approach for fall risk assessment and reduction in a pediatric dialysis population.

- Coordination of care (both as a priority itself and as a measurable component of other priority areas).
  - See section entitled "Coordination of Care: A Family-Centered Orientation" later in this chapter.

Pediatric CKD assessments must include:
- Growth and nutrition (see Figures 15-3 and 15-4).
- Developmental screening tests:
  - Denver Developmental Screening Test (DDST) is a widely used assessment for examining children 0 to 6 years of age (http://www.denverii.com).

- Health-Related Quality of Life (HRQoL) Measurement:
  - Tools:
    - ➤ Pediatric Quality of Life Inventory (PedsQL™) (http://www.pedsql.org).
    - ➤ Child Health and Illness Profile (CHIP) (http://www.childhealthprofile.org).
    - ➤ Child's Health Questionnaire (CHQ) (http://www.healthact.com/chq.html).

The ESRD *Conditions for Coverage* were released by the Centers for Medicare and Medicaid Services (CMS) on April 15, 2008. They require dialysis facilities to establish a written quality assessment and performance improvement (QAPI) program that is led by the medical director of the facility and designed to assist staff in achieving clinical performance excellence.
- Select criteria (What are you measuring?).

Figure 15-3
Example of a Checklist to be Used for Chart Review Prior to Patient Rounding

Patient Label	Cause of ESRD_____		Last Peritonitis_____
	Dialysis Start Date_____		Last ESI _____/_____
	Access Insertion_____		Access Revision_____

	freq	Jan	Feb	Mar	Apr	May	June	Comments
Laboratory Assessment								
Phosporus < 6	qmo							
Ca x P < 55 (65 if < 2yo)	qmo							
Potassium < 5	qmo							
Intact PTH	qmo							
Hemoglobin 11-13 g/dL	qmo							
Hematocrit (33-36%)	qmo							
Ferritin	q3mo							
Albumin	qmo							
CO_2	qmo							
Dialysis Adequacy	q3mo							
24-hour urine collection	q3mo							
Radiologic Studies								
Echocardiogram	qyr							
Hand/Wrist X-ray	qyr							
Clinical Assessment								
Blood Pressure (<_____)	qmo							
Growth (+/- HGH)	qmo							
Edema	qmo							
Access Site Eval	qmo							
Peritonitis	qmo							
School Status	qmo							
Transplant Status	qmo							
Use the boxes for absolute numbers, dates, Y/N or listed, in work up, scheduled for TX status. Highlight outliers.								

Source: Used with permission from Deborah Miller, Inova, Fairfax Hospital for Children.

Figure 15-4
Example: Quality Indicator Tracking Tool (Pediatric)

Indicator Audit % of Medical Records (MR)	Action Thres hold	Jan	Feb	Mar	Apr	May	Jun	Jul	Aug	Sep	Oct	Nov	Dec
Hospital admissions (morbidity) (% of total # of pts)													
Access (PD catheter; HD vascular access)													
Electrolyte Imbalance													
Hypertension/over hydration													
Hypotension/dehydration													
Infection													
Transfusion													
Dose of dialysis: Management of volume status Lower of 90% of normal for age/ht/wt or 130.80; euvolemic													
Dose of dialysis: Minimal delivered Kt/V greater than or equal to eKt/V 1.2 HD greater than or equal to 1.8/week PD													
Nutritional; Albumin greater than or equal to 4.0 g/dL(BCG)													
Mineral metabolism & renal bone disease Calcium greater than 8.4 mg/dL & less than 10.2 mg/dL Phosphorus 3.5-5.5 mg/dL Intact PTH q 3 months: 200-300 pg/mL													
Anemia Management: Hgb on ESAs less than 12 g/dL greater than 10 g/dL Transferrin Saturation greater than 20% Serum ferritin HD greater than 200 ng/mL; PD greater than 100 ng/mL; HD/PD less than 500 ng/mL													

Source: Adapted from CMS, 2008b. Used with permission from Helen Currier and Billie Axley.

- Identify metrics (How are you measuring it?).
- Determine frequency of measurement (How often are you measuring it?).
- Collect data results (What are the results?).
  - Identify the gaps between present performance and your organization's vision and goals.
- Plan for any needed performance interventions, such as process improvement.
- Evaluate program impact (What is the impact to your program?) (CMS, 2008a).

The QAPI program should also identify those measures that are *nursing-sensitive*. Such indicators reflect the structure, process, and outcomes of nursing care. Examples include nursing turnover, patient falls, staff skill mix, education/certification of nursing staff, and job satisfaction (American Nurses Association [ANA], 2009).

Common Challenges in Managing the Child with ESRD on Dialysis
Dialysis Dose
Children should receive at least the delivered dialysis dose as recommended for the adult population. For younger pediatric patients, prescription of higher dialysis doses and higher protein intakes at 150% of the recommended nutrient intake for age may be important (see Figures 15-5 through 15-16) (National Kidney Foundation [NKF], 2006a).

Mineral Metabolism and Bone Disease
The ESRD Program Interpretive Guidance (Version 1.1) (CMS, 2008a) notes that "Pediatric patients present significant special needs in the areas of growth and development and CKD mineral and bone disorder. A facility treating pediatric patients should follow current professionally accepted clinical practice standards for evaluating and monitoring the pediatric patient population in this area" (see Figures 15-17 through 15-20) (CMS, 2008a, p. 191).

Anemia
For an example of a Proactive Risk Assessment, see Figure 15-21. Associated data collection would include a patient's perspective pain measure and a monthly hemoglobin measure (see Figures 15-22 through 15-27).

Figure 15-5
HB Mean Facility URR

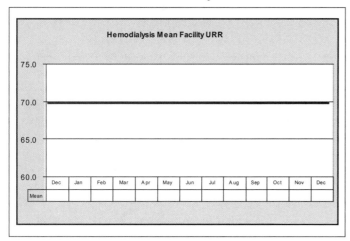

Figure 15-6
**Percentage of HD Patients with Equal
to or Greater Than 65 and 70 URR**

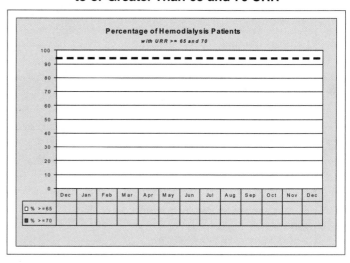

Figure 15-7
HD Mean Facility spKt/V

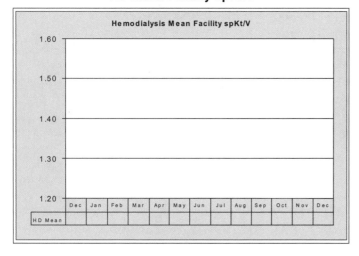

Figure 15-8
HD Mean Facility spKt/V

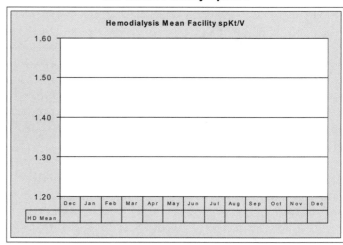

Figure 15-9
**Percentage of Patients with spKt/V Equal
to or Greater Than 1.2**

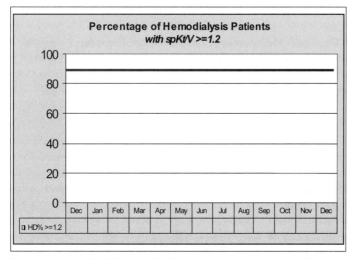

Figure 15-10
Frequent HD Mean Facility stdKt/V

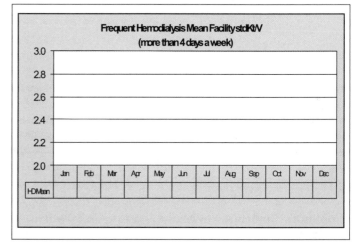

Source: Figures 15-5 through 15-10 used with permission from Helen Currier, Texas Children's Hospital.

Figure 15-11
Mean Albumin

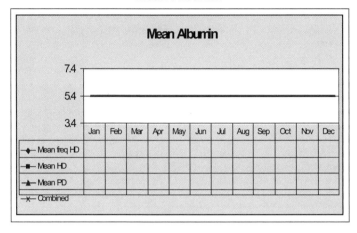

Figure 15-12
Percentage of Patients with Albumin Equal to or
Greater Than 3.4, 3.5, 3.8, and 4.0

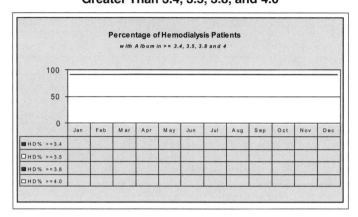

Figure 15-13
Percentage of Patients with Albumin Equal to or
Greater Than 3.4, 3.5, 3.8, and 4.0

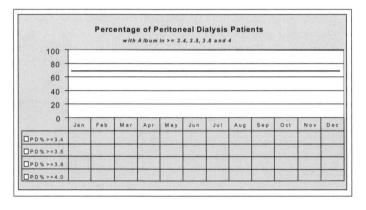

Figure 15-14
HD uPCR

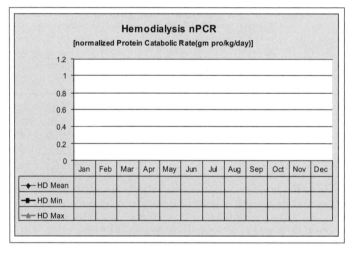

Figure 15-15
Percentage of HD uPCR Equal
to or Greater Than 1.2 and 1.0

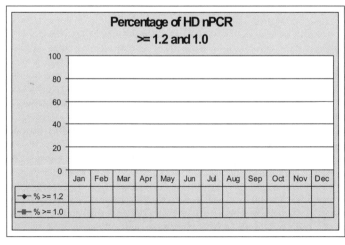

Figure 15-16
Percentage of Adol/YA nPCR Equal
to or Less Than 1.0

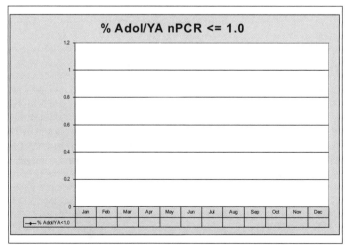

Source: Figures 15-11 through 15-16 used with permission from Helen Currier, Texas Children's Hospital.

Figure 15-17
Mean Phosphorus

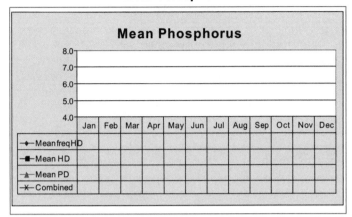

Figure 15-18
Mean Calcium

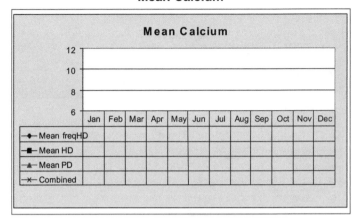

Figure 15-19
Mean Ca x Phos Product

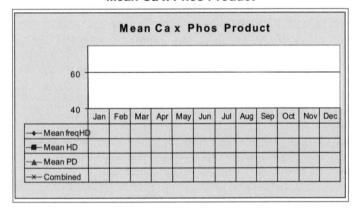

Figure 15-20
Mean Ca x Phos Percentages by Age

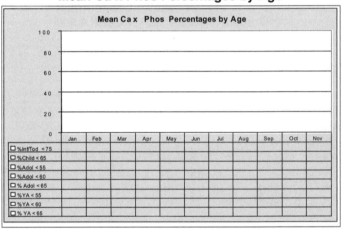

Source: Figures 15-17 through 15-20 used with permission from Helen Currier, Texas Children's Hospital.

Habilitation

The interdisciplinary team must assist the patient in achieving and sustaining an appropriate level of productive activity, as desired by the patient. This includes the educational needs of pediatric patients (patients under the age of 18 years), and rehabilitation and vocational rehabilitation referrals as appropriate (CMS, 2008a). Strategies to improve health-related quality of life (HRQoL) include drawing on psychological and social services and exercise intervention. Additionally, arts in health care can enhance and support the experience of health care for patients, families, and caregivers by incorporating the arts in all forms into a wide variety of settings for therapeutic, educational, and recreational purposes.

Vascular Access

Permanent access in the form of a fistula or graft is the preferred form of vascular access for most pediatric patients on maintenance HD therapy.

Circumstances in which a central venous catheter may be acceptable for pediatric long-term access include:

- Lack of local surgical expertise to place permanent vascular access in small children.
- Patient size too small to support a permanent vascular access.
- Bridging HD for PD training or PD catheter removal for peritonitis.
- Expectation of expeditious kidney transplantation.

Figure 15-21
Proactive Risk Assessment 2008

Title: Anemia Medication Management (ESAs/Iron)
Reason for selecting topic: Despite improvements in dialysis care, anemia remains a problem in pediatric patients on dialysis.
Explain how effectiveness of plan will be measured: Clinical data (hgb).

Process	Potential Failure	Likelihood of Failure	Effect on Patient	Causes	Strategies
Medication Selection	Multiple drug choice/physician preference	5	5	Pharmacokinetics Physician familiarity	Conversion chart Add/change formulary OR change Rx inventory
Ordering	Incorrect dose Incorrect frequency Incorrect route ordered	2 2 2	4 4 2	Dosing varies with age and modality of dailysis Ineligible handwriting Unfamiliarity with medication, preparation, and half-life Pharmacist error	Aranesp dispensed in pre-filled syringe Pharmacist calls unit for clarification
Dispensing	Incorrect concentration (multi-dose vs. single dose vial) Pharmacy resistance to routine dispensing	3 4	4 5	Pharmacist error Lack of understanding of Medicare Part B ESRD benefit	Educate front-end pharmacy staff
Administration	Incorrect route of administration Non-adherence with self-administration	1 5	2 5	Infrequency leads to missed doses Pain deters administration	Administer at clinic
Patient Education	Parent comprehension Incomplete or no education Lack of care reminders	3 1 5	4 4 3	Language barrier Literacy barrier	Utilize child life specialists for communicating to patients at appropriate level Utilize translator services
Monitoring	Lack of timely identification of signs and symptoms (iron deficiency, hyperparathyroidism, active infections, blood loss) Missed labs Lack of timely rsponse Physician notification in timely manner Patient not available	3 1 4 3 4	5 3 5 4 4	Causes include surgery, lab sampling, extracorporeal blood volume	Train RN(s) to function as *Anemia Managers*

Source: Used with permission from Helen Currier, Texas Children's Hospital.

Blood Pressure and Fluid Management

Accurate assessment of patient intravascular volume during the HD treatment should be provided to optimize ultrafiltration (NKF, 2006b). For pediatric patients weighing less than 35 kg, blood volume monitoring during HD should be available in order to evaluate body weight changes for gains in muscle weight vs. fluid overload (CMS, 2008a).

Annotations can be added to histograms that help to explain interventions or trends.

Coordination of Care: A Family-Centered Orientation

Care for the pediatric patient is characterized by both complex clinical conditions and complex regulatory requirements unique to the renal population. Aggregating clinical services (such as CKD, dialysis, and transplant) and support services in a service line model can streamline and improve the coordination of care. Programs that reap the most benefit from a service line model are those that involve care delivery at sites across the entire care continuum (Tesch & Levy, 2008). Emphasis is on the coordination of care – looking for opportunities to create protocols, standardize processes, and leverage information technology – so that the patient/family experience is consistent regardless of where care is delivered. Care coordination opportunities are included in Table 15-1.

Figure 15-22
Mean Hemoglobin

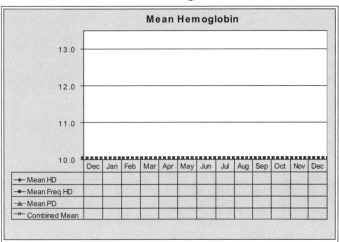

Figure 15-25
Percentage of Peritoneal Dialysis
Patients with Hemoglobin Equal
to or Greater Than 13, 11, 10.5, and 10

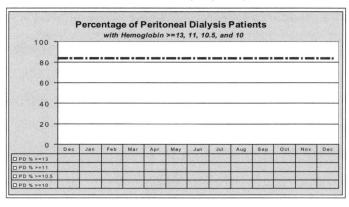

Figure 15-23
Percentage of Hemodialysis Patients with Hemoglobin
Equal to or Greater Than 13, 11, 10.5, and 10

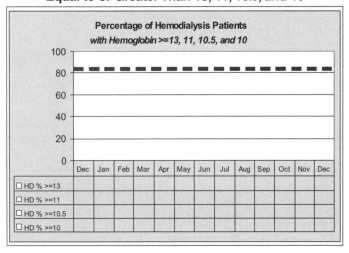

Figure 15-26
Mean T-Sat

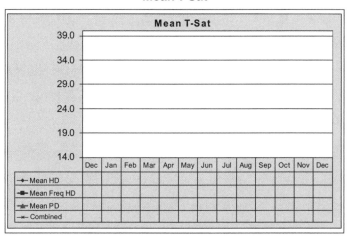

Figure 15-24
Percentage of Frequent Hemodialysis Patients with
Hemoglobin Equal to or Greater Than 13, 11, 10.5, and 10

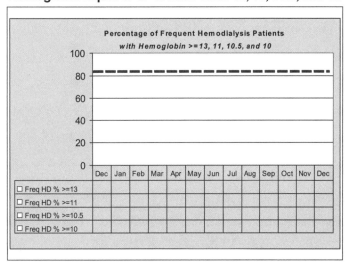

Figure 15-27
Percentage of Patients with T-Sat Equal
to or Greater Than 20

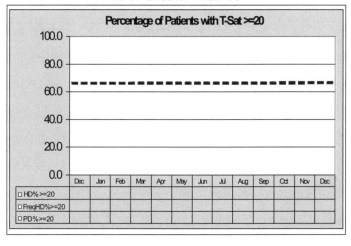

Source: Figures 15-22 through 15-27 used with permission from Helen Currier, Texas Children's Hospital.

Table 15-1
Renal Service Care Coordination

Other Opportunities for Care Coordination Across an Integrated Delivery System Include:
Space planning
Value stream mapping to identify waste and streamline the process • Activity • Management and information systems that support processes
Combined support for ESRD initiatives • Regulatory/accreditation • Outcomes • Process • Written protocols/policies and procedures • Research • Quality assessment/performance improvement • Patient/family education • Caregiver education • Information technology

Source: Used with permission from Helen Currier, Texas Children's Hospital.

An example is a facility developing a service line for coordinating the care of pediatric nephrology patients. Analysis of the service line can be examined in a QAPI program by tracking aspects of care (see Tables 15-2 through 15-5).

Service line benefits can include improved care outcomes, improved operational efficiencies, improved patient satisfaction, fostering alignment with medical director(s), improved physician relations, market differentiation, and reduced duplication of services.

Challenges for the Small Pediatric Program

The new conditions of coverage regarding QAPI present unique challenges to the small pediatric facility. Smaller programs have fewer staff and often rely on part-time nurses, registered dietitians, and social workers to fill many different roles The pediatric nurse is likely to have responsibility across modalities (PD and HD, or CKD and transplant) in the care of the child with CKD. Rather than running clinics several half days per week, these facilities may use traditional doctors' office scheduling, leaving no blocks of time for team meetings. Data entry and retrieval for programs without an electronic medical record require reading the medical record for data points and recording these manually. These challenges require ingenuity to develop tools meeting CMS requirements for quality initiatives in all dialysis and transplant programs.

As an example, an interdisciplinary team meeting held weekly on the designated "PD day" allows for a chart review on each of the patients on dialysis to be seen that day. Using a simple checklist, the chart is reviewed to ascertain laboratory values related to anemia, adequacy, calcium/phosphorous (Ca/Phos) balance, recent infections, hospitalizations, trans-

plant status, and growth. These parameters are then discussed by the interdisciplinary team to formulate priorities for this particular patient. Data are then pooled for a quarterly picture of quality. A small program will have fewer data points that can skew the aggregate data, so it is more accurate to look at these data quarterly. The interdisciplinary team, whose leader may be any of the disciplines represented on the team, can then examine trends and formulate a plan for improvement. This same method can be used for the child with CKD Stage 4 or 5. A chart review tool that looks at anemia, growth, immunizations, Ca/Phos balance, and transplant status is helpful for the individual patient as well as for looking at trends in care amenable to QAPI team action.

Meetings between nephrology and transplant teams will provide an opportunity for documentation of collaboration as well as offer a forum for discussion of complex patients and treatment protocols. The highest quality of care is the goal in all settings; approaching QAPI in a small program requires creative methods to adapt the process to the setting. While children are *no more unstable than adults* with CKD, children will often require more intense follow up since they are in a static state relative to growth and development.

Lessons Learned

Breaking the insular bubble of some pediatric CKD programs is critical to building a quality program. Professional isolation of nurses can result in habits that are not consistent with best practices. Avoid building a pediatric program solely on single-center experience. There is much professional insight to glean from nephrology colleagues who care for adults (for example, water treatment and infection control). The breadth and depth of experience in the adult community can assist pediatric programs in developing systems for QAPI. Pediatric nephrology teams need to network with others in the renal community – both pediatric and adult colleagues. Discussions do not have to be about specific work or current projects. Exploration of trends, questions regarding areas you want to learn more about, and sitting down with people outside of your daily and professional radar broadens the perspective and stimulates creativity. The key to success is an integrated, networked, and curious community that can leverage itself. Additionally, some hospital-based programs can benefit from contracting with independent consultants (experts in their field) for comprehensive program assessments, audits, and QAPI evaluations.

Best Practice

Best practice settings integrate curiosity, innovation, and collaboration into everyday practice – they are cultures that encourage spontaneity and consistent gatherings for discussion. Talented individuals are drawn to excellent programs. If the importance of the change is understood by all, then the greatest achievements will follow. A commitment from executives is a **must**. It is, in fact, the driving force. Woods (1998) writes on values that can provide guidelines for executives and team members looking to build a quality culture.

The Six Values of a Quality Culture

Value 1: We're all in this together: the health care organization, staff, patients, and their families.

Value 2: No subordinates or superiors allowed.

Renal Service Line Metrics Development

Table 15-2
Clinical Outcomes

Clinical Outcomes Include:
CKD Clinic • Slowing progression to ESRD • Improved status at ESRD incidence • Anemia • Access in place • Patient/family education • 2728 labs
Transplant • 1, 3, 5-year allograft survival • Acute rejection rates • ATN rates • Surgical outcomes • Infection • Thrombosis • Reflux
For All Programs • Relevant vaccination rates • HRQoL/adherence • QAPI • ANNA Nephrology Nursing Standards of Practice and Guidelines for Care
Disease Management • Patient educational programs

Source: Used with permission from Helen Currier, Texas Children's Hospital.

Table 15-4
Financial Performance

Financial Performance Includes:
Charges/Revenue • Gross charges • Hold bills (service department/billing) • Days in accounts receivable • Denials • Collections • Net margin
Costs • Average supply costs/patient • FTE salaries and overtime
Payer Mix Trends
Market Share
Vendor Contracts • Performance vs. service expectations

Source: Used with permission from Helen Currier, Texas Children's Hospital.

Table 15-3
Patient Service

Patient Service Includes:
Patient Satisfaction Survey Results
Patient Complaints
Patient Appointments • Bumped appointments • Delay in visit start time • Visit length exceeds appointment schedule • Next available appointment (new/existing)
Coordination of Care • Verification of relevant patient information (such as patient's care, treatment, services, current condition, medications)
Transition to Adult Care

Source: Used with permission from Helen Currier, Texas Children's Hospital.

Table 15-5
Operations

Operations Include:
Resource Allocation • Change in level of care required • Scheduling changes after original assignments • Efficacy of skill mix
Activity/Census • Average LOS • Inpatient discharges after Friday afternoon • Visit/treatment counts • Transplant referrals • Pre-transplant workup days
Inventory Management • Overnight/weekend shipments • Expired supplies
Medical Records • Timely completion of documentation • Unsigned documents > 24 hours
Staff Satisfaction/Retention • Staff surveys (nursing, technical, administrative, ancillary, medical) • Frontline leader performance • Standardize performance criteria (nursing, ancillary, administrative support)

Source: Used with permission from Helen Currier, Texas Children's Hospital.

Value 3: Open, honest communication is vital.

Value 4: Everyone has access to all the information he needs.

Value 5: Focus on processes.

Value 6: There are no successes or failures, just learning experiences.

Partnerships among physicians and nurses can improve multiple aspects of care and outcomes. Knowledge and communication must flow both horizontally and vertically. The over-arching goal is to improve pediatric health care and patient outcomes in the community through evidence-based practice, education, and research.

Conclusion: Improved Quality for Children Makes a Difference

Whatever your facility's quality management model (quality control, quality assurance, quality improvement) or problem-solving process, it is meant to be dynamic. In order to define a problem or opportunity, you must know your practice – *evaluating aggregate data is essential*. A multifaceted, collaborative QAPI program can result in important discoveries that help us create the best methods to evaluate and manage children with CKD. Prioritize your performance improvement goals, develop methods to measure and manage the *whole system performance* across the renal service, commit to transparency, data drive the improvement of chronic care emphasizing care coordination, and finally, share your performance results.

References

Agency for Healthcare Research and Quality (AHRQ). (2007). *Highlights of AHRQ children's health care quality findings.* Retrieved March 19, 2009, from http://www.ahrq.gov/child/qfindings.htm

American Academy of Pediatrics (AAP). (2003). AAP policy statement: Prevention of medication errors in the pediatric inpatient setting. *Pediatrics, 112*(2), 431-436. Revised May 2007.

American Nurses Association (ANA). (2009). *Nursing-sensitive indicators.* Retrieved March 19, 2009, from http://www.nursingworld. org/MainMenuCategories/ThePracticeofProfessionalNursing/Patient SafetyQuality/NDNQI/NDNQI_1/NursingSensitiveIndicators.aspx

Andreoli, S.P., Brewer, E.D., Watkins, S., Fivush, B., Powe, N., Shevchek, J., et al. (2005). American Society of Pediatric Nephrology position paper on linking reimbursement to quality of care. *Journal of the American Society of Nephrology,16,* 2263-2269.

Centers for Medicare and Medicaid Services (CMS). (2008a). *End-stage renal disease facilities.* Retrieved March 19, 2009, from http://www.cms.hhs.gov/CFCsAndCoPs/13_ESRD.asp

Centers for Medicare and Medicaid Services (CMS). (2008b). *Measures assessment tool.* Retrieved March 19, 2009, from http://www. esrdnetworks.org/resources-conditions-for-coverage/esrd-update-transitioning-to-new-esrd-conditions/MAT-Basic-Ver1% 200%20FINAL%209-11-08%20-2.pdf

Children's Hospital and Research Center Oakland. (2009). *Emergency department: Frequenty asked questions.* Retrieved March 15, 2009, from http://www.childrenshospitaloakland.org/healthcare/ depts/emergency_faq.asp

CRRTOnline.com. (2009). *Continuous renal replacement therapies.* Retrieved March 18, 2009, from http://crrtonline.com

Dieckmann, R.A., Gausche-Hill, M., Brownstein D., & the American Academy of Pediatrics (AAP). (2006). *Pediatric education for pre-hospital professionals (PEPP)* (2nd ed.). Boston, MA: Jones and Bartlett Publishers.

Goldstein, S.L., Somers, M.J., Brophy, P.D., Bunchman, T.E., Baum, M., Blowey, D., et al. (2004). The Prospective Pediatric Continuous Renal Replacement Therapy (ppCRRT) Registry: Design, development and data assessed. *International Journal of Artificial Organs*, 27(1), 9-14.

National Kidney Foundation (NKF). (2006a). *K/DOQI clinical practice guidelines for hemodialysis adequacy. Guideline 8. Pediatric hemodialysis prescription and adequacy.* Retrieved March 19, 2009, from http://www.kidney.org/Professionals/kdoqi/ guideline_upHD_PD_VA/hd_guide8.htm

National Kidney Foundation (NKF). (2006b). *K/DOQI Clinical practice guidelines for vascular access. Recommendation 8. Vascular access in pediatric patients.* Retrieved March 14, 2009, from http://www.kidney.org/Professionals/kdoqi/guideline_upHD_PD_ VA/va_rec8.htm

North American Pediatric Renal Trials and Collaborative Study (NAPRTCS). (2008). *NAPRTCS 2008 annual report.* Retrieved March 19, 2009, from http://spitfire.emmes.com/study/ped/ annlrept/Annual%20Report%20-2008.pdf

Pediatric CRRT. (2008). *Welcome to the PCRRT web site.* Retrieved March 19, 2009, from http://www.pcrrt.com

Tesch, T., & Levy, A. (2008). Measuring service line success: The new model for benchmarking. *Healthcare Financial Management, 62*(7), 68-74.

The Joint Commission. (2008). *Joint Commission alert: Prevent pediatric medication errors.* Retrieved March 19, 2009, from http://www.jointcommission.org/NewsRoom/PressKits/Preventing +Pediatric+Medication+Errors/nr_4_11_08.htm

Woods, J.A. (1998) The six values of a quality culture: Building a culture to develop committed employees, delighted customers, and continuous improvement. Retrieved March 19, 2009, from http://my. execpc.com/~jwoods/6values.htm

Zadrozny, S., Power, E.J., Nishimi, R.Y., & Kizer, K.W. (2004). *Child healthcare quality measurement and reporting, Workshop proceedings.* Washington, D.C.: National Quality Forum.

Additional Readings

Burrows-Hudson, S., & Prowant, B. (Eds.) (2005). *ANNA nephrology nursing standards of practice and guidelines for care.* Pitman, NJ: American Nephrology Nurses' Association.

Goldstein, S.L,, Smith, C.M., & Currier, H. (2003). Noninvasive interventions to decrease hospitalization and associated costs for pediatric patients receiving hemodialysis. *Journal of the American Society of Nephrology, 14,* 2127-2131.

Goldstein, S.L., Graham, N.M., Burwinkle, T.M., Warady, B., Farrah, R, & Varni, J.W. (2006). Health-related quality of life in pediatric patients with ESRD. *Pediatric Neprhology, 21,* 846-850.

Jain, S.R., Smith, L., Brewer, E.D., & Goldstein, S.L. (2001) Non-invasive intravascular monitoring in the pediatric hemodialysis population. *Pediatric Nephrology, 16,* 15-18.

Michael, M., Brewer, E.D., & Goldstein, S.L. (2004) Blood volume monitoring to achieve target weight in pediatric hemodialysis patients. *Pediatric Nephrology, 19,* 432-437.

United States Renal Data System (USRDS). (2001). United States Renal Data System's annual report: Pediatric end stage renal disease. *American Journal of Kidney Disease, 38*(Suppl.), S107-S116.

United States Renal Data System (USRDS). (2003). United States Renal Data System's annual report: Pediatric end stage renal disease. *American Journal of Kidney Disease, 42*(Suppl 5), S129-S140.

Chapter 15	CONTINUING NURSING EDUCATION EVALUATION FORM	1.4 Contact Hours

Clinical Application: Improving Quality for Children with Kidney Disease: Unique Dimensions

ANNP0915

Applying Continuous Quality Improvement in Clinical Practice contains 22 chapters of educational content. Individual learners may apply for continuing nursing education credit by reading a chapter and completing the Continuing Nursing Education Evaluation Form for that chapter. Learners may apply for continuing nursing education credit for any or all chapters.

Please photocopy this test page, complete, and return to ANNA.
You can also download this form from www.annanurse.org (choose Education - CNE Activities - Publications)
Receive continuing nursing education credit (CNE) immediately by completing the CNE evaluation process in ANNA's Online Library. Go to www.annanurse.org, and click on the Online Library icon for more information.

Name: _____

Address: _____

City: _____ State: _____ Zip: _____

E-mail:_____ Preferred telephone: ☐ Home ☐ Work_____

State where licensed and license number: _____

CNE application fees are based upon the number of contact hours provided by the individual section. CNE fees per contact hour for ANNA members are as follows: 1.0-1.9 – $15; 2.0-2.9 – $20; 3.0-3.9 – $25; 4.0 and higher – $30. Fees for nonmembers are $10 higher.

CNE application fee for Chapter 15: ANNA member $15   Nonmember $25

ANNA Member: ☐ Yes ☐ No   ☐ Member # (if available) _____

☐ Check or money order enclosed   ☐ American Express   ☐ Visa   ☐ MasterCard

Total amount submitted:_____

Credit card number _____ Exp. Date _____

Name as it appears on the card: _____
NOTE: Your evaluation form can be processed in 1 week for an additional rush charge of $5.00.
☐ **Yes, I would like this evaluation form rush processed. I have included an additional fee of $5.00 for rush processing.**

Instructions

1. To receive continuing nursing education credit for an individual study after reading the chapter, complete this evaluation form.

2. Detach, photocopy, or download (www.annanurse.org) the evaluation form and send along with a check or money order payable to **American Nephrology Nurses' Assocation** to: ANNA, East Holly Avenue Box 56, Pitman, NJ 08071-0056.

3. Test returns must be postmarked by **April 30, 2011**. Upon completion of the answer/evaluation form, a certificate will be sent to you.

This chapter was reviewed and formatted for contact hour credit by Sally S. Russell, MN, CMSRN, ANNA Director of Education Services.

> **CNE Application Fee for Chapter 15**
> **ANNA member = $15**
> **Nonmember = $25**

---

1. I verify that I have read this chapter and completed this education activity. _____ Date _____
   Signature

2. What would be different in your practice if you applied what you have learned from this activity? (Please use additional paper if necessary.)
   _____
   _____
   _____
   _____

		Strongly disagree				Strongly agree
3. The activity met the stated objectives.						
a. Explain how children differ clinically from adults.		1	2	3	4	5
b. Discuss benchmarking methodologies for assessing and treating chronic kidney disease and end stage renal disease in children.		1	2	3	4	5
c. Describe one way to build a quality culture of care in a pediatric setting.		1	2	3	4	5
4. The content was current and relevant.		1	2	3	4	5
5. The content was presented clearly.		1	2	3	4	5
6. The content was covered adequately.		1	2	3	4	5

7. How would you rate your ability to apply your learning to practice? ☐ diminished ability ☐ no change ☐ enhanced ability

Comments _____
_____

8. Time required to read the chapter and complete this form: _____ minutes

This educational activity is provided by the American Nephrology Nurses' Association (ANNA).
ANNA is accredited as a provider of continuing nursing education (CNE) by the American Nurses Credentialing Center's Commission on Accreditation (ANCC-COA).
ANNA is a provider approved of continuing nursing education by the California Board of Registered Nursing, provider number CEP 00910.
This CNE offering meets the Nephrology Nursing Certification Commission's (NNCC's) continuing nursing education requirements for certification and recertification.

Clinical Application:
Advanced Practice Nurses:
Monitoring Outcomes to Improve Care
To Patients with Chronic Kidney Disease

Patricia McCarley, MSN, RN, ACPN, CNN

Objectives

Study of the information presented in this chapter will enable the learner to:
1. Identify patient outcomes.
2. Describe the process of outcomes measurement.
3. Explain the challenges of delivering quality healthcare outcomes.
4. Discuss ways to improve outcomes in the nephrology setting and in patients with chronic kidney disease.

Introduction

"Outcomes matter most" (Nelson & Greenfield, 1994, p. 9). Variations in outcomes have been monitored consistently through the years. The importance of evaluating outcomes dates back to Florence Nightingale's documentation of morbidity and mortality statistics in the Crimean War. Under Ms. Nightingale's leadership and the new approaches she implemented, the high death rate of soldiers from wounds, infections, and lack of adequate care dropped to 2.2% over a 6-month period (Donahue, 1985).

Current healthcare outcomes monitoring was established in 2 major initiatives in the 1980s. The Joint Commission on Accreditation of Hospitals (JCAH) introduced clinical and organizational indicators in their agenda for change. Additionally, the demonstration of efficacy and appropriateness of healthcare outcomes was legislated by the Health Care Finance Administration (HCFA). The Agency for Health Care Policy (AHCPR) was established by Congress in 1989 to improve the quality of care and how that care is organized and delivered. The AHCPR has become the clearinghouse for the development of clinical practice guidelines and research in the area of medical effectiveness and patient outcomes (Urden, 1999).

Identify the Outcome

What is an outcome? It is the end result of a treatment or intervention. Different types of outcomes may be evaluated, including clinical, psychosocial, functional, fiscal, and patient satisfaction (Urden, 1999). Outcomes provide a focus for the identification of areas for improvement. The foundation for outcomes to measure should be based on clinical practice guidelines and standards of practice (Burrows-Hudson & Prowant, 2005).

"Standards are authoritative statements by which the nursing profession describes the responsibility for which its practitioners are accountable" (American Nurses' Association [ANA], 2004, p. 1). Standards provide a framework for identification of outcomes and evaluation of practice. Clinical practice guidelines are "systematically developed statements that address the care of specific patient populations" and "are based on the best available scientific evidence and/or expert opinion" (Burrows-Hudson & Prowant, 2005, p. 1). Guide-

lines describe a process of care that has the potential to improve patient outcomes. The National Guideline Clearinghouse (NGC) is a comprehensive database of evidence-based clinical practice guidelines available to nurses and other health professionals (NGC, 2008).

In the 2005 edition of *Nephrology Nursing Standards of Practice and Guidelines for Care*, the authors incorporated available clinical practice guidelines and identified desired healthcare outcomes for patients with chronic kidney disease (CKD) (Burrows-Hudson & Prowant, 2005). Using this document and the available guidelines from the NGC, samples of outcomes that might be measured for different areas of nephrology practice are found in Tables 16-1 through 16-4. While these lists are not meant to be comprehensive, they are intended to help practitioners identify outcomes that might serve to improve the health of patients. Targets are not included and should be identified by clinicians based on outcomes measures available from the best clinical practices.

Measure the Outcome

Measurement of outcomes provides evidence for assessment. The goal of data collection is to produce data that can be used in a timely manner (Endsley, 2003). Data that are used in everyday practice and important for patient care should be collected. Available measurements through quality monitoring within the facility can be used, and further analysis of the information can provide direction for measuring outcomes. In areas where data must be collected, basic measurement guidelines should be followed.
- Keep measurements simple.
- Start with one measurement or a small set of measurements.
- Measure from different angles to give you the most complete picture.
- Select a sampling strategy, such as every tenth patient, to provide a representative sample.
- Finally, incorporate data collection into daily work rather than duplicating efforts. Collecting data on a day-to-day basis from readily available clinical information also leads to the most current perspective of the clinical outcome (Endsley, 2003).

Table 16-1
Optimizing Disease Control and Minimizing Complications in Patients with CKD
Stage 5 on Hemodialysis (HD) or Peritoneal Dialysis (PD)

Outcome	Percent of Patients	Target
spKt/V equal to or greater than 1.2 (HD).		
Kt/Vurea equal to or greater than 1.7 (PD).		
Albumin equal to or greater than 4.0 g/dL.		
Phosphorous 3.5 to 5.5, mg/dL.		
Hemoglobin 11 to 12 g/dL.		
Patients with catheter on HD.		
Patients using fistulas on HD.		
Blood pressure less than 140/90 mm/Hg pre-HD.		
Blood pressure less than 130/80 mm/Hg post-HD or PD.		
Hb_{A1C} less than 7.0%.		
Patients referred to transplant.		
Echocardiogram in first 3 months of renal replacement therapy (RRT).		
Echocardiogram performed every 3 years.		
Cardiovascular risk reduction addressed: • Smoking cessation if smoker. • Weight loss if BMI greater than 25. • Exercise discussed. • Sodium restriction addressed. • Lipids measured.		
Wellness maintenance (age and sex-appropriate): Immunizations, mammogram, bone density, pap smear, PSA testing, colonosocpy, eye examination, dental examination.		
Maintain quality of life (optimal physical, social, emotional, psychosocial and role function.		

Sources: Alleman et al., 2008d; Burrows-Hudson & Prowant, 2005; NKF, 2002, 2003a, 2003b, 2004, 2005, 2006a, 2006b, 2007, 2008.
Adapted and used with permission from Patricia McCarley.

Identify an Area of Improvement

Once an area for improvement has been identified through analysis of the data and comparison to quality targets, advanced practice nurses (APNs) have the opportunity to take the lead in formulating quality improvement recommendations to the interdisciplinary team. Many challenges are apparent as the clinician strives to improve outcomes in patients with chronic illness.

Quality Initiative Resistance

In the current hectic clinical arena, there can be resistance to work on quality improvement initiatives. This may in part be due to skepticism that attainment will lead to meaningful improvement in health and other outcomes. In a national prospective cohort study, ESRD Quality (or EQUAL) (Platinga et al, 2007), the authors examined whether attainment of mul-

tiple targets in 668 incident hemodialysis treatments were associated with better outcomes. The patients represented 74 U.S. not-for-profit dialysis clinics. The targets were based on accepted clinical practice guidelines in care of patients with CKD. The targets measured were as follows: albumin (equal to or greater than 4.0 g/dl), hemoglobin (equal to or greater than 11 g/dl), calcium-phosphate product (less than 55 mg^2/dl^2), dialysis dose (Kt/V equal to or greater than 1.2), and vascular access type (arteriovenous fistula). The study showed that attainment of each individual target was strongly associated with better outcomes, including decreased mortality, fewer hospitalizations, and fewer days in the hospital. The results support the idea that efforts to improve clinical outcomes through continuous quality improvement are linked to improved health outcomes (Platinga et al., 2007).

Table 16-2
Outcomes – Patients with CKD Stages 3 through 5 Who Are Not on Renal Replacement Therapy

Outcome	Percentage of Patients	Target
Patients start dialysis with permanent vascular access.		
Treatment Option Education for patients with eGFR less than 30 ml/min/1.73m^2.		
Patients with eGFR les than 20 ml/min/1.73m^2 referred to transplant.		
Hemoglobin 11 to 12 g/dL.		
Phosphorous 2.7 to 4.6, g/dL.		
iPTH 35-79 pg/mL – Stage 3 CKD 80 to 110 pg/mL – Stage 4 CKD.		
Hb$_{A1c}$ less than 7.0 %.		
Lipids: LDL less than 100 mg/dL. HDL greater than 40 mg/dL. Triglyerides less than 150 mg/dL.		
BP less than 130/80 mmHg.		
Hepatitis B vaccination completed prior to renal replacement therapy.		
Cardiovascular risk reduction addressed: • Smoking cessation discussed if smoker. • Weight loss discussed if BMI greater than 25. • Exercise discussed. • Sodium restriction addressed. • Lipids measured.		
Education concerning avoidance of nephrotoxic drugs and agents.		
Education concerning vein preservation.		
Maintain quality of life (optimal physical, social, emotional, psychosocial and role function).		
Communicate status of patient with primary care provider.		
Wellness maintenance (age and sex appropriate): Immunizations, mammogram, bone density, pap smear, PSA testing, colonosocpy, eye examination, dental examination.		
Preserve kidney function: Patient on ACE inhibitor or ARB.		

Sources: Alleman et al., 2008d; Burrows-Hudson & Prowant, 2005; NKF, 2002, 2003a, 2003b, 2004, 2005, 2006a, 2006b, 2007, 2008.
Adapted and used with permission from Patricia McCarley.

Table 16-3
Outcomes – Hospitalized Patients with CKD

Outcome	Percentage of Patients	Target
Nephrotoxic drugs and agents are avoided.		
Drugs are dosed based on eGFR.		
Outpatient medications are continued if appropriate.		
Outpatient dialysis prescription is continued if appropriate.		
Access plan activated for patients with temporary dialysis access.		
Patients access site protected during hospitalization.		
Treatment option education for patients with eGFR less than 30 ml/min/1.73m^2.		
Patients with eGFR less than 20 ml/min/1.73m^2 referred to transplant.		
Education concerning vein preservation.		

Sources: Alleman et al., 2008d; Burrows-Hudson & Prowant, 2005; NKF, 2002, 2003a, 2003b, 2004, 2005, 2006a, 2006b, 2007, 2008. Adapted and used with permission from Patricia McCarley.

The Challenge of Chronic Illness

There are many challenges of delivering quality healthcare outcomes in chronic illness care. As practitioners in the medical community, nurses find themselves with a rapidly aging population who live longer and suffer from many chronic conditions, including CKD (Wagner et al., 2001). Recent surveys indicate that many U.S. patients are not receiving appropriate care (Balas, 2001; Chobanian et al., 2003; Clark et al., 2000). Deficiencies in the current management of chronic conditions may be due in part to:

- Rapid increases in chronic disease prevalence.
- Rushed practitioners who do not follow established guidelines.
- Complexity of disease treatments.
- Lack of care coordination.
- Absence of active follow up to ensure best outcomes.
- Patients not adequately trained to manage their disease.
- Poorly organized delivery systems (Wagner et al., 2001).

What characterizes effective chronic illness care? According to Edward Wagner, director of the Improving Chronic Illness Care (ICIC), a person with a chronic illness should have a primary care team led by the primary care physician (PCP), APN, or medical specialist. The primary care team optimizes a patient's outcomes through reviewing patient data concerning the course and management of the condition, helping patients self-manage their chronic illness, applying clinical initiatives that prevent complications and optimize disease control, and ensuring follow up (Wagner et al., 2001).

Improving Outcomes in Chronic Illness Care

APNs in nephrology settings are members of the primary care team for patients with CKD and are often uniquely positioned to see the "bigger picture." Familiarity with patient data allows APNs a valuable perspective of the current level of care. This perspective, combined with each APN's experience and knowledge of evidence from research and clinical practice guidelines, allows her or him to evaluate current clinical practice. Changes to nursing practice and healthcare delivery can be formulated by the APN, who can then facilitate the examination of proposed changes through the interdisciplinary quality improvement system (Burrows-Hudson & Prowant, 2005).

APNs in nephrology settings have the opportunity to assess and design strategies to meet the multifaceted needs of the patient with CKD. A review by the Cochrane Collaboration of interventions to improve care for patients with diabetes showed that interventions targeting a provider's behavior did not change outcomes unless accompanied by interventions directed at patients (Renders et al., 2001). Empowering patients to become more focused on and involved in their care, educating patients about lifestyle and daily behavior change, and emphasizing each patient's role and responsibility is a focus of the APN. Additionally, the Cochrane Review showed that enhancement of the role of the nurse led to improvement in outcomes and process of care for patients with diabetes (Renders et al., 2001). Effectiveness of APNs is related to their ability to foster changes in patients through knowing their patients well, understanding their goals, and motivating them to more effectively care for themselves (McCauley, Bixby, & Naylor, 2006).

The challenge of integrating other providers and community resources is critical to improve outcomes in patients with chronic illness (World Health Organization [WHO], 2002). APNs can provide leadership in strengthening the patient's support systems to enhance care by coordinating multidisciplinary health care from community systems and resources (Burrows-Hudson & Prowant, 2005).

Table 16-4
Outcomes – Recipients of Transplants with CKD

Outcome	Percentage of Patients	Target
Hemoglobin 11 to 12 g/dL.		
Blood pressure less than 130/80 mmHg.		

Lipids: LDL less than 100 mg/dL.
        HDL greater than 40mg/dL.
        Triglycerides less than 150 mg/dL.		

Hb_{A1c} less than 7.0%.		
Diabetes screening.		
Polyoma virus screening at 3/6/9/12 months post-transplant		
Wellness maintenance (age and sex-appropriate): Immunizations, eye examination, dental examination.		
Avoidance of nephrotoxic drugs or agents.		
Evaluate for malignancy: • Skin cancer surveillance/referral. • Colonoscopy. • PAP smear. • Mammography. • PSA.		
Osteoporosis screening.		
Cardiovascular risk reduction: • Smoking cessation discussed. • Weight loss discussed if BMI is greater than 25. • Activity/exercise discussed. • Sodium restriction addressed. • Lipids measured		
Maintain quality of life (optimal physical, social, emotional, psychosocial and role function).		
Communicate status of patient with primary care provider and/or nephrologist.		
Education concerning self-management of medications and adverse effects.		
Education concerning signs and symptoms of infection and transplant rejection.		
Level of immunosuppressive drugs maintained.		

Sources: Alleman et al., 2008d; Burrows-Hudson & Prowant, 2005; NKF, 2002, 2003a, 2003b, 2004, 2005, 2006a, 2006b, 2007, 2008.
Adapted and used with permission from Patricia McCarley.

APNs Improving Outcomes

McCauley and colleagues (2006) provide an excellent example of how APNs can measure outcomes, implement change, and improve care to patients with chronic illness. Their study initially examined whether APNs could improve outcomes to "vulnerable elders with heart failure" (p. 302). The first interventions involved APNs coordinating care with the healthcare team while the patient with congestive heart failure was hospitalized and during the immediate post-discharge period. This intervention was found to be effective in increasing the length of time between hospital discharge and readmission or death, and in reducing readmissions. Improved patient outcomes also included quality of life and physical function (Naylor et al., 1999). However, initial APN interventions that delayed or prevented hospitalizations in patients with heart failure did not extend beyond 1 month (Naylor et al., 1999).

The identified improvement project was to extend the previous outcomes beyond 1 month. APNs lengthened home care interventions to a 3-month period. Based on clinical practice heart failure guidelines and principles of effective chronic illness care, APNs' interventions focused on improving patient and family caregivers effectiveness in managing their illness. Their initiatives in this area included patient education about chronic illness, practical solutions to the management of medications and diet, and symptom recognition and management. Other interventions targeted strengthening the provider-patient relationship, improving access to community resources, and improving overall health outcomes. This comprehensive APN intervention resulted in increasing the length of time between hospital discharge and readmission or death, and in reducing readmissions and extended the outcomes for a 52-week period (Naylor et al., 2004).

This study provides an excellent example of APNs improving outcomes of patients with chronic illness. It demonstrates the effectiveness of an integrated approach by APNs to improve care. It exemplifies quality improvement principles that appear critical to improving care in patients with chronic illness, including:

- Knowledge and focus on clinical practice guidelines.
- Empowering patients to care for themselves.
- Integrating utilization of community resources.
- Enhancement of the role of the nurse.

APNs Improving Care in Patients with CKD

An access quality improvement plan was developed, implemented, coordinated, and managed in the Netherlands by three vascular access coordinators (VACs) (van Loon et al., 2007). The goal was to increase awareness of and commitment to the National Kidney Foundation (NKF) Kidney Disease Outcomes Quality Initiative (KDOQI) Vascular Access Clinical Practice Guidelines focusing on increased use of arteriovenous fistulas (AVFs) and prevention of access dysfunction (NKF, 2006a). Quality improvement outcomes monitored included types of access in incident and prevalent patients, surgical and radiology interventions, and thrombosis rates. Forty-six percent (24 clinics) of all Dutch facilities participated (van Loon et al., 2007).

An interdisciplinary taskforce, including nephrologists, radiologists, vascular access surgeons, and the 3 VACs, was convened. They defined and developed standardized procedures and interdisciplinary protocols for the construction and maintenance of vascular access, and for monitoring and intervention in vascular access malfunction. The VACs led the formation of an interdisciplinary team within each unit to participate in the clinic's access improvement program. The quality improvement program within each clinic focused on the establishment of pre-dialysis care, implementation of a continuous vascular access care education program aimed at the staff and patients, and introduction of vascular access monitoring protocols (van Loon et al., 2007).

Outcomes from the program coordinated and managed by the VACs included a significant increase in the number of incident and prevalent patients with AVFs and a decrease in the percent of patients with non-tunneled subclavian catheters. The percent of patients undergoing radiology and surgical interventions of malfunctioning access increased, signaling the success of the monitoring protocols (van Loon et al., 2007). The VACs in this study provide another example of APNs improving outcomes of patients with chronic illness. Through an integrated approach, critical quality improvement principles including knowledge and focus on clinical practice guidelines, education of patients, coordination of the community resources, and enhancement of the nurse's role, led to improved outcomes for the patients.

Conclusion

APNs in nephrology are positioned to have an impact on the outcomes of patients with CKD. Identifying and measuring outcomes, APNs can lead the planning, implementation, and evaluation of new integrated approaches. The outcome is improvement in the health of patients with CKD.

References

Alleman, K., Brooks, D.H., Campoy, S., Dinwiddie, L.D., Easom, A., Healy Houle, K., et al. (2008a). APN role in chronic kidney diease Stages 3 and 4. In C.S. Counts (Ed.), *Core curriculum for nephrology nursing* (5th ed., pp. 416-425). Pitman, NJ: American Nephrology Nurses' Association.

Alleman, K., Brooks, D.H., Campoy, S., Dinwiddie, L.D., Easom, A., Healy Houle, K., et al. (2008b). APN role in chronic kidney disease Stage 5 and hemodialysis. In C.S. Counts (Ed.), *Core curriculum for nephrology nursing* (5th ed., pp. 426-430). Pitman, NJ: American Nephrology Nurses' Association.

Alleman, K., Brooks, D.H., Campoy, S., Dinwiddie, L.D., Easom, A., Healy Houle, K., et al. (2008c). APN role in acute care. In C.S. Counts (Ed.), *Core curriculum for nephrology nursing* (5th ed., pp. 431-439). Pitman, NJ: American Nephrology Nurses' Association.

Alleman, K., Brooks, D.H., Campoy, S., Dinwiddie, L.D., Easom, A., Healy Houle, K., et al. (2008d). APN role in transplantation. In C.S. Counts (Ed.), *Core curriculum for nephrology nursing* (5th ed., pp. 440-444). Pitman, NJ: American Nephrology Nurses' Association.

Alleman, K., Brooks, D.H., Campoy, S., Dinwiddie, L.D., Easom, A., Healy Houle, K., et al. (2008e). APN care of vascular access. In C.S. Counts (Ed.), *Core curriculum for nephrology nursing* (5th ed., pp. 445-448). Pitman, NJ: American Nephrology Nurses' Association.

American Nurses' Association (ANA). (2004). *Nursing: Scope and standards for practice.* Washington, DC.: Author.

Balas, E.A. (2001). Information systems can prevent efforts and improve quality (comment). *Journal of the American Medical Informatics Association, 8*(4), 398-399.

Burrows-Hudson, S., & Prowant, B. (Eds). (2005). *ANNA nephrology nursing standards of practice and guidelines for care.* Pitman, NJ: American Nephrology Nurses' Association.

Chobanian, A.V., Bakis, G.L., Black, H.R., Cushman, W.C., Green, L.A., Izzo, J.L., et al. (2003). The seventh report of the Joint National Committee on Prevention, Detection, Evaluation, and Treatment of High Blood Pressure. *Journal of the American Medical Association, 289,* 2560-2562.

Clark, C.M., Gradkin, J.E., Hiss, R.G., Lorenz, R.A. Vincor, F., & Warren-Boulton, E. (2000). Promoting early diagnosis and treatment of type 2 diabetes. The National Diabetes Education Program. *Journal of the American Medical Association, 284*(3), 363-365.

Donahue, M.P. (1985). *Nursing: The finest art and illustrated history* (pp. 241-248). St. Louis, MO: C.V. Mosby Co.

Endsley, S. (2003). Putting measurement into practice with a clinical instrument panel. *Family Practice Medicine, 10*(2), 43-48.

McCauley, K.M., Bixby, M.B., & Naylor, M.D. (2006). Advanced practice nurse strategies to improve outcomes and reduce cost in elders and heart failure. *Disease Management, 9*(5), 302-310.

National Guideline Clearinghouse (NGC). (2008). *NGC guideline syntheses.* Retrieved January 6, 2009, from http://www.guideline.gov/compare/synthesis.aspx

National Kidney Foundation (NKF). (2002). K/DOQI clinical practice guidelines for chronic kidney disease: Evaluation, classification and stratification. *American Journal of Kidney Disease, 39*(Suppl1), S1-S266.

National Kidney Foundation (NKF). (2003a). K/DOQI clinical practice guidelines for bone metabolism and disease in chronic kidney disease. *American Journal of Kidney Disease, 42*(Suppl 3), S1-S201.

National Kidney Foundation (NKF). (2003b). K/DOQI clinical practice guidelines for managing dyslipidemias in chronic kidney disease. *American Journal of Kidney Disease, 41*(Suppl 3), S1-S91.

National Kidney Foundation (NKF). (2004). K/DOQI clinical practice guidelines on blood pressure management and use of antihypertensive agents in chronic kidney disease. *American Journal of Kidney Diseases, 43*(Suppl 1), S1-S268.

National Kidney Foundation (NKF). (2005). K/DOQI clinical practice guidelines for cardiovascular disease in chronic kidney disease. *American Journal of Kidney Disease, 45*(Suppl 13), S1-S153.

National Kidney Foundation (NKF). (2006a). K/DOQI Clinical practice guidelines and clinical practice recommendations: 2006 update – Hemodialysis adequacy, peritoneal dialysis adequacy, and vascular access. *American Journal of Kidney Disease, 48*(1, Suppl 1), S2-322.

National Kidney Foundation (NKF). (2006b). K/DOQI Clinical practice guidelines and clinical practice recommendations for anemia in chronic kidney disease update. *American Journal of Kidney Disease, 47*(Suppl 3), S1-S145.

National Kidney Foundation (NKF). (2007). K/DOQI Clinical practice guidelines and clinical practice recommendations for diabetes and chronic kidney disease. *American Journal of Kidney Disease, 49*(2, Suppl 2), S12-154.

National Kidney Foundation (NKF). (2008). *Elements of excellence: A team approach to chronic kidney disease care.* New York: Author.

Naylor, M.D., Brooten, D.A., Campbell, R.L., Maislin, G., McCauley, K.M., & Schwartz, J. S. (1999). Comprehensive discharge planning and home follow-up of hospitalized elderly: A randomized clinical trial. *Journal of American Medical Association, 281,* 613-620.

Naylor, M.D., Brooten, D.A., Campbell R.L., Maislin, G,, McCauley, K.M., & Schwartz, J.S. (2004). Transitional care of older adults hospitalized with heart failure: A randomized controlled trial. *Journal of American Geriatric Society, 52*(5), 675-684.

Nelson, E.C., & Greenfield, S. (1994). Outcomes matter most (Editorial). *Journal of Clinical Outcomes Management, 1,* 9-10.

Plantinga, L.C., Fink, N.E., Jaar, B.G., Sadler, J.H., Levin, N.W., Coresh, J., et al. (2007). Attainment of clinical performance targets and improvement in clinical outcomes and resource use in hemodialysis care: A prospective cohort study. *BMC Health Service Research.* Retrieved January 6, 2009, from http://www.biomedcentral.com/content/pdf/1472-6963-7-5.pdf

Renders, C.M., Valk, G.D., Griffin, S.J., Wagnes, E.H., Erick Van, J.T., & Assendelft, W. (2001). Interventions to improve management of diabetes in primary care, outpatients, and community settings. *Diabetes Care, 24*(10), 1821-1833.

Urden, L.D. (1999). Outcome evaluation: An essential component for CNS practice. *Clinical Nurse Specialist, 13,* 39-46.

van Loon, M., van der Mark, W., Beukers, N., de Bruin, C., Blankestijn, P.J., Huisman, R., et al. (2007). Implementation of a vascular access quality programme improves vascular access care. *Nephrology Dialysis Transplantation, 22*(6), 1628-1632.

Wagner, E.H., Austin, B.T., Davis, C., Hindmarsh, M., Schaefer, J., & Bonomi, A. (2001). Improving chronic illness care: Translating evidence into action. *Health Affairs, 20*(6), 64-78.

World Health Organization (WHO). (2002). *Innovative care for chronic conditions: building blocks for action.* Retrieved January 6, 2009, from http://www.who.int/diabetesactiononline/about/icccreport/en/index.html

Chapter 16	CONTINUING NURSING EDUCATION EVALUATION FORM	1.4 Contact Hours

Clinical Application: Advanced Practice Nurses: Monitoring Outcomes to Improve Care to Patients with Chronic Kidney Disease

ANNP0916

Applying Continuous Quality Improvement in Clinical Practice contains 22 chapters of educational content. Individual learners may apply for continuing nursing education credit by reading a chapter and completing the Continuing Nursing Education Evaluation Form for that chapter. Learners may apply for continuing nursing education credit for any or all chapters.

Please photocopy this test page, complete, and return to ANNA.
You can also download this form from www.annanurse.org (choose Education - CNE Activities - Publications)
Receive continuing nursing education credit (CNE) immediately by completing the CNE evaluation process in ANNA's Online Library. Go to www.annanurse.org, and click on the Online Library icon for more information.

Name: _____
Address: _____
City: _____ State: _____ Zip: _____
E-mail:_____ Preferred telephone: ☐ Home ☐ Work_____
State where licensed and license number: _____

CNE application fees are based upon the number of contact hours provided by the individual section. CNE fees per contact hour for ANNA members are as follows: 1.0-1.9 – $15; 2.0-2.9 – $20; 3.0-3.9 – $25; 4.0 and higher – $30. Fees for nonmembers are $10 higher.
CNE application fee for Chapter 16: ANNA member $15   Nonmember $25
ANNA Member: ☐ Yes ☐ No   ☐ Member # (if available) _____
☐ Check or money order enclosed   ☐ American Express   ☐ Visa   ☐ MasterCard
Total amount submitted:_____
Credit card number _____ Exp. Date _____
Name as it appears on the card: _____
NOTE: Your evaluation form can be processed in 1 week for an additional rush charge of $5.00.
☐ **Yes, I would like this evaluation form rush processed. I have included an additional fee of $5.00 for rush processing.**

Instructions

1. To receive continuing nursing education credit for an individual study after reading the chapter, complete this evaluation form.

2. Detach, photocopy, or download (www.annanurse.org) the evaluation form and send along with a check or money order payable to **American Nephrology Nurses' Assocation** to: ANNA, East Holly Avenue Box 56, Pitman, NJ 08071-0056.

3. Test returns must be postmarked by **April 30, 2011.** Upon completion of the answer/evaluation form, a certificate will be sent to you.

This section was reviewed and formatted for contact hour credit by Sally S. Russell, MN, CMSRN, ANNA Director of Education Services.

> **CNE Application Fee for Chapter 16**
> **ANNA member = $15**
> **Nonmember = $25**

1. I verify that I have read this chapter and
   completed this education activity. _____Date _____
   Signature

2. What would be different in your practice if you applied what you have learned from this activity? (Please use additional paper if necessary.)
   _____
   _____
   _____
   _____

	Strongly disagree				Strongly agree
3. The activity met the stated objectives.					
a. Identify patient outcomes.	1	2	3	4	5
b. Describe the process of outcomes measurement.	1	2	3	4	5
c. Explain the challenges of delivering quality healthcare outcomes.	1	2	3	4	5
d. Discuss ways to improve outcomes in the nephrology setting and in patients with chronic kidney disease.	1	2	3	4	5
4. The content was current and relevant.	1	2	3	4	5
5. The content was presented clearly.	1	2	3	4	5
6. The content was covered adequately.	1	2	3	4	5

7. How would you rate your ability to apply your learning to practice?   ☐ diminished ability   ☐ no change   ☐ enhanced ability

Comments _____
_____

8. Time required to read the chapter and complete this form: _____ minutes

This educational activity is provided by the American Nephrology Nurses' Association (ANNA).
ANNA is accredited as a provider of continuing nursing education (CNE) by the American Nurses Credentialing Center's Commission on Accreditation (ANCC-COA).
ANNA is a provider approved of continuing nursing education by the California Board of Registered Nursing, provider number CEP 00910.
This CNE offering meets the Nephrology Nursing Certification Commission's (NNCC's) continuing nursing education requirements for certification and recertification.

Clinical Application:
CQI in Conservative Management

Debra Hain, DNS, ARNP, GNP-BC

Objectives

Study of the information presented in this chapter will enable the learner to:
1. Discuss the concept of self-management for the patient with chronic kidney disease.
2. Describe The Model for Improvement as proposed by the Institute for Healthcare Improvement.

Introduction

Over the next several decades, there will be a significant growth in the number of older adults (65 years of age or older) who will experience chronic kidney disease (CKD) (Fried et al., 2006). Existing estimates indicate that there are about 20 million people living with CKD (Coresh, Astor, Green, Eknoyan, & Levey, 2003). The associated social and economic burden of CKD has led to the declaration of CKD as a public health problem requiring further attention (Schoolwerth et al., 2006). As a public health problem, CKD meets the following criteria:
- The disease has a significant social and economic burden.
- The disease has unequal distribution with more socioeconomic disadvantaged individuals and minorities with CKD.
- Strategies that target economic, political, and environmental factors may affect the outcomes of the disease burden.
- Preventative strategies are not in place (Schoolwerth et al., 2006).

Concerns regarding this serious public health problem led to the development of the National Kidney Foundation (NKF) Kidney Disease Outcomes Quality Initiative™ (KDOQI) Clinical Practice Guidelines for CKD (NKF, 2002a).

Historically, there has not been a clear definition of CKD; often, it is identified as chronic renal insufficiency or chronic renal failure. The CKD Clinical Practice Guidelines provide a much needed definition for CKD (see Table 17-1), as well as an established classification system (see Table 17-2), which includes stages of CKD based on estimated glomerular filtration rate (eGFR). These guidelines have been a significant resource in clinical practice by providing stages and treatment goals for each stage as depicted in the American Nephrology Nurses' Association (ANNA) (2006) *CKD Fact Sheet.*

CKD and Self-Management

In CKD Stages 1 and 2, individuals are usually asymptomatic, and they may begin to experience the complications of CKD at Stage 3. These manifestations may include anemia, hypertension, proteinuria, protein-energy malnutrition, dysplipidemia, disturbances in mineral and bone disorder, and decreased quality of life (NKF, 2002a). Current evidence indicates that as the glomerular filtration rate declines, the risk of death, cardiovascular events, and hospitalization increase (Sarnak et al., 2003). Early identification and treatment of CKD, therefore, is imperative (Costantini et al., 2008). The goals of treatment are focused on slowing the progression of the disease and reducing the associated complications. Even

Table 17-1
Definition of Chronic Kidney Disease

Definition
1. Kidney damage for 3 months, as defined by structural or functional abnormalities of the kidney, with or without decreased GFR (glomerular filtration rate), manifested by either: • Pathological abnormalities.   • Markers of kidney damage, including abnormalities in the composition of the blood or urine, or abnormalities in imaging tests.   2. GFR < 60 ml/min/1.73 m^2 > 3 months, with or without kidney damage.

Source: NKF, 2002b.
Adapted and used with permission from Debra Hain.

Table 17-2
Stages of Chronic Kidney Disease (Adapted from the National Kidney Foundation CKD Clinical Guidelines)

Stage	Description	eGFR (mL/min/1.73 m^2)
1	Kidney damage with normal or increase GFR	≥ 90
2	Kidney damage with mild decreased in GFR	60 to 89
3	Moderate decreased GFR	30 to 59
4	Severe decreased GFR	15 to 29
5	Kidney failure	< 15 or on dialysis

Source: Adapted from NKF, 2002a.
Adapted and used with permission from Debra Hain.

though there are evidence-based treatment recommendations for meeting these goals, an essential component of any treatment plan is patient adherence. Self-management may be one possible way to improve adherence to the prescribed regimen.

Self-management can be defined as the "positive efforts [of patients] to oversee and participate in their health care in order to optimize health, prevent complications, control symptoms, marshal medical resources, and minimize the intrusion of the disease into their preferred lifestyles" (Curtin & Mapes, 2001, p. 386). Self-management of a chronic disease can be challenging for some older adults, but with the proper guidance and support, it can become a reality. There are many ways to promote self-management; however, before implementing any strategies, initiation of an interdisciplinary quality improvement project would be beneficial.

Interdisciplinary Approach to Quality Improvement

In the current healthcare arena, it is crucial to improve quality of care while reducing healthcare costs. One way to accomplish this is to engage in the quality improvement process. As health care evolves, nurses must maintain an active voice in the quality improvement process, which includes performing as a leader or team member of an interdisciplinary team. The challenges of caring for older adults with CKD who were not adhering to the prescribed regimen was of great concern in nephrology nursing practice. In order to address this important clinical issue, the advanced registered nurse practitioner (ARNP) and one of the nephrology fellows in a large physician group practice decided to initiate the quality improvement process by identifying key stakeholders and then establishing an interdisciplinary team. The interdisciplinary team consisted of a nephrologist, a nephrology fellow, an ARNP, an LPN, and a renal dietitian who was employed in a community dialysis setting. The continuous quality improvement (CQI) team selected the Model for Improvement (see Figure 17-1) to guide the quality improvement process (Institute for Healthcare Improvement [IHI], 2008).

The Model for Improvement

Following the steps of The Model for Improvement (IHI, 2008), the team engaged in dialogue about the subsequent questions: 1) What are we trying to accomplish?, 2) How will we know that a change is an improvement?, and 3) What change can we make that will result in improvement (see Figure 17-1)?

Question #1: What are we trying to accomplish?

The team developed the aim statement, which was clear with specific numerical goals. The statement was: "To fully integrate, by August, an interdisciplinary innovative approach to medical care and patient education with the outcome measure of improving patient satisfaction and increasing knowledge of self-management strategies in a population of older adults diagnosed with CKD Stages 3 and 4." The team decided to first conduct a pilot project (test of change) with the goal of achieving the following results: 1) improve self-management knowledge as evidenced by patient verbalization of self-management strategies, and 2) achieve 90% or higher patient satisfaction of medical care and CKD education that was provided during the program as compared to the traditional office visit they had experienced.

Question #2: How do we know that a change is an improvement?

It was important to assure all members of the team that 1) the purpose of measurement was for learning and not as a method of judgment of whether they were doing their jobs, 2) all measurements have limitations, and 3) there is a need to balance the set of measurements to determine if the process has improved. The team needed to develop an operational definition that according to Lloyd (2008) provided:

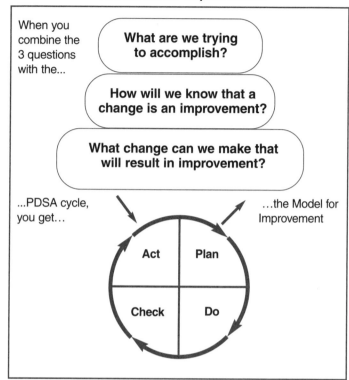

Figure 17-1
The Model for Improvement

Source: Langley, Nolan, Nolan, Norman, & Provost, 1996.
Adapted and used with permission from Debra Hain.

- A description in quantifiable terms.
- What to measure.
- Steps to follow to measure it consistently.

The plan for measurement will be discussed later in this chapter.

Question #3: What change can we make that will result in improvement?

Changes considered by the team were intended to increase the odds that the intervention will lead to long-term improvement results. To boost the chances of achieving this goal, the team addressed all possible predictions as to how and why the intervention will achieve the goals as identified. Once these questions were answered, the team used the Plan-Do-Study-Act (PDSA) cycle to guide the quality improvement process.

Plan-Do-Study-Act

The PDSA cycle, an adaptation of the Shewhart PDCA Model promoted by W. Edward Deming (Walton, 1986) and as part of the Model for Improvement, was used to guide the quality improvement process (see Figure 17-2).

Plan

The ARNP and nephrology fellow identified that CKD Stages 3 and 4 in a population of older adults was a high-risk problem that warranted further investigation. A quality

Figure 17-2
Plan-Do-Study-Act Cycle

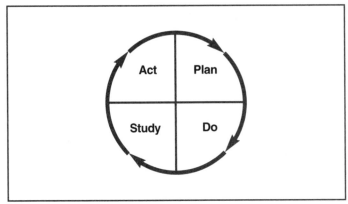

Note: Guide to using the PDSA Model:
- *Act:* What changes need to be made?
- *Plan:* Objective, questions and predications (why); plan to carry out the cycle (who, what, where, when).
- *Do:* Carry out the plan document problems and unexpected observations; begin analysis of the data.
- *Study:* Complete the analysis of the data, compare the data to predictions, and summarize what was learned.

Source: Adapted from IHI, 2008.
Used with permission from Debra Hain.

Table 17-3
Following the Concepts of the Cause and Effect Diagram

Identified Problem: Older adults were experiencing challenges following the prescribed medical regimen as evidenced by missed medical appointments, inconsistent self-administration with medication and not following dietary instructions.

Actual or Potential Causes	Related Factors
Medical History	• Co-morbidity factors • Length of time diagnosed with CKD • Past health experience
Social History	• Lack of strong family support • Need assistance in the home
Medication Factors	• No formal system for medication administration, such as a pre-pour divided container or routine • Does not understand reason for medication and how to take the medications • Forgets to take medication
Adherence Factors	• Lack of knowledge of how to engage in self-management strategies • Does not feel the prescribed regimen can fit into his/her lifestyle • Does not think the prescribed regimen is important or necessary • Poor health habits • Low-self-efficacy • Locus of control, external • Belief that one does not have a health problem • Not satisfied with current model of care
Interdisciplinary Team Factors	• Inconsistent approach to care • Non-supportive program • Poor communication among team members • Lack of coordination in care plan/intervention • High level of frustration related to patient not following the prescribed regimen
Other	• Transportation problems • Forgetting appointment

Note: Following the concept of the cause and effect diagram (see Office of Organizational Excellence, 2002, for an example), the interdisciplinary team developed a list of actual to potential causes for the problem and related factors.
Source: Used with permission from Debra Hain.

improvement project may provide the most appropriate method to address this issue. They selected the members of the interdisciplinary team and developed a formal plan for data collection, trending, and analyzing the data. Based on the information that was obtained, the team was able to identify and document actual or potential causes for the problem and related factors (see Table 17-3) and then develop a plan of action. The plan of action incorporated the improvement that was identified, the specific goals of the project, the timeframe to complete it, each person's role, and how and when outcome(s) would be measured (see Table 17-4). The ultimate goal was to develop a "best practice" plan. The interdisciplinary team concluded that conducting a small pilot project would be the most effective and efficient way to determine the feasibility of the proposed practice change.

The following represents the plan:

- Develop a shared medical appointment program. Shared medical appointments, also known as group visits, are a new concept in patient care. Multiple patients volunteer to be seen in an interactive group session with an interdisciplinary team for follow-up or routine care (American Academy of Family Physicians [AAFP], 2009). Positive results have been reported with their use in the care of patients with diabetes mellitus and post-bariatric surgery (Kaidar-Person et al., 2006; Kirsh et al., 2007). The role of the APRN is evolving as a potential way to increase provider productivity and improve patient satisfaction (Sanders, 2008). It was believed that this type of appointment could meet psychosocial and educational needs of older adults in order to enhance their ability to engage in self-management activities.

- Two groups of older adults diagnosed with CKD Stages 3 and 4 (10 in each group) were selected as possible participants in the shared medical appointments (they were informed that they could decline to participate without experiencing penalties).

- Participants were asked to sign a confidentiality statement that requested they didn't discuss the medical and personal information about other people in the group unless they received approval from that person.

- An interdisciplinary team approach was used to discuss various relevant topics, such as management of anemia, mineral and bone disorder, and strategies to slow the progression of the disease.
- Pertinent medical data, CKD education, and counseling were provided.
- Verbal support was offered to promote desired behavior.
- Recommended dietary changes were reinforced by providing nutritious snacks at each meeting.
- Family members were invited as active participants.
- Laboratory studies from patients seen in the nephrology department and who were diagnosed with CKD Stages 3 and 4 were collected once a month for a total of three months. The results of these laboratory studies guided the discussion about CKD and self-management strategies. The labs were documented in electronic medical records (EMRs) and were available for retrieval throughout the project. Some monthly labs of interest included hemoglobin, hematrocrit, albumin, serum phosphorus, and calcium. Other laboratory studies evaluated as part of their care were lipid panel, vitamin D, and intact parathyroid hormone. Patients and family member(s) were provided a copy of the laboratory studies for review and discussion during the session.
- Group dialogue was initiated regarding laboratory studies, and recommended dietary and medications to treat CKD; individuals were encouraged to discuss effective strategies that they had successfully used to achieve established goals.
- Even though this was a group setting, an individual approach was taken as the nephrologist initiated the dialogue with each patient before group discussion occurred. Issues of concern that participants wanted to discuss privately with the physician were addressed after the session.
- All individuals were encouraged to set realistic goals that could fit into their lifestyle.
- Individuals were encouraged to engage in self-management activities once they left the session and report their successes and make recommendations for change at the next session; support was provided to assist them in achieving this goal.
- A participant satisfaction survey was completed at the beginning and end of the project.
- Monthly review of medications included a brown bag evaluation of medications (having the patients bring all their medications – prescribed and over-the-counter – that they were taking).

The team met after each session to review the goals and make appropriate changes. Post-session team meetings included discourse regarding evidence-based practice strategies for persons with CKD Stages 3 and 4.

Do

Everyone involved in the implementation of the plan was educated and trained. This included those at the front desk, schedulers, and individuals performing the billing. The following steps were implemented:

- Findings were communicated to all members of the interdisciplinary team.
- Education was provided for other staff members (including the other nephrologists and nurses in the nephrology department).

Table 17-4
Plan of Care for the Pilot Project

	Plan of Care
Improvement Need	• Increase adherence to prescribed regimen
Specific Goals of Project	• Increase patient satisfaction • Improve self-management activities
Timeframe to Complete	• Pilot project over three months
Role of Interdisciplinary Team Members (All team members were engaged in education of participants; however, nephrology fellow, nurse practitioner, and dietitian presented educational information to the entire group as well as individually.)	• Nephrologist: Leads the medical team in the health assessment • Nephrology fellow and APRN assist the nephrologist and provide CKD education • LPN: Directs patient care; records vital signs and concerns of patient, and pertinent information to assist the other members of the health care team • Office coordinator: Registers participants, assures medical insurance information is correct, and guides the participants to assigned room for shared medical appointment • Dietitian: Assesses current dietary habits, evaluated laboratory studies and provide dietary education that considers the person's preference
How and When Outcomes Will Be Measured	• Monthly laboratory studies were obtained prior to each shared medical appointment session and were ready for review at the shared medical appointment • Patient satisfaction was measured before and at the end of the shared medical appointment pilot project • Self-management strategies were measured by self-report and comparing laboratory studies on a monthly basis for total of three months

Source: Used with permission from Debra Hain.

- Health professionals were encouraged to consider this model of care to meet the needs of an aging CKD population.
- The intervention and findings were documented for further evaluation and recommendations for change.
- The planned strategies were reviewed after every session and at the end of the pilot project to assess the continued effectiveness of this model of care.

Study

Results were analyzed to determine if the plan achieved the desired outcomes. The findings were presented after the pilot project was completed.

Table 17-5
Self-Report Evidence of Increased Knowledge of
Self-Management Strategies to Improve Health and Slow Progression of CKD

		Evidence of Improvement
Participant 1	History of hyperkalemia that was not responsive to medical intervention and repetitive instructions to decrease potassium dietary intake.	During shared medical appointments, the patient was able to determine dietary habits that included coconut milk (something he enjoyed). After an individual approach to CKD education, he was able to reduce his intake of coconut milk, stating he was unaware this was a problem. He was able to continue to drink it but in the recommended amount. His serum potassium level over the next two months was within acceptable range.
Participant 2	History of missed appointments.	During shared medical appointments, it was determined that she lived alone and often forgot about her appointment. After establishing self-management strategies, she was present for the scheduled shared medical appointments. These include putting a calendar near the phone where she could record and frequently review the scheduled appointments, and the office coordinator called her the day before the scheduled appointment.
Participant 3	History of not understanding what strategies to engage in to slow the progression of CKD.	During shared medical appointments, it was determined that an older couple was unaware that the male patient had CKD Stage 4. The team used a group and an individual approach to CKD education for them. At the final shared medical appointment, they both reported increased knowledge and were able to discuss self-management strategies that they could implement to slow the progression of CKD.

Source: Used with permission from Debra Hain.

- Older adults who participated in this project were very satisfied. Ninety-four percent (94 %) of the participants graded the experience as good or excellent, as compared to 75% patient satisfaction with the traditional medical office visit. They were able to discuss self-management strategies for living with CKD as compared to reports of limited understanding of potential strategies. Patient satisfaction, as one outcome indicator, supports the need for this type of model of care as an alternative for patients.
- Review of laboratory results indicated stabilization of the disease as evidenced by stable eGFRs. Speculation suggests that this may be due to participants' engagement in self-management strategies.
- Camaraderie increased among interdisciplinary team members, who continued to discuss other possible quality improvement projects.

Act

During this phase, the interdisciplinary team reviewed the data and determined what changes were needed. While the team had data indicating improved clinical outcomes, factors that included organizational mission, economical risks, and benefits, had to be considered before this model of care could be implemented.

- The model of care was adopted on a small scale to determine feasibility; however, at this time, the organization has determined that it is not feasible and will re-evaluate it at a later time. They thought the implementation of shared medical appointments once a month for select patients with CKD would be a viable and worthwhile option.

- Patient satisfaction increased, and they felt empowered to engage in self-management activities that promote health.
- While this type of appointment is not appropriate for all patients, it offers an alternate avenue to provide care to a complex group of patients.

Evaluation of the Quality Improvement Project

Overall, patient satisfaction ranged from good to excellent. Several patients expressed a desire to continue with this type of visit. They thought the information they received enhanced their ability to manage medications and follow the recommended diet (see Table 17-5 for self-reports of engagement in self-management activities). In addition, the program instilled hope to some of the participants as they witnessed examples of the success of others in managing their chronic disease. One male, 70 years of age, arrived at each session stating, "I need to be the first person seen. I have to leave because I have things to do." We would honor his request only later to see that he remained there for the entire session. It is believed that he felt cohesiveness with his peers who offered encouragement.

This quality improvement project provided a way to evaluate a new model of care as a "test of change." The evidence from this pilot project lays the foundation for further development of this innovative model of care. Outcomes indicate that there are challenges to this type of care, but they are not insurmountable. Some of the challenges are as follows:

- Lack of adequate resources needed to run the program (the renal dietitian was funded by grant money; funding would become an issue for a future program; time, limited space, and staff (such as the LPN and ARNP).

- Some patients felt they preferred the privacy of the traditional physician office visit.
- Currently, the nephrology department has few access problems, so the organization's administrative team chose not to continue this model of care until the practice had a wait list for patients wanting an appointment.

Despite these obstacles, the team continues to be enthusiastic about the project with hopes that it will be feasible at a later date. What was learned from this project? Healthcare providers must make a commitment to put the process and systems in place to measure quality in order to achieve "best practice." The group decided to continue seeking quality improvement projects to improve clinical outcomes.

Implications for Nephrology Nursing Practice

A dynamic CKD environment requires innovative action. Nephrology nurses are called upon to consider alternative methods of delivering health care and CKD education. Quality improvement projects can be one method of planning, implementing, and evaluating effective and individualized strategies that promote adherence. In a dynamic healthcare arena, it is critical to establish cost-effective and efficient models of care that improve clinical outcomes. "Outcomes of care are gaining increased attention and will be of particular interest to providers as the healthcare industry continues to move toward a 'pay-for-performance' reimbursement model" (Parisi, 2008, p. 9). To meet this objective, it is crucial that nephrology nurses consider implementing a successful quality improvement program as they provide care to persons with CKD.

References

American Academy of Family Physicians (AAFP). (2009). *Shared medical appointments/group visits*. Retrieved March 10, 2009, from http://www.aafp.org/online/en/home/policy/policies/s/sharedmedapptsgrpvisits.html

American Nephrology Nurses' Association (ANNA). (2006). *Chronic kidney disease fact sheet*. Retrieved January 26, 2009, from http://www.annanurse.org/download/reference/practice/ckd_fact.pdf

Coresh, J., Astor, B.C., Greene, T., Eknoyan, G., & Levey, A.S. (2003). Prevalence of chronic kidney disease and decreased kidney function in the U.S. population: Third national health and nutrition examination survey. *American Journal Kidney Disease, 41*, 1-12.

Costantini, L., Beanlands, H., McCay, E., Cattran, D., Hladunewich, M., & Francis, D. (2008). The self-management experience of people with mild to moderate chronic kidney disease. *Nephrology Nursing Journal, 35*(2), 147-155.

Curtin, R.B., & Mapes, D.L. (2001). Health care management strategies of long-term dialysis survivors. *Nephrology Nursing Journal, 28*(4), 385-394.

Fried, L.F., Lee, J.S,, Shlipak, M., Chertow, G.M., Green, C., Ding, J., et al, (2006). Chronic kidney disease and functional limitations in older people: Health aging and body composition study. *Journal of American Geriatrics Society, 54*, 750-756.

Institute for Healthcare Improvement (IHI). (2008). *How to improve: Improvement methods*. Retrieved March 10, 2009, from http://www.ihi.org/IHI/Topics/Improvement/ImprovementMethods/HowToImprove/

Kirsh, S., Watts, S., Pascizzi, K., O'Day, M.E., Davidson, D., Strauss, G., et al. (2007). Shared medical appointments based on chronic care model: A quality improvement project to address the challenges of patients with diabetes mellitus with high cardiovascular risk. *Quality and Safety in Health Care, 16*(5), 349-353.

Langley, G.L., Nolan, K.M., Nolan, T.W. Norman, C.C., & Provost, L.P. (1996). *The improvement guide: A practical approach to enhancing organizational performance*. San Francisco: Jossey-Bass Publishers.

Lloyd, R.C. (2008) *An introduction to the model for improvement*. Retrieved March 10, 2009, from http://www.ihi.org/IHI/Programs/AudioAndWebPrograms/OnDemandPresentationMFI.htm

National Kidney Foundation (NKF). (2002a). K/DOQI clinical practice guidelines for chronic kidney disease: Evaluation, classification, and stratification. *American Journal of Kidney Disease, 39*(Supp.), S1-S266.

National Kidney Foundation (NKF). (2002b). *K/DOQI clinical practice guidelines for chronic kidney disease: Evaluation, classification, and stratification*. Retrieved January 27, 2009, from http://www.kidney.org/professionals/KDOQI/guidelines_ckd/p1_exec.htm

Office of Organizational Excellence. (2002). *Fishbone diagram: A problem-analysis tool*. Retrieved March 10, 2009, from http://quality.enr.state.nc.us/tools/fishbone.htm

Parisi, L. (2008). Measuring performance improving quality. In E. Capezuti, D. Zwicker, M. Mezey, & T. Fulmer (Eds.), *Evidence-based geriatric nursing protocols for best practice* (3rd ed.). New York: Springer Publishing Company.

Person-Kaidar, O., Swartz-Wong, E.W., Lefkowitz, M., Conigliaro, K., Fritz, N., Birne, J., et.al. (2006). Shared medical appointments: New concept for high volume follow-up in baratric patients. *Surgery for Obesity and Related Disease, 2*(5), 509-512.

Sanders, D. (2008). Shared medical appointments: An innovation for advanced practice. *Clinical Nurse Specialist, 22*(2), 102-103.

Sarnak, M.J., Levey, A.S, Schoolwerth, A.C. Coresh, J., Culleton,B., Hamm, L.L., et al. (2003). Kidney disease as a risk factor for development of cardiovascular disease: A statement from the American Heart Association Councils on kidney in cardiovascular disease, high blood pressure, clinical cardiology and epidemiology and prevention. *Circulation, 108*, 2154-2169,

Schoolwerth, A.C., Engelgau, M.M., Hostetter, T.H., Rufo, K.H., Chianchiano, D., McClellan, W.M., et al. (2006). Chronic kidney disease: A public health problem that needs a public health action plan. *Preventing Chronic Disease: Public Health Research, Practice and Policy, 3*(2), 1-6.

Walton, M. (1986) *The Deming management method*. New York: Putman Publishing Group.

Chapter 17

CONTINUING NURSING EDUCATION EVALUATION FORM

1.1 Contact Hours

Clinical Application: CQI in Conservative Management

ANNP0917

Applying Continuous Quality Improvement in Clinical Practice contains 22 chapters of educational content. Individual learners may apply for continuing nursing education credit by reading a chapter and completing the Continuing Nursing Education Evaluation Form for that chapter. Learners may apply for continuing nursing education credit for any or all chapters.

Please photocopy this test page, complete, and return to ANNA.
You can also download this form from www.annanurse.org (choose Education - CNE Activities - Publications)
Receive continuing nursing education credit (CNE) immediately by completing the CNE evaluation process in ANNA's Online Library. Go to www.annanurse.org, and click on the Online Library icon for more information.

Name: _____

Address: ___/_____

City: _____ State: _____ Zip: _____

E-mail:_____Preferred telephone: ☐ Home ☐ Work_____

State where licensed and license number: _____

CNE application fees are based upon the number of contact hours provided by the individual section. CNE fees per contact hour for ANNA members are as follows: 1.0-1.9 – $15; 2.0-2.9 – $20; 3.0-3.9 – $25; 4.0 and higher – $30. Fees for nonmembers are $10 higher.

CNE application fee for Chapter 17: ANNA member $15   Nonmember $25

ANNA Member: ☐ Yes ☐ No   ☐ Member # (if available) _____

☐ Check or money order enclosed   ☐ American Express   ☐ Visa   ☐ MasterCard

Total amount submitted:_____

Credit card number _____ Exp. Date _____

Name as it appears on the card: _____

NOTE: Your evaluation form can be processed in 1 week for an additional rush charge of $5.00.

☐ **Yes, I would like this evaluation form rush processed. I have included an additional fee of $5.00 for rush processing.**

Instructions

1. To receive continuing nursing education credit for an individual study after reading the chapter, complete this evaluation form.

2. Detach, photocopy, or download (www.annanurse.org) the evaluation form and send along with a check or money order payable to **American Nephrology Nurses' Assocation** to: ANNA, East Holly Avenue Box 56, Pitman, NJ 08071-0056.

3. Test returns must be postmarked by **April 30, 2011**. Upon completion of the answer/evaluation form, a certificate will be sent to you.

This chapter was reviewed and formatted for contact hour credit by Sally S. Russell, MN, CMSRN, ANNA Director of Education Services.

CNE Application Fee for Chapter 17
ANNA member = $15
Nonmember = $25

---

1. I verify that I have read this chapter and completed this education activity. _____Date _____

   Signature

2. What would be different in your practice if you applied what you have learned from this activity? (Please use additional paper if necessary.)

   _____
   _____
   _____
   _____

	Strongly disagree				Strongly agree
3. The activity met the stated objectives.					
a. Discuss the concept of self-management for the patient with chronic kidney disease.	1	2	3	4	5
b. Describe The Model for Improvement as proposed by the Institute for Healthcare Improvement.	1	2	3	4	5
4. The content was current and relevant.	1	2	3	4	5
5. The content was presented clearly.	1	2	3	4	5
6. The content was covered adequately.	1	2	3	4	5

7. How would you rate your ability to apply your learning to practice?   ☐ diminished ability   ☐ no change   ☐ enhanced ability

Comments _____

_____

8. Time required to read the chapter and complete this form: _____ minutes

This educational activity is provided by the American Nephrology Nurses' Association (ANNA).
ANNA is accredited as a provider of continuing nursing education (CNE) by the American Nurses Credentialing Center's Commission on Accreditation (ANCC-COA).
ANNA is a provider approved of continuing nursing education by the California Board of Registered Nursing, provider number CEP 00910.
This CNE offering meets the Nephrology Nursing Certification Commission's (NNCC's) continuing nursing education requirements for certification and recertification.

Clinical Application: Quality Improvement In Hemodialysis – Patient Safety

Barbara Cortes, RN
Billie Axley, MS, RN, CNN

Objectives

Study of the information presented in this chapter will enable the learner to:
1. Identify patient safety resources.
2. Discuss application of continuous quality improvement for patient safety initiatives in the clinical setting.

Overview

The Institute of Medicine (IOM) released a report in 1999 that targeted errors occurring within the healthcare field as being a leading factor jeopardizing patient safety. The reported mortality statistics that resulted from errors were staggering (IOM, 1999). One of the report's main conclusions was that the majority of errors that occur in health care are not a result from "individual recklessness" or the actions of any particular group. Rather, the source of errors is the systems, processes, and conditions that lead people to make mistakes or fail to prevent mistakes (IOM, 1999). Recommendations were made for methods to identify errors, evaluations, and the actions needed to be taken for improvement. Continuing in its framework calling for improvement in the healthcare system, the IOM released a document in 2001 entitled, *Crossing the Quality Chasm: A New Health System for the 21st Century*. In this document, the IOM identified "Six Aims for Improvement" as core needs for health care:
- "Safe: Avoiding injuries to patients from the care that is intended to help them."
- "Effective: Providing services based upon scientific knowledge."
- "Patient-centered: Providing care that is respectful of and responsive to the individual patient."
- "Timely: Reducing waits and harmful delays."
- "Efficient: Avoiding waste (equipment, supplies, ideas, energy)."
- "Equitable: Providing care that does not vary" (IOM, 2001, p. 3).

In 2001, the Forum of End Stage Renal Disease (ESRD) Networks, the National Patient Safety Foundation (NPSF), and the Renal Physicians Association (RPA) joined forces to develop a National ESRD Patient Safety Initiative (ESRD Networks, NPSF, & RPA, 2001). The mission of the initiative was to improve patient safety through the reduction of healthcare errors while identifying ways to measure the improvements made with patient safety. *The National ESRD Patient Safety Initiative: Phase II Report* (ESRD Networks et al., 2001) indicated that while the treatment of ESRD is one of the success stories of modern medicine, challenges in patient safety continue. As with any quality improvement effort, the first step must look at the facts. It was determined by participants in the initiative that further information was needed on what the primary patient safety issues were for patients with ESRD and nephrology professionals. Several "Action Teams" were formed, and one team was charged with conducting interviews with patients on dialysis and healthcare professionals within the dialysis community who could discuss errors occurring in the field. The causes or contributing factors for errors were explored. Opportunities for improvement were identified from the large range of issues reported. As a result, a ranked list of patient safety issues ("Top Patient Safety Issues, Compiled Ranked List") was compiled:
- "Patient falls."
- "Medication errors: Includes deviation from dialysis prescription, allergic reaction, omissions."
- "Access-related events: Includes clots, infiltrates, difficult cannulation, poor blood flow."
- "Dialyzer errors: Includes incorrect dialyzer, incorrect line, incorrect dialysate, dialyzer or dialysis equipment-related sepsis."
- "Excess blood loss/prolonged bleeding" (ESRD Networks et al., 2001, p. 25).

Addressing challenges in patient safety in the nephrology community can be seen in ongoing educational efforts by professional organizations. The RPA and ESRD Networks adopted five patient safety concerns from key patient safety events identified in the document, "Health and Safety Survey to Improve Patient Safety in End Stage Renal Disease" (RPA, 2007). The patient safety concerns identified included:
- Hand hygiene.
- Patient falls.
- Incorrect dialyzer or dialyzing solution.
- Medication omissions or errors.
- Non-adherence to procedures.

Having identified these opportunities for improvement, the RPA has offered education modules addressing these topics to promote patient safety. These modules contain slideshows offering nephrology professionals a method with which to explore effective practices to reduce the occurrence of adverse safety events. These can be accessed on the RPA's "Keeping Kidney Patients Safe" Web site (RPA, 2009).

Nurse-Sensitive Outcomes

The American Nurses Association (ANA) (1991) defines nurse-sensitive quality indicators as those that capture care, or the outcomes of care, most affected by nursing. ANA's identified prevalent patient safety issues are mirrored in nephrology nursing:

- Patient falls.
- Medication errors.
- Access-related events.
- Dialyzer errors.
- Excess blood loss.
- Treatment complications.

Nurses can have an impact on safety issues as measured by these nurse-sensitive quality indicators. In order to discover why or what may have contributed to the issues, one must look closely at the processes involved. Examining processes in care can lead to the identification of the root causes of problem areas, creating new opportunities for improvement.

Could under-reporting of potential events be one barrier to improve patient safety? When one considers event reporting, "close-calls" or "near-misses" seems to be lacking. The IOM defined a near miss (close call) as "an event or situation in the patient care environment that could have resulted in an accident, injury, or illness but did not, either by chance or through timely intervention" (ESRD Networks et al., 2001, p. 14). Under-reporting of near-misses can be unfortunate, since these represent potential events or situations from which information can be gleaned and actions taken to prevent an actual event from occurring. Rather than waiting for an event or error to occur to intervene, could the tracking, evaluation, and acting on a close call or near miss have a significant impact on the reduction of incidences that compromise patient safety? Under-reporting may prevent an awareness of potential threats that nurses could use proactively for patient safety initiatives.

Under-reporting of near-miss events could occur for a number of reasons. These include fear of criticism or corrective action, a lack of understanding about process improvement, or an inefficient structure in place for the reporting process. The continuous quality improvement (CQI) process can be used to address the challenges of near misses to identify and report barriers, create a positive change in the culture within the dialysis unit, and create an environment that fosters a focus on learning rather than on blame. Educating the patient care staff on the processes of quality improvement, opening safe avenues for the sharing of information, and support for action are vital to a proactive CQI environment.

National Focus on Patient Safety

The National Patient Safety Goals (NPSG) is a valuable resource to develop safety initiatives, as outlined by the Joint Commission and updated in late 2008 (The Joint Commission, 2008). The NPSG helps identify areas that need to have routine processes in place and methods for ongoing monitoring and evaluation. Although these were initially developed with a focus on the inpatient setting, they can be applicable to all patient care environments, including nephrology.

NPSG Related to Nephrology

Goal 1: Improve the accuracy of patient identification through:
- A patient identification system that uses at least 2 patient identifiers when providing care, treatment, and services.
- A check system to eliminate transfusion errors related to patient misidentification.
- Prior to the start of any invasive procedure, conduct a final verification process to confirm the correct patient; use a check system to eliminate errors related to patient misidentification (correct patient, correct dialyzer).

Goal 2: Improve the effectiveness of communication among caregivers through:
- A read-back process when receiving telephone or verbal orders to ensure accuracy; the person receiving the result reads back the complete order.
- A read-back process with telephone reporting of critical test results; the person receiving the order "reads back" the test complete test result.
- Displaying a standard "do not use" list of abbreviations, acronyms, symbols, and dose designations; for standard, use throughout the organization.
- Timely reporting and receipt of critical tests and critical test results/values.
- A standardized approach to "hand off" communication between or among caregivers, including opportunities to ask and answer questions about the patient.

Goal 3: Improve the safety of using medications by:
- Reviewing annually, at a minimum, a list of look-alike/sound-alike medications that are available at the facility and taking action(s) to prevent errors involving the interchange of these medications.
- Labeling all prepared medications, medication containers, and mixed solutions.
- Reducing the potential for patient harm that may be associated with the use of anticoagulation therapy.

Goal 7: Reduce the risk of health care associated infections through:
- Compliance with the World Health Organization (WHO) hand hygiene guidelines and/or the Centers for Disease Control and Prevention (CDC) hand hygiene guidelines.
- Implementation of best practice or evidence-based guidelines to prevent healthcare-associated infections; evidence-based practices to preventing infection due to multiple drug-resistant organisms; preventing access infections and septicemia.
- Unanticipated death or permanent loss of function related to a healthcare-associated infection to be treated as a sentinel event.
- Implementation of evidence-based practices for preventing central venous catheter associated blood stream infections.

Goal 8: Accurately and completely reconcile medications across the care continuum by:
- Ensuring a process exists to review and compare the patient's current medications with those recently ordered for the patient.

- Ensuring that a patient is transferred to another location or organization with a complete and up-to-date list of medications that is communicated to the next provider, and that the communication is documented.
- Ensuring that when a patient is transferred to another location or organization, the patient receives a copy of the complete and up-to-date list of medications that is explained to the patient and/or family.

Goal 9: Reduce risk of patient harm from falls by implementation of a fall reduction program; includes evaluation of program's effectiveness.

Goal 13: Encourage patient's active involvement in self care as a safety strategy by identifying ways in which the patient and family members can report concerns about safety and encourage them to do so (The Joint Commission, 2008).

Quality Improvement/Root Cause Analysis for Patient Safety: Learning from Adverse Events

Data Tracking

Numerous formats and tools have been used for collecting and tracking data. An important factor in collecting and tracking data is consistency. Once a method of tracking is determined, change should be discouraged without significant cause and careful consideration. How data are collected and trended can affect how the data are interpreted or the picture they present. Consider collecting data on incidents that have already happened within a chosen time frame. For example, initial data collection may begin with yesterday and track back though the last 3 months. This will get the process of collection, trending, and analysis started. Current and prospective incidents must also begin to be collected, providing a means by which to measure the impact of improvement efforts.

Key Tools

It is often unnecessary to struggle to create the tools needed to collect and trend the data. The nephrology community has multiple networking opportunities, resources, success stories, and best practices. At least three key tools are recommended:

- An individual incident reporting form to encourage thorough documentation of facts leading to, during, and after the incident.
- An incident investigation form that triggers further detailed investigation through a list of specific questions to be answered about the event. Questions should relate to the specific type of event and can be customized based on what root causes may be suspected.
- A summary form that collects specific information from each incident within a block of time, which assists with summarizing and trending multiple incidents for the quality improvement committee. Multiple incidents with similar circumstances may trigger an even more in-depth comparison and trending.

Application of Key Tools

- After a cardiac arrest occurs during a hemodialysis treatment, documentation of what took place prior to, during, and post-

arrest is needed. An incident report or adverse event report (two names for the same type of form), or an electronic report should be submitted to summarize the event and actions that occurred.
- An incident investigation form or checklist can be helpful. This can prompt staff to perform an investigational evaluation of the machine and equipment used for the patient who arrested. This should be accomplished before discarding the disposable equipment. Consider if the machine should be pulled from service for inspection per unit policy, rather than preparing it for use for the next patient. This form would contain a specific checklist of items to evaluate and questions to answer that may identify contributing factors to the arrest or rule them out.
- An event tracking summary form allows facility management to list all incidents that occurred in the facility during the month. At a minimum, the summary should include the date of occurrence, type of event, and outcome for superficial trending and quality improvement review. A summary tool can be customized to include other key pieces of information gathered from the events for more in-depth trending of similarities between events. Examples of information gathered could include whether the same equipment was involved, the same dialyzer type was used, or similar hypotensive episodes were experienced prior to the arrest.
- Additional resources for assistance with quality improvement data methods and data collection tools are provided in the "Additional Readings" section at the end of this chapter's "Reference" list.

Analysis of Data

Accurate and thorough reporting on a regular basis is crucial to data collection. One method to promote the flow of information in the dialysis facility is to initiate open discussions about patient safety with patient care staff. Another method to promote the flow of information is to encourage patient care staff to accurately report any events, including near misses and any safety concerns they may have. Explain the importance of reporting and detailed investigations, and how the information obtained will be used (for example, used for event analysis and not for punitive action). Provide facility staff with general guidelines to identify errors that may assist in their understanding of reporting. The IOM (2001) provided definitions of Error Severity Codes:

- "Did not reach the patient, potential injury."
  - Example: Nursing station keeps all multidose medication vials in the same location.
- "Reach the patient – No injury or effect on the patient."
  - Example: Missed antibiotic.
- Emotional injury.
  - Example: Fright.
- "Minor temporary" – Required "...increased patient monitoring or change in treatment plan..."
  - Example: Error in setting or monitoring heparin levels; abrasions, skin tear.
- "Major temporary" – "Temporary injury" that does not compromise basic functions of daily living.
  - Example: "Severe drug reaction."

Figure 18-1

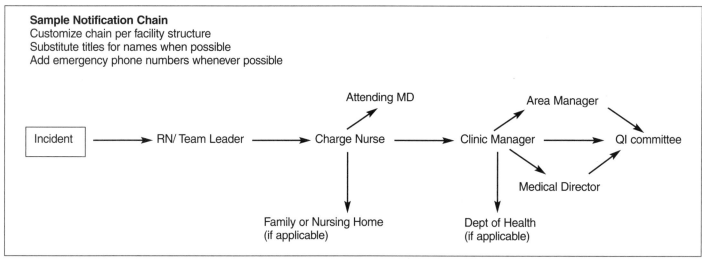

Sample Notification Chain
Customize chain per facility structure
Substitute titles for names when possible
Add emergency phone numbers whenever possible

Source: Used with permission from Barbara Cortes.

- "Minor permanent – Permanent injury that does affect basic functions of daily living."
  ○ Example: Hip fracture.
- "Extreme injury.
  ○ Example: Brain damage, severe paralysis, death" (IOM, 2001, p. 21).

Sharing the outcome of error investigations with facility staff and using the facts collected allow an opportunity for those involved in the processes to provide input into the solutions. What effect could staff members consistently reporting near misses or concerns have on patient safety?

To be successful in learning from errors and near misses, the facility staff must have a step-by-step system for reporting and documenting. A diagram that displays the appropriate notification chain and contact information, and required forms being accessible could enhance staff adherence for reports. Ongoing staff education is a key element to ensure that staff members understand the process of form completion and submission. See Figure 18-1 for a sample notification chain diagram.

A Quality Improvement Approach

Quality improvement can be approached as a continuous learning process. Change occurs routinely within the dialysis unit, creating new challenges and interruptions in any processes set in place. Learning where breaks in process steps occurred after investigating an adverse event provides the opportunity to revise or apply new strategies using the CQI process. Teamwork is a crucial quality improvement component regarding patient safety. Active participation from those involved in daily process steps, in combination with having a problem-solving CQI culture in place, will result in more positive outcomes. These include ideas for improvement strategies, a collaborative focus toward change, and the potential for cre-

ating an environment more receptive to change. Patient care staff who are empowered and challenged to affect change could be self-motivated to incorporate their strengths, knowledge, and support into improvement efforts.

Eisenhauer, Hurley, and Dolan (2007) conducted a study on the nurse-sensitive outcome of medication errors. The study focused on medication administration and what thought processes nurses use to prevent harm or promote therapeutic responses. The authors wrote that nurses' thinking processes extend beyond just the rules and procedures of the process, and they concluded that the nurses' thinking processes are based on patient data and professional knowledge to provide safe and effective care (Eisenhauer et al., 2007). Through education and professional development, nurses use a CQI approach in the critical aspects of their professional practice.

Building a Safety Culture

Benjamin Franklin once said, "An ounce of prevention is worth a pound of cure." That summarizes what is applicable here. The IOM indicated that healthcare organizations must develop a "culture of safety," and that the culture should be such that the workforce and processes are "focused on improving the reliability and safety of care for patients" (IOM, 1999, p 4). As data are collected and reviewed, root causes are found, and prevention can become the goal. A methodical approach for daily monitoring and routine inspection rounds in the facility, especially patient care areas, can be advantageous. The rounds can identify and provide the opportunity to correct safety hazards before they become a patient safety event. Preventative measures and heightened awareness of potential safety hazards can assist with accident/error prevention.

Building a culture of safety includes education for all facility staff because they are responsible for the safety of themselves, co-workers, patients, and visitors. Continuing education, regular communication through staff meetings, and involvement in

CQI activities build knowledge, teamwork, and accountability. Strategizing toward best practice must involve all patient care staff to improve the delivery of safe patient care. Managers who foster accountability will expect participation from many staff members in the CQI process and assure them of the value of their involvement and contributions. Sharing positive outcomes of the CQI initiatives with the entire team assists in spreading an improvement culture in the facility.

Strategizing best practice processes may need creativity to find what works best in each facility. Once a process path is chosen, team leaders must maintain consistency, continuously evaluating adherence. If a needed change is determined in the implemented process path, it should be changed with all participating caregivers as a whole. Deviations from a planned process path by an individual(s), known as "short cuts," can be potentially deleterious to the initiative. Routine and frequent observational monitoring can quickly identify if non-standard processes are evolving. Deviations should be corrected before they become adopted as poor practices.

A planned process path must include a goal, steps needed to reach the goal, assigned person(s) to perform the steps, and an assigned leader who can monitor and evaluate the process. Review of the success and/or failures within the process path must be reviewed frequently to determine if reinforcement of participants or changes are needed within the path.

Regulations Pursuing a Safety Culture

The Centers for Medicare Services (CMS) *Conditions for Coverage* provide guidance to the dialysis facility team for using CQI as a problem-solving method to improve patient safety (CMS, 2008). The *Conditions for Coverage* 494.110 condition regarding quality assessment and performance improvement (QAPI) states, "Dialysis facility must develop, implement, maintain, and evaluate an effective data-driven, quality assessment and performance improvement program with participation by the professional members of the interdisciplinary team" (CMS, 2008, V626). This condition looks at facility aggregate data and requires facility-based assessment and improvement of care (Kari & Payne, 2008). The program scope indicates that it is to be an "ongoing program" that continuously looks at indicators, trends, outcomes, and develops an improvement plan when indicated (CMS, 2008).

The *Conditions for Coverage* also address the monitoring of performance improvement. The requirement is that the facility must continuously monitor its performance and take actions that result in performance improvements (CMS, 2008). An additional charge to the facility in its performance improvement program is to have a mechanism to ensure that improvements are sustained over time. This charge for sustained improvement ensures actions that resulted in improvements during a focus of a project (such as a CQI project) are incorporated into the facility's routine, and improvement will not be at risk of being lost over time. Mechanisms by which the facility may track an improved process could include practice audits, review of records, repeat patient satisfaction surveys, and designating the improvement as part of the facility's routine monitoring activities. By including an improvement focus as an indicator assigned for periodic monitoring in the facility's

QAPI program, the facility staff can determine that the improved process has been adopted into the facility's safety culture.

Prioritizing improvement activities is addressed by CMS as a standard for setting priorities based upon prevalence and severity of identified problems (CMS, 2008). The facility must give priority to improvement activities that affect clinical outcomes and patient safety. Considerations in prioritization include:
• Prevalence of problem.
• Severity of problem.
• Impact on clinical outcomes.
• Impact on patient safety.

Internal reviews that are routinely performed assist the facility in identifying opportunities for improvement:
• Unacceptable variation in key quality indicators.
• Client complaints.
• Adverse occurrences.

Resources for comparing a facility's outcomes are available:
• Literature – Evidence-based practice, clinical practice guidelines.
• Benchmarking – Measure of what is occurring compared to best clinical practice.
• Actual clinical practices compared to professional standards of practice.

Integrating Continuous Quality Improvement into Clinical Outcomes

Patient Falls

Evidence exists in the literature that patient falls can present a major threat to patients' state of health, quality of life, morbidity, and mortality. Data from the Centers for Disease Control and Prevention (CDC) (2007) indicate falling as a leading cause of accidental injury and death among older adults in the U.S. In the Mayo Clinic Proceedings, Dr. Allan Tencer (2005) describes a fall as presenting a serious risk of injury in the elderly. Falls can lead to permanent changes in the person's lifestyle, from an inability to function independently to resulting in a further decline in the older adult's physical health status.

Outcomes linked to falls reviewed by the CDC (2007) as moderate-to-severe injury outcomes include hip fractures or head traumas that reduce the mobility and independence of individuals aged 65 and older. Of all fall-related fractures, the CDC's (2007) National Center for Injury Prevention and Control reports hip fractures as causing the most severe health problems, reducing quality of life for older adults and increasing the risk of premature death. More than one-third of adults aged 65 years or older fall each year in the United States. An estimated 20% to 30% of older adults who fall suffer moderate-to-severe injuries, resulting in reduced mobility and independence, increasing their risk of premature death (CDC, 2007).

Poe, Cvach, Gartrell, Radzik, and Tameria (2005) indicate falls are a nursing quality indicator because the nurse's role is to assess, coordinate, implement, and evaluate patient care. A review of the literature concerning patient falls in the acute healthcare setting reveals that fall prevention strategies utilizing evidence-based practices are identified in nursing research. The Joint Commission's *National Patient Safety Goals* can be used as a guide to reducing the risk of patient falls, and one nurse wrote of her facility's experience (Salyer, 2005). Salyer's facility developed a patient-safety team to work with staff focusing on patient safety as a shared responsibility. The team learned to become comfortable talking about errors, concerns, and suggestions for improvement. A risk scale was utilized to assess each patient on admission and then again on a scheduled basis. When a patient's score on the risk assessment reached an identified level, the patient was placed on a fall prevention program. Salyer (2005) reported that her facility's fall prevention program resulted in a decrease in the incidence of patient falls.

The Joint Commission's identified root causes of fall-related sentinel events at The Johns Hopkins Hospital in Baltimore guided a group of nursing leaders in the development of a fall safety initiative using an evidence-based approach (Poe et al., 2005). The nursing administration leader, Stephanie Poe, describes falls as being particularly challenging where an older adult population having physical and cognitive limitations is exposed to unfamiliar surroundings. Nursing leaders from Johns Hopkins incorporated patient assessment, care planning, physical environment, and communication in their evidence-based protocol. Orientation and training of staff members were reported as key strategies in implementing the fall prevention protocol. Patient assessment was accomplished using a Fall Risk Factor Category that assigned a progressive score for the patient's age, fall history, level of mobility, elimination needs, mental status change, and medications.

A different outcome and learning experience concerning implementation of a fall safety program can be found in a study from the Academic Medical Center in Amsterdam. Nursing guidelines for fall prevention were implemented and tracked for one year. Despite the use of a model upon which the changes were based, there was no enduring improvement in the number of falls experienced (Semin-Goossens, Van Der Helm, & Bossuyt, 2003). Upon re-examination of the project, the nursing leaders found the daily practice of staff nurses differed from the fall prevention protocols. The authors concluded the possibility that they underestimated the amount of behavioral change required by the nurses to successfully implement the improvement project. Semin-Goossens and colleagues (2003) indicate that researchers did not even discover a "Hawthorne effect" within the project, where improvement is seen as a result of the focus itself, lending further evidence to having failed to change the attitude of the nurses. Three action items were identified to change the result of the project.

- Investigate at the start of the project to what extent the nurses experienced patient falls to be troublesome to ensure the target group would welcome a change.
- Investigate the extent to which a nursing unit is accustomed to working with evidence-based guidelines and protocols. The process can be expected to be more complicated and time-consuming without previous experience of working according

to standards.
- Organization is needed to create an environment in which it is easier to implement change (Semin-Goossens et al., 2003).

Dempsey (2004) perceives nurses as having an important role in developing a fall prevention program. This study evaluated a fall prevention program 5 years after its initiation to determine if the effects were sustainable. The program showed initial attempts to implement evidence-based nursing guidelines for fall prevention were successful, with fall rates significantly reduced in one year, from 73 to 40 falls, constituting a 50% reduction (Dempsey, 2004). The study revealed that the fall rate worsened in the following 5 years and increased to levels prior to the initiation of the program (Dempsey, 2004). Although studies have demonstrated that it is possible for a nursing evidence-based prevention program to reduce the rate of patient falls, the success of programs appears to depend on the nurses themselves, according to Dempsey (2004). In Dempsey's (2004) study, a number of nurses expressed the belief that falls were inevitable. A review revealed that diminished adherence to the program was associated with a rise in the incidence of reported falls. The challenge to change a system is to empower the workers to make change (Dempsey, 2004).

Example of a Fall Reduction Program

Integrating CQI concepts and fall prevention into the nephrology setting is demonstrated in the following scenario. A nurse manager within a dialysis provider organization had been exploring methods to prevent falls. The nurse indicated the potential for collaboration for development of a CQI project, asking the question of whether nurses can have an impact on the fall rate in outpatient hemodialysis facilities. Data collection prior to the initiation of the project served as baseline data, with collection and analysis occurring again at selected intervals during the project and at the end of the project. Information learned from the search for resources revealed that the CDC's Web site contains resources for education on fall prevention in older adults (CDC, 2007; Fall Prevention Center of Excellence, 2005). This well-known, credible resource for healthcare concerns would be very useful to the CQI team in designing a fall reduction program adapted for the outpatient dialysis facility.

- Baseline data from facility trend report guided the CQI team:
  - Trending the data revealed 29 fall reports had been submitted over a 1-year time frame.
- The facility QAPI team identified "Reducing Patient Falls" as an opportunity for improvement:
  - Initiation of fall prevention improvement project:
    - ➤ Staff members expressing interest in the improvement project were provided team meeting time and resources to implement the improvement project; the project leader was chosen.
    - ➤ Goal – 50% reduction in falls in 6 months.
- Root cause analysis would reveal multiple potential contributing safety hazards:
  - Leaks and spills.
  - Unnecessary obstacles.
  - Insufficient lighting.

○ Uneven floors and/or flooring defects.
- Fall prevention activities for the dialysis facility included:
  ○ Patient and family education on fall risks and fall prevention.
  ○ Regular evaluation of patients' ambulatory status and balance, noting any changes.
  ○ Implemented policy for escorting patients at identified risk to scale and to lobby after treatment.
  ○ Facility administration placed work order to modify patient areas to include grab bars and handrails in areas of ambulation.
  ○ The education department to provide mandatory education program for staff members on prompt cleaning of fluid spills and reporting of fluid leaks.
  ○ Worked with a sub-committee to remove obstacles from the patient environment. These included identifying a location for storage of wheelchairs during treatments.
  ○ Placed work request with administrator for physical plant repairs.
  ○ Requested physician-approved physical activities and referrals to strength improvement resources.
- Closing the loop.
  ○ The CQI team completed their action plan with an evaluation:
    ➤ Answer the question:
      - Did outcomes improve as a result of the action steps?
        ✔ If improvement did occur: Were the successful actions incorporated into the facility routine?
        ✔ If actions did not create improvement: Did the team go back to select new 1 to 2 root causes and develop a new actions steps?
- Outcomes: 5 fall event reports during the 6 months of the project – Goal exceeded!!
  ○ Facility celebrated success.
  ○ Facility staff members incorporated successful action steps into daily routine.
  ○ QAPI team continued to monitor indicator on regular schedule.

Example of a Device Safety Program

A staff member became concerned over a sudden increase in the number of dialyzers used over a few days compared to the number of treatments provided. The staff member went to the clinic manager with the information, and the manager quickly formed a CQI team consisting of the nurse staff member, a technician, and the facility charge nurse. After discussion and brainstorming for possible causes of the problem, the team decided there was a need to initially gather data to determine primary root causes.
- A staff meeting was held to review:
  ○ How to complete an event form.
  ○ Instructions given to complete an event form for each clotted dialyzer.
  ○ Completed event forms are given directly to the charge nurse.
  ○ Charge nurse provided the patient care staff with an investigational tool that listed required questions to answer when documenting a clotted dialyzer.

○ Questions included:
  ➤ Was heparin administered? How much? When? What route? By Whom?
  ➤ How soon before the treatment was the dialyzer primed?
  ➤ Dialyzer type.
  ➤ Day of week and shift.
  ➤ How far into the treatment did the dialyzer clot?
  ➤ Was any sign of clotting noted prior to the dialyzer failure?
  ➤ Whether the clotted dialyzer had been a reuse or new?

The charge nurse logged each dialyzer each day that were discarded due to clotting. This was recorded onto a customized summary log that listed each event with the requested information. The clinical manager, charge nurse, and staff member reviewed the results together. The summary identified some similarities in the data among events, but the number of clotted dialyzers reported did not account for the number of the additional dialyzers being used from the supply room.

The clinical manager, charge nurse, and staff member then brainstormed to identify other sources for the problem. Possibilities included an increase in the number of patients missing scheduled treatments or a device issue causing a specific type of dialyzer to be discarded either after removal from its packaging or after priming. The knowledge of the existence of a system problem could have been delayed with under-reporting dialzyer problems if observed by individuals at separate times. The clinical manager and charge nurse repeated the process steps as before but with several changes:
- First, they congratulated staff on their documentation of clotted dialyzer events and shared the outcome of data collected with them.
- The need to continue the search for the primary root cause was presented. Staff members were instructed to complete an event report for any dialyzer that was discarded for any reason.
- The team asked to add additional questions to the investigation tool to address different types of reasons for an unplanned disposal of a dialyzer.
- The summary tool was updated to include additional information to be collected.
- Two staff members were assigned to assist with monitoring on alternate schedule days and encouraging adherence to the new daily process.

Expanding their initial work, tracking all discarded dialyzers, and collecting data on the type and reason for the discards provided more data with which to identify root causes of the problem to improvement team members.

If data revealed that dialyzers were being discarded due to defects, the team would be in a position to proceed with their root cause analysis. This process would explore the existence of commonalities in the reported defects. As the scope of the problem was identified, the clinical manager would report the findings to the facility's medical director and the QAPI team. If the root cause analysis suggested a product defect, the remaining product would immediately be removed from use, along with immediate notification of the facility's administrative staff of findings. The facility's policy and procedures for notification of other organizations as indicated would be followed. Using the CQI process in which all staff members work as a team, problems can be identified quickly, data gathered for root causes, and actions taken to keep patients safe.

Conclusion

A 2004 report by IOM entitled, *Keeping Patients Safe: Transforming the Work Environment of Nurses,* which addressed the safety of patients and concluded that nursing is inseparably linked to patient safety (IOM, 2004). The report indicated safeguards in the nurses' work environment should focus on safety, evidence-based processes, effective nursing leadership, and adequate staffing. The ultimate goal of improvement efforts always centers on patients and their needs. Dialysis facilities and patient care staff provide a service to patients with ESRD who expect and deserve a safe environment and delivery of care. A facility culture of CQI provides an environment where each employee can be part of improvement teams, be involved in identifying opportunities for improvement, and be a part of the solutions for patient safety.

References

American Nurses Association (ANA). (1991). *Nursing-sensitive indicators for acute care settings and ANA's safety and quality initiative.* Washington, DC: Author.

Centers for Disease Control and Prevention (CDC). (2007). *CDC fall prevention studies: Research, Translating research into programs, Dissemination.* Retrieved January 31, 2009, from http://www.cdc.gov/ncipc/duip/FallsPreventionActivity.htm

Centers for Medicare and Medicaid Services (CMS). (2008). *Conditions for coverage for end stage renal disease facilities: Final rule.* Retrieved March 6, 2009, from http://www.cms.hhs.gov/CFCsAndCoPs/downloads/ESRDfinalrule0415.pdf

Dempsey, J. (2004). Falls prevention revisited: A call for a new approach. *Journal of Clinical Nursing, 13*(4), 479-485.

Eisenhauer, L., Hurley, A., & Dolan, N. (2007). Nurses' reported thinking during medication administration. *Journal of Nursing Scholarship, 39*(1), 82-87.

End Stage Renal Disease (ESRD) Networks, National Patient Safety Foundation (NPSF), & Renal Physicians Association (RPA). (2001). *National ESRD patient safety initiative: Phase II report.* Retrieved March 6, 2009, from http://www.renalmd.org/publications/downloads/ESRDreport2.pdf

Fall Prevention Center of Excellence. (2005). *Welcome to Stopfalls.org.* Retrieved March 6, 2009, http://www.stopfalls.org/

Institute of Medicine (IOM). (1999). *To err is human: Building a safer health system.* Retrieved March 6, 2009, from http://www.iom.edu/Object.File/Master/4/117/ToErr-8pager.pdf

Institute of Medicine (IOM). (2001). *Crossing the quality chasm: A new health system for the 21st century.* Retrieved March 6, 2009, from http://www.iom.edu/Object.File/Master/27/184/Chasm-8pager.pdf

Institute of Medicine (IOM). (2004). *Keeping patients safe: Transforming the work environment of nurses.* Washington, DC: National Academies Press.

Kari, J.. & Payne, G. (2008). *Transition to surveys with new ESRD regulations.* Symposium conducted at the meeting of the American Nephrology Nurses' Association, Philadelphia, PA.

The Joint Commission. (2008). *National patient safety goals.* Retrieved March 6, 2009, from http://www.jointcommission.org/PatientSafety/NationalPatientSafetyGoals/

Poe, S., Cvach, M.M., Gartrell, D.G., Radzik, B.R., & Tameria, J. (2005). An evidence-based approach to fall risk assessment, prevention, and management. *Journal of Nursing Care Quality, 20*(2), 107-116.

Renal Physicians Association (RPA). (2007). *Health and safety survey to improve patient safety in end stage renal disease.* Retrieved March 6, 2009, from http://www.kidneypatientsafety.org/pdf/healthsafetysurveyreports/HSSProfessionalSurveyReport_FNL_3-21-07.pdf

Renal Physicians Association (RPA). (2009). *Keeping kidney patients safe. Patient safety education modules.* Retrieved March 6, 2009, from http://www.kidneypatientsafety.org/modules.cfm

Salyer, R. (2005). Improving medical/surgical practice with JCAHO's 2005 National Patient Safety Goals. *Med/Surg Insider, 35*(Suppl), 12-13.

Semin-Goosens, A., Van Der Helm, J.M., & Bossuyt, P.M. (2003). A failed model-based attempt to implement an evidence-based nursing guidelines for fall prevention. *Journal of Nursing Care Quality, 18*(3), 217-226.

Tencer, A.F. (2005). Biomechanics of falling. *Mayo Clinic proceedings.* Retrieved March 6, 2009, from http://mayoclinicproceedings.com/content/80/7/847.full.pdf+html?sid=8f0c198f-dae0-40ff-9ba8-fe801c8d2be5

Additional Readings

Healthcare Improvement Project. (n.d.). *U.S. aid from the American people.* Retrieved January 11, 2009, from www.hciproject.org

Hill, K., Black, K., Haines, T., Walsh, W., & Vu, M. (2005). Commentary on Dempsey, J. (2004); Falls prevention revisited: A call for a new approach. *Journal of Clinical Nursing,13,* 479-485.

Institute for Healthcare Improvement (IHI). (n.d.) *Homepage.* Retrieved March 6, 2009, from http://www.ihi.org/ihi

National Institute for Health and Clinical Excellence (NICE). (2007). *Falls: The assessment and prevention of falls in older people.* Retrieved January 30, 2009, from http://www.nice.org.uk/nicemedia/pdf/word/CG021NICEguideline.doc

Renal Physicians Association. (n.d.). *Dialysis safety: What dialysis patients need to know.* Retrieved January 28, 2009, from http://www.kidneypatientsafety.org/pdf/toolkit/RPA_dialysis_safety.pdf

Renal Physicians Association. (n.d.). *Staff activity planning guide.* Retrieved January 28, 2009, fromhttp://www.kidneypatientsafety.org/pdf/toolkit/Staff%20Activity%20Planning%20Guide.pdf

Chapter 18	CONTINUING NURSING EDUCATION EVALUATION FORM	1.4 Contact Hours

Clinical Application: Quality Improvement in Hemodialysis – Patient Safety

ANNP0918

Applying Continuous Quality Improvement in Clinical Practice contains 22 chapters of educational content. Individual learners may apply for continuing nursing education credit by reading a chapter and completing the Continuing Nursing Education Evaluation Form for that chapter. Learners may apply for continuing nursing education credit for any or all chapters.

Please photocopy this test page, complete, and return to ANNA.
You can also download this form from www.annanurse.org (choose Education - CNE Activities - Publications)
Receive continuing nursing education credit (CNE) immediately by completing the CNE evaluation process in ANNA's Online Library. Go to www.annanurse.org, and click on the Online Library icon for more information.

Name: _____
Address: _____
City: _____ State: _____ Zip: _____
E-mail:_____ Preferred telephone: ☐ Home ☐ Work _____
State where licensed and license number: _____

CNE application fees are based upon the number of contact hours provided by the individual section. CNE fees per contact hour for ANNA members are as follows: 1.0-1.9 – $15; 2.0-2.9 – $20; 3.0-3.9 – $25; 4.0 and higher – $30. Fees for nonmembers are $10 higher.

CNE application fee for Chapter 18: ANNA member $15   Nonmember $25

ANNA Member: ☐ Yes ☐ No   ☐ Member # (if available) _____
☐ Check or money order enclosed   ☐ American Express   ☐ Visa   ☐ MasterCard
Total amount submitted:_____
Credit card number _____ Exp. Date _____
Name as it appears on the card: _____
NOTE: Your evaluation form can be processed in 1 week for an additional rush charge of $5.00.
☐ **Yes, I would like this evaluation form rush processed. I have included an additional fee of $5.00 for rush processing.**

INSTRUCTIONS

1. To receive continuing nursing education credit for an individual study after reading the chapter, complete this evaluation form.

2. Detach, photocopy, or download (www.annanurse.org) the evaluation form and send along with a check or money order payable to **American Nephrology Nurses' Assocation** to: ANNA, East Holly Avenue Box 56, Pitman, NJ 08071-0056.

3. Test returns must be postmarked by **April 30, 2011.** Upon completion of the answer/evaluation form, a certificate will be sent to you.

This chapter was reviewed and formatted for contact hour credit by Sally S. Russell, MN, CMSRN, ANNA Director of Education Services.

CNE Application Fee for Chapter 18
ANNA member = $15
Nonmember = $25

1. I verify that I have read this chapter and completed this education activity. _____Date _____
Signature

2. What would be different in your practice if you applied what you have learned from this activity? (Please use additional paper if necessary.)
_____
_____
_____
_____

	Strongly disagree				Strongly agree
3. The activity met the stated objectives.					
a. Identify patient safety resources.	1	2	3	4	5
b. Discuss application of continuous quality improvement for patient safety initiatives in the clinical setting.	1	2	3	4	5
4. The content was current and relevant.	1	2	3	4	5
5. The content was presented clearly.	1	2	3	4	5
6. The content was covered adequately.	1	2	3	4	5

7. How would you rate your ability to apply your learning to practice?   ☐ diminished ability   ☐ no change   ☐ enhanced ability

Comments _____
_____

8. Time required to read the chapter and complete this form: _____ minutes

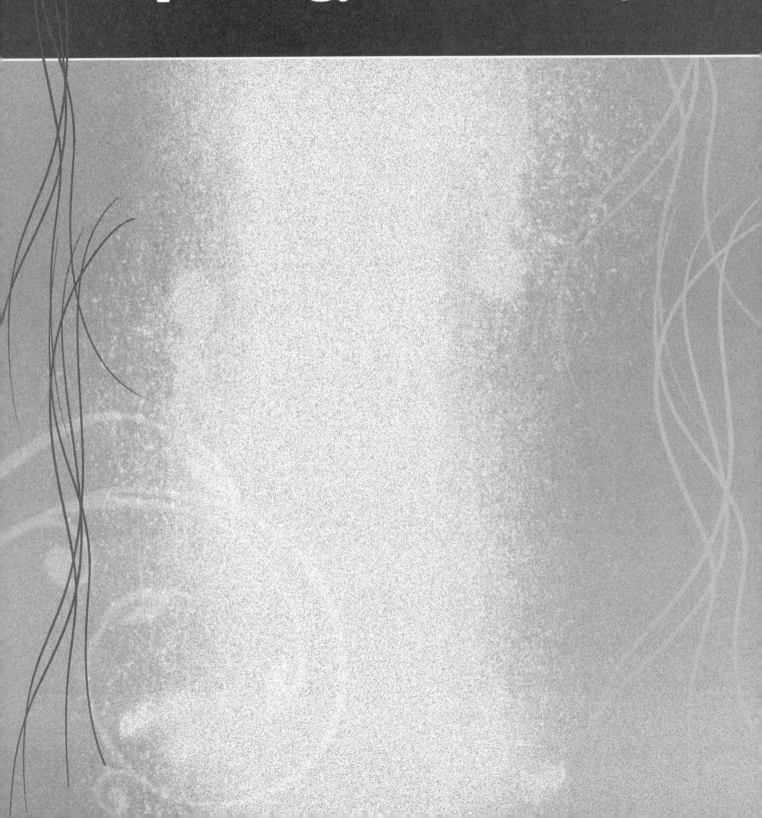

Section 3:
Nephrology Community

Quality Assurance and Performance Improvement in the Outpatient Setting

Bonnie Greenspan, BSN, RN, MBA

Objectives

Study of the information presented in this chapter will enable the learner to:
1. Identify opportunities to close quality gaps through quality assessment performance improvement (QAPI) activities in the outpatient setting.
2. List nine QAPI indicators mandated for review by the 2008 ESRD *Conditions for Coverage.*
3. Identify two relevant strategies to keep QAPI on track in the outpatient setting.

Introduction

Every dialysis facility needs an effective quality assurance and performance improvement (QAPI) program. The Centers for Medicare and Medicaid Services (CMS) provided their basic expectations for the content of such a program in the 2008 *Conditions for Coverage for End Stage Renal Disease (ESRD) Facilities* (CMS, 2008). These regulations charge the facility medical director with the responsibility of developing and maintaining an effective, data-driven QAPI program that requires participation of the professional members of the interdisciplinary team. The QAPI program must focus on indicators related to improved health outcomes and the prevention and reduction of medical errors. With the interdisciplinary team in place, QAPI programs face opportunities and challenges to meet the unique improvement needs of their patients, as well as the requirements of the *Conditions for Coverage.*

The Nephrology Nurse and QAPI

No matter which specific function a nurse routinely performs in nephrology, its performance improvement elements can be found within the framework of Shewhart's Modified Check-Plan-Do-Check-Act (CPDCA) performance improvement cycle (Walton, 1986). The nurse's role in continuous quality improvement (CQI) is to:
- Contribute to the identification of any errors and opportunities for improvement and effectively report them for follow up (Check).
- Participate in analyzing and developing strategies for improvement (Plan).
- Implement and assist others in execution of improvement strategies (Do).
- Observe for success or barriers to effectiveness of the strategies (Check).
- Implement and assist others in the implementation of revised strategies (Act) (Walton, 1986).

The hemodialysis facility could be thought of as an almost perfect laboratory for QAPI activities. The technical processes of hemodialysis care are repeated many times every day. Specific clinical standards, such as those developed by the National Kidney Foundation's (NKF) Kidney Disease Outcomes Quality Initiative™ (KDOQI) have been developed and broadly accepted by the kidney care community to address standards for patient outcomes (NKF, 2009). Patients on hemodialysis are diverse in age, gender, and co-morbidities, but they share common health challenges. The frequency of the elements of care in the dialysis setting is so high that the facility care team can often quickly observe the effects of adjustments to improve safety. Nurses have access to patients who are in their facility 4 to 5 hours at a time, generally 3 times a week. Thus, when errors or other clinical challenges are communicated to formal QAPI teams, they have the opportunity to identify significant improvement challenges and to formulate, implement, evaluate, and revise plans to address them.

The pivotal element of the process is the consistent incorporation of communication of QAPI opportunities to the interdisciplinary team. QAPI opportunities arise when obstacles exist that relate to the elements of safe and therapeutic care, which nurses must continuously monitor to assure patient safety, such as:
- Medical errors.
- A higher than expected percentage of patients failing to meet community clinical outcome standards.
- Infection control alerts.
- Procedural breaks.
- Decreasing patient satisfaction.

In order to take advantage of this opportunity, nurses must go beyond the immediate response to the problem and ensure that an occurrence receives critical review. This must be done in the context of the overall facility status at that time to determine if or what follow up is needed.

All staff members must be involved to assure there is progress and improved safety. They must be attentive and tenacious, and participate in a QAPI structure that consistently captures and focuses on the errors and observations of facility staff. The structure must be robust enough to overcome varied obstacles to an effective QAPI program. Those obstacles can sometimes be the same attributes that provide observational advantages to QAPI. Erroneous assumptions about the source of an error may occur due to the frequent repetition of dialysis tasks and the team's familiarity with each other. These assumptions, if not carefully analyzed, can short circuit the critical, objective search for root causes. In order for QAPI to succeed, it must become part of the facility's culture. The facility structure must provide support and continuously reinforce the basic value for and commitment to a CQI process. Failure to acquire and maintain this commitment may result in addressing symptoms of the problem rather than identifying the root causes of the problem itself. Addressing only symptoms can result in lost time and energy for staff and potential injury to patients, and it reinforces the self-perpetuating cycle of crisis management.

How Important Is QAPI?

In 1996, the Institute of Medicine (IOM) undertook an investigation of the quality of care in the United States. The alarming results, first published in the 2000 report, *To Err Is Human: Building a Safer Health System,* revealed medical errors findings (IOM, 2000). Having discovered what they described as a gap between the quality of care often provided in clinical settings and the care that was identified as best practice by the professional community, they began phase 2 of their effort with *Crossing The Quality Chasm: A New Health System for the 21st Century* (IOM, 2001). This publication describes broad goals for correcting system problems identified as contributing significantly to the quality gap. In phase 3 of the quality initiative, specific areas are targeted for improvement.

Although the hemodialysis setting has not yet been specifically incorporated into the study, the 2004 IOM and Board of Healthcare Services report, *Keeping Patients Safe: Transforming the Work Environment of Nurses,* provides important guidance in its message. "Improving patient safety requires more than relying on the workforce and well-designed work processes; it requires an organizational commitment to vigilance for potential errors and the detection, analysis, and redressing of errors when they occur" (IOM, 2004, p. 286). It is important for nephrology professionals to assess the practices in their facilities for the same sort of improvement opportunities. The QAPI gap in chronic hemodialysis represents the difference between the care that is given in the average facility today and the care that would be given if best practices were consistently and universally applied. Nurses and their teams can lead the way in finding solutions to challenges. These include the elements of safe and therapeutic care using formal and informal QAPI activities that identify and correct systemic causes and incorporate best practices. Nurse managers can assess what may be gained in their own facility by determining:

- Where the facility stands in clinical outcomes as compared to the highest performers through the Dialysis Facility Report or comparable sources (University of Michigan Kidney Epidemiology and Cost Center, 2008).
- What errors have occurred.
- What deficits exist in the resources of the healthcare team to address the needs of its patients (such as staff knowledge, skill sets, constraints on time, tracking and communication, physical plant).

When the results of the facility's assessment for their potential to improve the health and safety of its patients is understood, the process of closing the quality gap can be pursued with the needed energy. The application of simple, targeted organizational tools and systems can help reconcile the requirements of this important goal with real time and resource constraints.

Safety, Efficacy, and Satisfaction: Mastering All You Survey

Effective clinical management in the hemodialysis facility requires monitoring and responding to a wide array of data. These activities must address safety, efficacy of treatments, and ancillary patient management, as well as patient and staff satisfaction. Information technology has facilitated making data relevant and timely, generating critical information for analysis.

One method in which businesses have addressed the challenge of managing data is by creating "dashboards." Applied in health care, this method could provide a dashboard consisting of a set of critical performance indicators selected and monitored by facility managers. The dashboard can be a useful tool for managers to maintain focus on key performance indicators and to communicate status and progress toward multiple goals to the rest of the team. Without some form of a "dashboard," a facility may operate by routinely backpedaling from crisis to crisis rather than progressing toward excellence.

CMS released the *Conditions for Coverage for ESRD Facilities* effective October 14, 2008 (CMS, 2008). In the release of the *Conditions for Coverage,* the CMS also provided a dynamic tool entitled the *Measurements Assessment Tool (MAT)* (see Table 19-1) (Witten et al., 2008). The tool lists specific community-accepted targets for significant indicators in each area of the regulations and is a useful source in designing a facility dashboard (CMS, 2008).

The QAPI Program

Technology alone cannot make the voluminous data generated each month meaningful. The *Conditions for Coverage* charges the medical director with the responsibility for an effective, data-driven QAPI program (CMS, 2008). That program must involve professional members of the interdisciplinary team participating collaboratively rather than sequentially or in silos. They are focused on indicators related to improved health outcomes, and the prevention and reduction of medical errors (CMS, 2008). The clinical performance indicators the QAPI program is required to address include:

- Adequacy of dialysis.
- Nutrition.
- Chronic kidney disease-mineral bone disorder (CKD-MBD).
- Anemia.
- Vascular access management.

These are also required elements of the patient assessment and plan of care per the *Conditions for Coverage.* However, the effective QAPI program is differentiated from individual patient assessment and care planning activities (CMS, 2008).

The QAPI program provides a forum for reviewing the facility's aggregate success in achieving the desired standard for these indicators in the facility population. Its success is compared to the facility trend and targets in each area, and to the performance in facilities in the same state, ESRD network, and the U.S. This comparison is available annually, through the Dialysis Facility Report generated by the University of Michigan and distributed by the ESRD Networks (The University of Michigan Kidney Epidemiology and Cost Center, 2008). These data will ultimately be available on a real-time basis more often than annually.

The Web-based application, Consolidated Renal Operations in a Web-Enabled Network (CROWNWeb) system, was developed to create more uniform data entry and retrieval for all dialysis units participating in the Medicare program (CMS, 2008). Each interdisciplinary team is expected to review its facility's comparative performance. If a facility finds itself in the lowest quintile or "worse than expected" category, this should be viewed as a dashboard "warning light." The interdisciplinary team would need to explore the quality gap between its performance and that of the community at large. Identifying and effectively addressing that gap is an important

Table 19-1

MEASURES ASSESSMENT TOOL (MAT)

Tag	Condition/Standard	Measure	Values	Reference	Source
494.40 Water and dialysate quality:					
V196	Water quality	Max. chloramine (must determine)	≤0.1 mg/L daily/shift	AAMI RD52	Records
V196		Max. total chlorine (may determine)	≤0.5 mg/L daily/shift		
V178		Action / Max. bacteria – product water / dialysate	50 CFU/mL / <200 CFU/mL		
V180		Action / Max. endotoxin – product water / dialysate	1 EU/mL / <2 EU/mL (endotoxin units)		
494.50 Reuse of hemodializers and blood lines (only applies to facilities that reuse dializers &/or bloodlines)					
V336	Dialyzer effectiveness	Total cell volume (hollow fiber dializers)	Measure original volume Discard if after reuse <80% of original	KDOQI HD Adequacy 2006; AAMI RD47	Records Interview
494.80 Patient assessment: The interdisciplinary team (IDT), patient/designee, RN, MSW, RD, physician must provide each patient with an individualized & comprehensive assessment of needs					
V502	- Health status/comorbidities	- Medical/nursing history, physical exam findings	Refer to Plan of care & QAPI sections (below) for values	Conditions for Coverage	Chart
V503	- Dialysis prescription	- Evaluate: HD every mo, PD first mo & q 4 mo			
V504	- BP & fluid management	- Interdialytic BP & wt gain, target wt, symptoms		KDOQI Hypertension & Anti-Hypertensive Agents in CKD 2004 (BP)	
V505	- Lab profile	- Monitor labs monthly & as needed		KDOQI HD Adequacy 2006 (volume)	
V506	- Immunization & meds history	- Pneumococcal, hepatitis, influenza; med allergies			
V507	- Anemia (Hgb, Hct, iron stores, ESA need)	- Volume, bleeding, infection, ESA hypo-response			
V508	- Renal bone disease	- Calcium, phosphorus, PTH & medications			
V509	- Nutritional status	- Multiple elements listed			
V510	- Psychosocial needs	- Multiple elements listed			
V511	- Dialysis access type & maintenance	- Access efficacy, fistula candidacy			
V512	- Abilities, interests, preferences, goals, desired level of participation in care, preferred modality & setting, outcomes expectations	- Reason why patient does not participate in care, reason why patient is not a home dialysis candidate			
V513	- Suitability for transplant referral	- Reason why patient is not a transplant candidate			
V514	- Family & other support systems	- Composition, history, availability, level of support			
V515	- Current physical activity level & referral to voc &physical rehab	- Abilities &barriers to independent living; achieving educational & work goals			
494.90 Plan of care The IDT must develop & implement a written, comprehensive plan of care that specifies the services necessary to address the patient's needs as identified by the comprehensive assessment & changes in the patient's condition, & must include measurable & expected outcomes & estimated timetables to achieve outcomes. Outcome goals must be consistent with current professionally accepted clinical practice standards.					
V543	(1) Dose of dialysis: volume	Management of volume status	Euvolemic & BP 130/80 (adult); lower of 90% of normal for age/ht/wt or 130/80 (pediatric)	KDOQI HD Adequacy 2006	Chart
V544	(1) Dose of dialysis (HD adequacy)	Adult HD <5 hours 3x/week Adult HD 2x/week, RKF <2 mL/min HD 4-6x/week	Kt/V ≥1.2; Min. 3 hours/tx if RKF <2ml/min Inadequate treatment frequency Min. Kt/V ≥2.0/week	KDOQI HD Adequacy 2006	DFR
V544	(1) Dose of dialysis (PD adequacy)	Adult PD patient <100 mL urine output/day Pediatric PD patients, low urine urea clearance	Min. delivered Kt/V$_{urea}$ ≥1.7/week Min. delivered Kt/V$_{urea}$ ≥1.8/week	KDOQI PD Adequacy 2006	Chart
V545	(2) Nutritional status Monitored monthly	Albumin Body weight Other parameters in Patient assessment V509	≥4.0 g/dL bromcresol green (BCG) method % usual weight, % standard weight, BMI, estimated % body fat	KDOQI Nutrition 2000 KDOQI CKD 2003	Chart
V546	(3) Mineral metabolism & renal bone disease	Calcium Phosphorus Intact PTH q 3 months	All: >8.4 mg/dL & <10.2 mg/dL All: 3.5-5.5 mg/dL Adult: 150-300 pg/mL (16.5-33.0 pmol/L) Pediatric 200-300 pg/mL	KDOQI Bone Metabolism & Disease 2003	Chart
V547	(4) Anemia	Adult & pediatric Hgb on ESAs Adult & pediatric Hgb on ESAs Adult & pediatric Hgb off ESAs	Hgb: <12.0 g/dL[3] Hgb: 10-12.0 g/dL[4] Hgb: >10.0 g/dL[4]	[3]=FDA "black box" warning [4]=Medicare reimbursement policy	DFR
V548	Monitor Hgb/Hct monthly	Adult & pediatric Hgb on ESAs	Hgb: 11-12.0 g/dL, ≤13.0 g/dL[5]	[5]=KDOQI Anemia CKD 2007	
V549	Monitor iron stores routinely	Adult & pediatric: transferrin saturation Adult & pediatric: serum ferritin	>20% (HD, PD), or CHr >29 pg/cell[6] HD: >200 ng/mL, PD: >100 ng/mL[6]	[6]=KDOQI Anemia 2006	

Page 1 of 2

Source options: DFR=Dialysis Facility Reports **CW**=CROWNWeb **Chart**=Patient Chart **Records**=Facility Records **Interview**=Patient/Staff Interview
Abbreviations: *BMI* = Body mass index; *CFU*=colony forming units; *RKF*=residual kidney function; *CHr*=reticulocyte hemoglobin; *ESA*=erythropoiesis stimulating agent
Centers for Medicare & Medicaid Services – Interim Version 1.4

Source: Used with permission from Judith Kari, CMS, 2008.

Table 19-1 (continued)

MEASURES ASSESSMENT TOOL (MAT)

Tag	Condition/Standard	Measure	Values	Reference	Source
V550 V551	(5) Vascular access	Fistula Graft Central Venous Catheter	HD/PD: <500 ng/mL or evaluate if indicated[6] Preferred[1,2] Acceptable if fistula not possible[1,2] Avoid, unless bridge to fistula/graft or to PD, if transplant soon, or in small adult/peds pt[1]	[1]=KDOQI Vascular Access 2006 [2]=Fistula First	DFR Interview CW
V552	(6) Psychosocial status	Survey physical & mental functioning annually KDQOL-36 survey annually	Achieve & sustain average or lower case mix adjusted risk & no score declining ≥10 points	Conditions for Coverage CMS CPM; DOPPS	Chart Interview
V553 V554	(7) Modality	Home dialysis referral Transplantation referral	Candidacy or reason for non-referral	Conditions for Coverage	Chart Interview
V555	(8) Rehabilitation status	Productive activity desired by patient Pediatric: formal education needs met Vocational & physical rehab referrals as indicated	Achieve & sustain appropriate level, unspecified	Conditions for Coverage	Chart Interview
V562	(d) Patient education & training	Dialysis experience, treatment options, self-care, QOL, infection prevention, rehabilitation	Documentation of education in record	Conditions for Coverage CMS CPM 4/1/2008	Records Interview
	494.110 Quality assessment & performance improvement (QAPI): The dialysis facility must develop, implement, maintain, & evaluate an effective, data-driven QAPI program with participation by the professional members of the IDT. The program must reflect the complexity of the organization & services (including those under arrangement), & must focus on indicators related to improved health outcomes & the prevention & reduction of medical errors. The dialysis facility must maintain & demonstrate evidence of its QAPI program including continuous monitoring for CMS review.				
V629	(i) HD adequacy (monthly) (i) PD adequacy (rolling average each patient tested ≤4 months)	HD: Adult (patient with ESRD ≥3 mo) PD: Adult	% with spKt/V ≥1.2 or URR ≥65% (conventional 3 times/week dialysis) % with weekly Kt/V$_{urea}$ ≥1.7 (dialysis+RKF)	Conditions for Coverage CMS CPM 4/1/2008 (all)	DFR Records
V630	(ii) Nutritional status	Unspecified in Conditions for Coverage & CPMs Refer to parameters in Patient assessment V509	↑ % within target range	Conditions for Coverage	Records
V631	(iii) Mineral metabolism/renal bone disease	Calcium, phosphorus, & PTH	↑ % in target range monthly	Conditions for Coverage CMS CPM 4/1/2008	Records
V632	(iv) Anemia management Patients taking ESAs &/or Patients not taking ESAs	Mean hemoglobin (patient with ESRD ≥3 mo) Mean hematocrit Serum ferritin & transferrin saturation or CHr	↑ % with mean 10-12 g/dL ↑ % with mean 30-36% Evaluate if indicated	Conditions for Coverage CMS CPM 4/1/2008 (all)	DFR Records
V633	(v) Vascular access (VA) Evaluation of VA problems, causes, solutions	Cuffed catheters > 90 days AV fistulas for dialysis using 2 needles Thrombosis episodes Infections per use-life of accesses VA patency	↓ to <10%[1] ↑ to ≥65%[1] or ≥66%[2] ↓ to <0.25/pt/yr (fistula) or 0.50/pt/yr(graft) ↓ to <1% (fistula); <10% (graft) ↑ % with fistula >3 yrs & graft >2 yrs	[1]=KDOQI 2006 [2]=Fistula First CMS CPM 4/1/2008	DFR Records CW 2/09
V634	(vi) Medical injuries & medical errors identification	Medical injuries & medical errors reporting	↓ frequency through prevention, early identification & root cause analysis	Conditions for Coverage	Records
V635	(vii) Reuse	Evaluation of reuse program including evaluation & reporting of adverse outcomes	↓ adverse outcomes	Conditions for Coverage	DFR Records
V636	(viii) Patient satisfaction & grievances	Report & analyze grievances for trends CAHPS In-Center Hemodialysis Survey available Other surveys for pediatric & home patients	Prompt resolution of patient grievances ↑ % of patients satisfied with care	Conditions for Coverage CMS CPM 4/1/2008	Records Interview
V637	(ix) Infection control	Analyze & document incidence for baselines & trends	Minimize infections & transmission of same Promote immunizations	Conditions for Coverage	DFR Records
V637	Vaccinations	Hepatitis B, influenza, & pneumococcal vaccines Influenza vaccination by facility or other provider	Documentation of education in record ↑ % of patients vaccinated on schedule ↑ % of patients receiving flu shots 10/1-3/31	Conditions for Coverage CMS CPM 4/1/2008	Records
V627	Health outcomes: Physical & mental functioning	Survey adult/pediatric patients KDQOL-36 survey annually	Achieve & sustain appropriate status ↑ % completing survey	Conditions for Coverage CMS CPM 4/1/2008	Records
V627	Health outcomes: Patient survival	Standardized mortality ratio (1.0 is average, >1.0 is worse than average, <1.0 is better than average)	↓ mortality	Conditions for Coverage CMS CPM 4/1/08	DFR

Page 2 of 2

Source options: DFR=Dialysis Facility Reports **CW**=CROWNWeb **Chart**=Patient Chart **Records**=Facility Records **Interview**=Patient/Staff Interview
Abbreviations: BMI = Body mass index; **CFU**=colony forming units; **RKF**=residual kidney function; **CHr**=reticulocyte hemoglobin; **ESA**=erythropoiesis stimulating agent Centers for Medicare & Medicaid Services – Interim Version 1.4

Source: Used with permission from Judith Kari, CMS, 2008.

Table 19-2
Sample Conditions for Coverage Dashboard

Mandatory QAPI Categories Under Conditions for Coverage					
Plan of Care	**Errors**	**Vascular Access**	**Dialyzer Reprocessing**	**Patient Satisfaction**	**Infection Control**
Adequacy	Medication/ prescription errors	Percentage of catheters	Dialyzer error: Set up	Patient complaints	Septicemia
Nutrition	Falls	AVF/AVG infiltrations	Dialyzer error: Treatment	Complaints resolved	Percentage of patients HBsAg+
Chronic Kidney Disease/Mineral and Bone Disorders	Hypotension	Infections	Patient signs and symptoms	Annual ICH CAHPS* Survey	Percentage of patients HBsAb-
Anemia	Equipment malfunction	Access failures		Annual patient KDQOL 36™ survey	Percentage of known patients Hep C+
Mortality	Blood loss			Facility patient satisfaction survey	Percentage of patients vaccinated Influenza/pneumovax
	Needle sticks				Percentage of staff HBsAb+
	Intradialytic treatment problems				

Note: The first column lists the *Conditions for Coverage* QAPI review categories which relate to patients' plans of care (POC). The remaining column headers list the mandatory non-POC categories with examples of performance indicators within those categories.
*CAHPS In-Center Hemdodialysis Survey (AHQR, 2009a).
**Kidney Disease Quality of Life (KDQOL) 36™ (LifeOptions, n.d.).
Source: Used with permission from Bonnie Greenspan.

aspect of the QAPI review.

The *Conditions for Coverage* also require performance indicators in the QAPI review that are not directly related to a patient's plan of care (CMS, 2008). These include:
• Medical injuries and medical errors identification.
• Hemodialyzer reuse program review (if the facility reprocesses dialyzers).
• Patient satisfaction and grievances.
• Infection control factors.

A routinely monitored dashboard listing the safety and effectiveness outcome indicators will greatly assist a facility in assessing its status and progress. The dashboard in Table 19-2 captures the areas of monitoring and management addressed by the *Conditions for Coverage* (CMS, 2008).

The dashboard sample presented in Table 19-2 is a minimum guide to areas for QAPI monitoring and management. It could be challenging for an individual to effectively monitor and maintain oversight of these elements. They could be duplicative, as many of these areas are already being monitored by a uniquely qualified point person in most facilities. That is why the interdisciplinary team must coordinate the effort to move from monitoring to ensuring effective action. This can be done by operationalizing the dashboard and designating facility team members to be accountable for specified tracking, planning, and reporting responsibilities at pre-determined intervals. A

partial operationalized dashboard example is presented in Table 19-3.

Although the partially operationalized dashboard in Table 19-3 is by no means a prescription for any individual facility, it demonstrates several basic aspects of QAPI management. Several areas require more than one task, and those tasks have varying frequencies; for example, there may be a *daily* checklist with a *monthly* report. This is denoted in the chart by a number that links the frequency to the task. An important element is the identification of the expected tasks and the person accountable for each area of management. Identification of a lead staff member for each area provides the "expert" to present data and initial analysis to the interdisciplinary team. The lead member serves as the contact person to whom potential problems could be conveyed.

Some designations of roles may be generally applied. The social worker, for example, will often take the lead for tracking and reporting patient satisfaction. Some of this may be accomplished through annual or more frequently distributed surveys. In April 2008, CMS endorsed the use of the In-Center Hemodialysis Consumer Assessment of Healthcare Providers and Systems (ICH-CAHPS) survey instrument to measure incenter hemodialysis patient satisfaction as a clinical performance measure (Agency for Healthcare Research and Quality [AHRQ], 2009b). This survey is a standardized experience of care assessment tool appropriate for patients on in-center hemodialysis. Patients on home therapy and pediatric patients will require other tools. Another assessment required for the plan of care, the Kidney Disease Quality of Life (KDQOL) 36™ inventory, is a survey of physical and mental functioning that is predictive of hospitalization and mortality (Lifeoptions, n.d.). While this is not a measure of patient satisfaction with facility services, individual patient scores could be aggregated to provide additional information, which gives a consumer voice to action priorities. In addition to these surveys, the *Conditions for Coverage* require tracking responses to patient complaints and grievances (CMS, 2008). Encouraging patients to communicate their concerns helps to update and enrich the overall picture of patient satisfaction in the unit. Paying attention to patient reporting can also shorten response time to minor problems and prevent their escalation.

QAPI Roles

Biomedical staff, social workers, and dietitians often have clear roles in the QAPI process, but expanding the pool of potential QAPI contributors encourages participation at all clinical levels in the facility. Those staff members who demonstrate interest and competence can take some ownership of their areas of interest. The desired frequency of written or verbal communication with the nurse manager, whether daily or as needed, should be clearly defined, as should the reporting mechanism for the QAPI meeting. The tasks assigned to the responsible team or individual can range from a daily review of unit activities for specific occurrences to preparation of a quarterly support program.

The operationalized dashboard in Table 19-3, for instance, schedules a special team to design a support program each quarter for the purpose of addressing mineral and bone disorder management. The management of mineral and bone disorders requires ongoing inter-dialytic participation of patients to a greater degree than most other clinical measures followed. A number of studies have demonstrated the difficulty of attaining and maintaining KDOQI values in mineral and bone disorder management (Aly, Gellins, Gonzalez, & Martin, 2004; Bernstein, Lesperance, Raymond, & Wazny, 2008). Programs designed to encourage health-supporting behaviors in this area (diet, adherence to oral medication regimens, adequate dialysis) typically meet with temporary success. Maintenance of that success, however, is difficult in much the same way that maintaining weight control is challenging in the general population. Maintenance of successful outcomes requires ongoing support, and the success of any single strategy will vary. Unmet expectations of lasting correction of out-of-range values can produce disappointment and even fatigue-induced avoidance in staff members. Acknowledging and discussing the difficulty of lasting success and the value of persistence can lead to a rotational program. The facility can design a rotation of improvement team members to the QAPI interdisciplinary team. It is designed to refocus, support, and reward progress in this challenging management area, and incorporate more staff members in the QAPI process and its successes.

Assignment of tasks should reflect consideration of the interest and ability of the responsible person, and the efficiency and effectiveness of the choice. No dialysis facility can dedicate hours of staff time for painstaking lengthy daily reports, nor is that type of information easy to use. A technician skilled

Table 19-3
Sample Segment of Operationalized Dashboard

Plan of Care	Errors	Vascular Access
Adequacy R: V. Picky, RN F: Monthly T: Track, trend, present	**Medication/Prescription Errors** R: A. Observant, RN, CNN; N. Alternate, RN, CNN F: (1) Daily T: (1) Review, report as indicated F: (2) Monthly T: (2) Report to QAPI	**Percentage of Catheters** R: Spec tech, CCHT F: Monthly T: Track, trend, present
Nutrition R: Edie Well, RD F: Monthly T: Track, trend, present	**Falls** Same as medication/prescription errors	**Infiltrations** R: Spec tech, CCHT F: (1) Daily T: (1) Review, report as indicated F: (2) Monthly T: (2) Report to QAPI
Chronic Kidney Disease/Mineral and Bone Disease R: Edie Well, RD and bone team F: (1) Monthly T: (1) Trend F: (2) Quarterly T: (2) Develop program	**Hypotension** Same as medication/prescription errors	**Infections** R: IC Fan, RN, CNN F: (1) Daily T: (1) Review, report as indicated F: (2) Monthly T: (2) Track, trend, present to QAPI
Anemia R: N. Alternate, RN, CNN F: Monthly T: Track, trend, present	**Equipment Malfunction** R: Biomed F: (1) Daily T: (1) Review, report F: (2) Monthly T: (2) Track, trend, report to QAPI	**Failures** R: Spec Tech, CCHT F: (1) Daily T: (1) Review, report F: (2) Monthly T: (2) Report to QAPI
	Blood Loss Same as medication/prescription errors	
	Needle Sticks R: IC Fan, RN, CNN F: (1) Daily T: (1) Review, report F: (2) Monthly T: (2) Track, trend, report to QAPI	

Notes: R = responsible team member, F = frequency of task, T = task; some areas may have more than one task.
Source: Used with permission from Bonnie Greenspan.

Table 19-4
Fistula Log

October (Date)	Fistulas Pending (Numbers)	Fistulas New (Number)	Access Infiltrations (Number, Patient/Staff Initials)	All Failures (Number)
1	3	2	0	0
2	2	3	1 (BC)/(LR)	0

Source: Used with permission from Bonnie Greenspan.

in cannulation, for example, may play an expanded role in performance improvement in the area of vascular access with little time requirement. His or her clinical expertise could be used advantageously in many clinical situations, and a simple monthly grid with minimal daily data entry would suffice for tracking and reporting. An example of a fistula log is shown in Table 19-4.

Identifying a point person for infection control management provides an opportunity for another team member to participate. Similar concrete data collection points can contribute to a consistent focus on indicators, such as immunization rates, that deliver meaningful protection to the patient population.

Preventing Medical Errors

A critical goal of QAPI is the reduction and prevention of medical errors (CMS, 2008). Staff should have a clear understanding of what they are expected to report and the mechanism to use so that a reliable record of errors exists. QAPI relies heavily on a culture that does not seek to place blame, but rather, on advancing the effectiveness of the system to prevent medical errors. If the frequency or severity of errors is high or trending upward, a review and analysis of the systems contributing to those errors must be explored. Nurses should review and assess medical and prescription errors daily to determine what follow up is required. It is important to identify interventions, change in policies, or procedures needed to prevent the reoccurrence of the error(s). The attention given to recording and tracking errors provides the framework for the QAPI team to identify root causes and reduce errors. The quality improvement process is focused upon improving outcomes by identifying deficiencies and instituting corrective actions; it is not punitive.

If a nurse observes a dialysate set up error, she or he would take immediate action to correct the dialysate to the patient's prescription. Upon discovering an error for one patient, the nurse would then check the dialysate for all other patients and make any corrections as needed. That nurse would subsequently use the CQI process to explore possible root causes for the error. This allows the QAPI team to track and investigate problems, and implement corrective action(s) to prevent recurrence of the problem. Without this process, there would be no systematic correction that would prevent the reoccurrence of errors. Tracking systems provide oversight of activities for safety and quality purposes, and need to be simple in their design to foster efficient and appropriate use. The Renal Physicians Association [RPA] and the Forum of End Stage Renal Disease Networks (2008) developed *Keeping Kidney Patients Safe,* a Web site that includes a priority medical error list of dialysis facility patient safety concerns for which they provide strategic assistance. The areas of potential errors addressed are hand hygiene lapses, patient falls, incorrect dialyzer or dialyzing solution, medication omissions or errors, and non-adherence to procedures. In addition to specific approaches to the defined areas, the site provides a patient safety improvement tool kit with basic tactical approaches for improving patient safety (RPA & the Forum of ESRD Networks, 2008).

Personalized Performance Indicators

The *Conditions for Coverage* QAPI performance indicators are comprehensive and encourage nurses to begin to think in QAPI terms (CMS, 2008). Nurses who do so will identify indicators that pose unique threats in the facility, although they may not yet have resulted in injury or error. Staff turnover, for instance, can have profound implications that can be addressed before serious harm occurs to patients. Similarly, public patient transportation changes, security concerns within or near the facility, or other emerging threats can be effectively addressed through a functional QAPI program. An observation of a particular health opportunity, such as smoking cessation or exercise encouragement, may prompt a meaningful special QAPI task group. Table 19-5 provides an example of other dashboard measures that can be tracked to reduce specific facility indicators that contribute to patient safety, mortality or morbidity, and patient satisfaction.

Facility mortality, perhaps the ultimate QAPI indicator, may appear in any of a number of places on the dashboard, but it must be considered on two levels. The standardized mortality rate is provided annually in the Dialysis Facility Report (The University of Michigan Kidney Epidemiology and Cost Center, 2008). The report should be used to review the relationship between actual deaths as compared to expected deaths for one and three-year periods. A rolling annual mortality rate, while not as meaningful as the standardized mortality rate, can help alert the team to an increase in mortality despite the low monthly frequency. A cluster, or group of deaths occurring close together in time or location, should prompt an accelerated and more intense review. Additionally, each individual death should be reviewed promptly to determine if anything can be learned from it. The review should include treatment records and laboratory reports from the month prior to the patient's death, and should address these three issues:

- Was the death expected? If so, had the probability been discussed with the patient and/or family members? If not, why not?
- Was the death preventable? If so, what changes must be instituted to improve future preventive care?
- Did the care provided to the patient meet facility care goals? If not, what changes should be made?

Nurse managers have the benefit of the mandated interdisciplinary team. Within this framework, managers can make certain that important indicators receive the type and timely review required to ensure safety and progress in the facility. Other circumstances may arise that require prompt action. These may require immediate review, notification of the medical director, and/or action as set forth in the facility's policy prior to the next scheduled full QAPI team meeting. Typical examples would be routine testing that produced non-routine results (for example, unsafe water quality or culture results).

Table 19-5
Additional Facility-Initiated Dashboard Measures

Staffing	Security	Diabetes Management
Adequate total number of staff	Patient personal property losses	Percentage of patients excercising
Adequate number of RNs with appropriate skillset	Staff personal property losses	Percentage of patients with Hgb_{A1C} less than 7
Sufficient number of staff competent at cannulation of developing fistulas	Incidents	Percentage of patients with lipids in target range
Technician certification within CMS-defined timeframe	Training	Percentage of patients with monthly foot checks
Sharps exposure rate or frequency	Enforcement	Percentage of patients with annual eye examinations

Source: Used with permission from Bonnie Greenspan.

Other threats, such as infection control outbreaks or acute changes in routinely tracked outcomes, may require convening an unscheduled conference with the medical director and other appropriate QAPI team members.

The QAPI team may assign appropriate facility staff to a task force established to address a specific area that reports to the QAPI interdisciplinary team at designated intervals. The more familiar the QAPI team becomes with the trends within the facility and outcomes outside the facility, the better prepared they are to prioritize resources. This allows the interdisciplinary team to address the most widespread and serious problems while continuing to monitor and evaluate opportunities to improve the rest of the topics on the dashboard. As the well-functioning QAPI team develops strategies and timelines to address risks or deficiencies, the medical director has the responsibility to communicate with the facility's governing body about the resources that are required to implement those plans (CMS, 2008). Adherence to the commitments of a meaningful, operationalized dashboard is the basis of the healthy function of a QAPI program and provides the structure required to master all that is surveyed.

Finding Meaning in the Numbers: The QAPI Meeting

Performance indicators will drive and track the progress of the QAPI initiatives for the interdisciplinary team to progress toward closing the quality gap in those findings. The QAPI meeting should have excellent potential for problem solving, given the combined expertise of the interdisciplinary team members. However, the QAPI team meeting provides its own challenges. Time constraints present a challenge in exploring an objective review and analysis of issues. Taking short-cuts to reduce meeting time can lead to repeated deferral of problem indicators to later meetings. This postponement and indefinite delay can prevent meaningful action.

Alternatively, discussion can evolve into impromptu and narrowly constructed care plan meetings. Caution should be used when individual patients failing to meet the identified targets become the focus of the discussion. Addressing patient-specific needs may or may not be productive for individual patients, but it can jeopardize the QAPI program meeting objectives unit wide. When this occurs, the team is unable to focus on or loses sight of critical issues that are often closer to the root cause. This loss of focus uses up precious meeting time and makes it difficult to redirect attention to broader issues of maintaining a safe environment for care. Unlike patient care plans, error/safety issues have no other "home" except at the QAPI meeting. Some basic survival strategies for keeping the meeting on track are:

- Manage the logistics. Schedule the meeting for a regular, realistic time and duration. A fully focused 50-minute monthly meeting can be powerful with a calendar for rotating specialized QAPI teams and appropriate off-line collaboration of interdisciplinary team members as needed.
- Be prepared. Circulate reports and be familiar with them before the meeting. Review them with the person(s) responsible for generating the reports for any pertinent information and distribute to interdisciplinary team members as appropriate. This will foster more efficient and effective use of the meeting time.
- Assign specific review tasks to staff members prior to the meeting with the expectation that they will summarize findings for the group. For example, the following summary might introduce the case of a persistent and worsening problem with aggregate hemoglobin levels:

Hemoglobin results indicate that the number of patients in target range decreased for the sixth month in a row. We were in the bottom 20% of our Network in anemia management outcomes on the last Dialysis Facility Report.

Nurse Hero has broken the patient numbers into categories based on iron indices, appropriateness of erythropoietic stimulating agent (ESA) management, history of infection, and hospitalization over the last six months:

○ *The percentage of patients reaching the target range for serum ferritin and iron saturation has drifted slightly downward. This does, however, reflect some patients whose serum ferritin levels are above the upper limit as defined by the facility's protocol.*

○ *The rate of identified infections is unremarkable.*

○ *ESA protocols are being followed accurately.*

○ *The average unit ESA dose has increased by 800 units/treatment over last year's average, year to date.*

Biomedical technician Bob Tech reviewed the facility water logs (chlorine and chloramine checks) and the Association for the Advancement of Medical Instrumentation standards. He has rechecked the water quality to rule out any potential for water-linked hemolysis. The reports are within the range of the standards. Question: Where do we go from here to sort this out?

Notice the choice of words in the question: "Where do we go from here?" as opposed to "Why do you think we're doing so badly?" The latter question could lead to a defensive response. The former, more constructive question focuses on brainstorming for possible solutions. Could there be a higher than normal blood loss in dialyzers or lines during treatment termination? How could this be assessed? What other underlying causes might be linked to the problem? It is important to be objective and consider both the facility's strengths and vulnerabilities in formulating solutions. Care must be taken to ensure the team is challenged to become increasingly vigilant about improvement opportunities rather than to find rationalizations for or defending the actions leading to the disturbing data.

The information should be offered to:
- Present critical data as clearly and objectively as possible.
- Manage the team participation.

Presenting data may often be possible with simple reporting, but visual display of the data can focus attention on the elements of the problem and facilitate progress. For example, an anemia problem could be represented by a simple Excel graph as shown in Figure 19-1.

Maintaining objectivity during the root cause analysis can be challenging. To determine root causes, discussion needs to be participatory, interdisciplinary, data-driven, and solution-focused. The team can suggest more information for review. (Editor's Note: Please refer to Chapter 3, page 21, "Root Cause Analysis in Quality Improvement" for further discussion about this process.)

Using the example in Figure 19-1, there is an increasing percentage of patients who are not achieving the hemoglobin target range, even when considering the most obvious underlying sources. In addition to those questions suggested above, the interdisciplinary team's brainstorming questions could include:
- How many patients who are out of range have catheters?
- Have the patients who are affected had recent invasive procedures (such as vascular access procedures)?
- Protocols have been followed for ESA dosing and IV iron administration. Should the anemia team revisit these protocols? Review the most recent literature for evidence-based studies that may suggest a novel approach or dosing.
- Has the facility had any machine problems (such as blood pump occlusion or incorrect dialysate proportioning)?
- Are staff members confirming dialysate conductivity with an external conductivity meter?

Or they may suggest possible causes.
- Did this begin after a new water treatment loop was opened in the dialysis facility addition?
- Do the venous lines contain excessive residual blood, and could that be affecting the anemia management?
- Is the heparin protocol or dialyzer priming procedure in need of review?

These questions illustrate a useful direction for the QAPI discussion if the team is to brainstorm and explore possible causes and develop meaningful plans.

It may be necessary to elicit participation from knowledgeable team members who are reluctant to speak. Participants must be confident that the QAPI program's intent is not to establish blame, but rather, it is a positive commitment to identify problems, improve the system, and eliminate significant barriers. The QAPI team leader may be required to politely acknowledge an individual's assertion that the problem has been resolved while continuing to seek input from other team members on the issue. These meeting skills may require practice and experience. Resisting premature closure of an issue when other team mem-

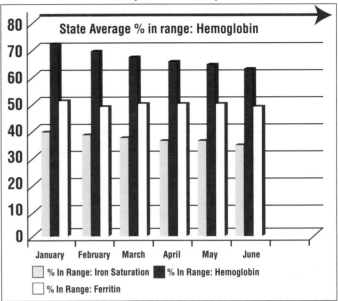

Figure 19-1
Sample Excel Graph

State Average % in range: Hemoglobin

% In Range: Iron Saturation   % In Range: Hemoglobin
% In Range: Ferritin

Source: Used with permission from Bonnie Greenspan.

bers would dismiss it may require self confidence or courage as well as objectivity to explore all relevant options.

Conflicting priorities for the indisciplinary team members' time must be acknowledged, underscoring the necessity to schedule and respect regular start and stop times for a standing QAPI meeting. Patients depend on the team's thoroughness to address problems that affect them. Having no plan will guarantee lack of success. The time spent identifying and preparing to eliminate errors or problems can save countless hours of dealing with recurrence of those problems. It is important to spend the time needed to prevent the potential injury imposed upon the patients when the quality gap persists.

Follow Through and Revision

An indisciplinary team may encounter challenges when QAPI evolves into the culture throughout the dialysis facility. It is exciting to find more staff members enthusiastically involved in projects and developing strategies to address various quality gaps that emerge. Making the most of this energy without reducing the effectiveness of QAPI efforts requires control as well as enthusiasm. In a classic *I Love Lucy* television episode, Lucy and Ethel find work on a candy assembly line. Lucy and Ethel ignore the training, and as a result, they are unable to manage the rapidly moving candies as the conveyor belt speeds up. Finally unable to cope, they stuff the excess chocolates into their mouths. While hilarious, the scene leaves an indelible impression of how quickly exceeding capacity can drive an unready team out of control. With that in mind, it is important that the indisciplinary team sets reasonable timelines and prioritizes the implementation of its strategies. They should do so anticipating the impact on patient health and safety (CMS, 2008). Once the indisciplinary team has established priorities and formulated a pathway to the resolution of critical issues, they must make a commitment to it, even if it requires abandoning comfortable, old habits (see Table 19-6).

Success in QAPI relies on more than the intellectual and

Table 19-6
Sample Annual QAPI Calendar

January 14 – 11:30 A.M.	February 11 – 11:30 A.M.	March 11 – 11:30 A.M.
Clinical outcomes report Access report BioMed/reuse report Error/grievance review Results of mineral and bone disorder Q1 report Staff turnover team	Clinical outcomes report Access report Infection control review Error/grievance review Hemoglobin team report Safety team	Clinical outcomes report Access report Patient status review Error/grievance review Preview of mineral and bone disorder Q2 effort Exercise team
April 8 – 11:30 A.M.	**May 13 – 11:30 A.M.**	**June 10 – 11:30 A.M.**
Clinical outcomes report Access report BioMed/reuse report Error/grievance review Results of mineral and bone disorder Q2 report Annual competence review	Clinical outcomes report Access report Infection control review Error/grievance review Hemoglobin team report TBD	Clinical outcomes report Access report Plant walk-through Error/grievance review Preview of mineral and bone disorder Q3 effort TBD
July 8 – 11:30 A.M.	**August 12 – 11:30 A.M.**	**September 9 – 11:30 A.M.**
Clinical outcomes report Access report BioMed/reuse report Error/grievance review Results of mineral and bone disorder Q3 report Staff turnover team	Clinical outcomes report Access report Infection control review Error/grievance review Focused indicator Safety team	Clinical outcomes report Access report Patient status review Error/grievance review Preview of mineral and bone disorder Q4 effort Exercise team
October 14 – 11:30 A.M.	**November 11 – 11:30 A.M.**	**December 9 – 11:30 A.M.**
Clinical outcomes report Access report BioMed/reuse report Error/grievance review Results of mineral and bone disorder Q4 report Employee awards	Clinical outcomes report Access report Infection control review Error/grievance review Focused indicator TBD	Clinical outcomes report Access report Plant walk-through Error/grievance review Preview of mineral and bone disorder Q1 effort TBD

Note: TBD = to be determined, Q = quarter.
Source: Used with permission from Bonnie Greenspan.

creative effort of the team; it requires diligent effort. Once the strategy is devised, implementation requires persistence and attention to logistics in meeting established timelines. The concept of intentional implementation might be useful in intensifying commitment to perform the required change in practice behaviors (Casper, 2008). When new procedures are a part of a performance improvement plan, staff members should discuss details about how and when these changes will be incorporated into existing routines. They should address any barriers to implementation of the strategy and refine the specifics accordingly. Accountability must always be clear, reinforced, and supported.

In *Fortune Magazine's* 1999 article, "Why CEOs Fail," Ram Charan stated that fewer than 10% of effectively formulated strategies are successfully completed. In an estimated 70% of cases, bad strategy is not the real problem, but instead, it is poor execution (Charan, 1999). "Key subordinates whose sustained poor performance deeply harms the company..." was associated with failure of the manager to effectively deal with their performance (Charan, 1999, p. 2). It is important to build a genuine belief in a culture where systemic errors are

acknowledged and evaluated to develop strategies for prevention. This places the emphasis on system issues rather than an individual problem. Capable key employees supportive of improving performance and open to increasing their own effectiveness are the link between a desire for improved outcomes and their achievement.

Nurses seeking improvement must be willing to persist in their efforts. Nasso (2006) described a project to reduce the incidence of peritonitis in patients on peritoneal dialysis. Twelve months after the team analyzed its data, established root causes, and implemented an array of remediations, their initiative showed no improvement. The team persisted in utilizing a more systematic search for identification of root causes. They used fishbone diagrams to identify their failed strategies and gathered input from more successful programs. They developed new action steps for reducing the peritonitis rate. Over the ensuing six months, peritonitis rates were reduced from 1 case per 16 to 20 patient months to the goal of 1 case per 36 patient months (Nasso, 2006).

Successful CQI Initiatives

The evidence of success in CQI projects can be found in the professional literature. Arnaout, Hamilton, and Steele (2007) added nursing case managers to their existing physician and staff model that led to a significant decrease in mortality, hospital days, catheter use, and an increase in dialysis adequacy. Glazer et al. (2006) reported on a multidisciplinary CQI program undertaken as a part of their participation in the Medicare End Stage Renal Disease Managed Care Demonstration Project in which:

- Primary use of arteriovenous fistulas (AVFs) increased from 27% in 1997 to 88% in 2003.
- Prevalence of AVFs increased from 30% in 1997 to 62% in 2003.
- Replacement AVF access increased from 26% in 1998 to 58% in 2003 (Glazer et al., 2006).

Conclusion

The examples cited in this chapter illustrate advancement in patient care that can be achieved through collaborative CQI efforts. It is the belief of this author that those successes and the many examples that have been shared by practicing nephrology nurses were a result of individuals or groups who:

- Believed it was their responsibility to improve the care and safety of their patients.
- Resisted the temptation to rationalize findings and approached improvement in an objective, data-based manner.
- Focused on issues that would have a significant impact on the patient group.
- Sought input from knowledgeable experts within or outside of their facility in identifying root causes and formulating and evaluating a plan.
- Followed through, despite setbacks, with implementation of all critical commitments and planned revisions as necessary.

The following comments summarize the rationale for continuous quality improvement activities in all areas of nursing: "So it is reasonable to ask whether there is any reason to change what health professionals have been trying to do for some time (if not forever). In fact, there are several differences of emphasis. The most important is the reminder to health professionals that patients are members of the community who do not deserve to die or to suffer injury as a result of mistakes that could have been avoided" (Braithwaite, Hindle, & Iedema, 2005, p. 46). Nephrology nurses are up to that challenge.

References

Agency for Healthcare Research and Quality (AHRQ) (2009a). *CAHPS Surveys and tools to advance patient-centered care.* Retrieved March 21, 2009, from https://www.cahps.ahrq.gov/default.asp

Agency for Healthcare Research and Quality (AHRQ). (2009b). *In-center hemodialysis consumer assessment of healthcare providers and systems.* Retrieved March 21, 2009, from http://www.cahps.ahrq.gov/content/products/ICH/PROD_ICH_Intro.asp

Arnaout, M.A., Hamilton, E., & Steele, D.J. (2007). A case management model to improve hemodialysis outpatient outcomes [Abstract]. *Hemodialysis International 11*(2), 247-251.

Aly, Z.A., Gellens, M.E., Gonzalez, E.A., & Martin, K.J. (2004). Achieving K/DOQI laboratory target values for bone and mineral metabolism: An uphill battle. *American Journal of Nephrology, 24*(4), 422-426.

Bernstein, K.N., Lesperance, E.M., Raymond, D.B., & Wazny, L.D. (2008). Are CSN and NKF-K/DOQI mineral metabolism guidelines for hemodialysis patients achievable? Results from a provincial renal program [Abstract]. *Canadian Association of Nephrology Nurses and Technicians Journal, 18*(2), 36-41.

Braithwaite, J., Hindle, D., & Iedema, R. (2005). *Patient safety research: A review of the literature.* Sydney, Australia: Centre for Clinical Governance Research in Health, University of New South Wales. Clinical Excellence Commission.

Casper, E.S. (2008). Using implementation intentions to teach practitioners: Changing practice behaviors via continuing education [Abstract]. *Psychiatric Services 59*(7), 747-52.

Centers for Medicare and Medicaid Services (CMS). (2008). *Conditions for coverage and conditions for participations: End-stage renal disease facilities.* Retrieved March 19, 2009, from http://www.cms.hhs.gov/CFCsAndCoPs/13_ESRD.asp

Charan, R. (1999). Why CEOs fail. *Fortune Magazine.* Retrieved March 19, 2009, from http://www.businessbuilders.bz/why-ceos-fail.pdf

Glazer, S., Diesto, J., Crooks, P., Yeoh, H., Pascual, N., Selevan, D., et al. (2006). Going beyond the kidney disease outcomes quality initiative: Hemodialysis access experience at Kaiser Permanente Southern California. *Annals of Vascular Surgery, 20*(1).

Institute of Medicine (IOM). (2000). *To err is human: Building a safer health system.* Washington: National Academy Press.

Institute of Medicine (IOM). (2001). *Crossing the quality chasm: A new health system for the 21st century.* Washington: National Academies Press.

Institute of Medicine (IOM) and Board of Healthcare Services. (2004). *Keeping patients safe: Transforming the work environment of nurses.* Washington: National Academies Press.

LifeOptions (n.d.). *Measuring dialysis patients' health-related quality of life with Kidney Disease Quality of Life (KDQOL-36™) Survey.* Retrieved on March 21, 2009, from http://www.lifeoptions.org/kdqol/pdfs/kdqol36_pros.pdf

Nasso, L. (2006). Our peritonitis continuous quality improvement project: where there is a will there is a way. [Abstract]. *Canadian Association of Nephrology Nurses and Technicians Journal, 16*(1), 20-23.

National Kidney Foundation (NKF). (2009). *NKF-KDOQI guidelines.* Retrieved March 21, 2009, from http://www.kidney.org/PROFESSIONALS/kdoqi/guidelines.cfm

Renal Physicians Association and the Forum of End Stage Renal Disease Networks. (2008). *Keeping kidney patients safe.* Retrieved March 21, 2009, from http://www.kidneypatientsafety.org

The University of Michigan Kidney Epidemiology and Cost Center. (2008). *Guide to the 2008 dialysis facility reports: Overview, methodology, and interpretation.* Retrieved March 18, 2009, from http://www.sph.umich.edu/kecc/assets/documents/facguide.pdf

Walton, M. (1986). *The Deming management method.* New York: Putnam Publishing Group.

Witten, B., Payne, G, Kari, J., Spencer, T., Frank, K., Miller, R., et al. (2008). *Measures Assessment Tool: Instructional material for surveyor training in 2008 ESRD conditions for coverage.* Presented at Roll Out of ESRD Regulations in Dallas,TX, and Cherry Hill, NJ, September 2008.

Additional Readings

Institute of Medicine (IOM). (2003). *Priority areas for national action: Transforming health care quality.* Washington: National Academies Press.

Institute of Medicine (IOM). (2004). Evidence-based review methodology for the closing the quality gap series. In *Closing the gap: A critical analysis of quality improvement strategies.* Washington: National Academies Press.

| Chapter 19 | CONTINUING NURSING EDUCATION EVALUATION FORM | 1.4 Contact Hours |

Quality Assurance and Performance Improvement in the Outpatient Setting

ANNP0919

Applying Continuous Quality Improvement in Clinical Practice contains 22 chapters of educational content. Individual learners may apply for continuing nursing education credit by reading a chapter and completing the Continuing Nursing Education Evaluation Form for that chapter. Learners may apply for continuing nursing education credit for any or all chapters.

Please photocopy this test page, complete, and return to ANNA.
You can also download this form from www.annanurse.org (choose Education - CNE Activities - Publications)
Receive continuing nursing education credit (CNE) immediately by completing the CNE evaluation process in ANNA's Online Library. Go to www.annanurse.org, and click on the Online Library icon for more information.

Name: _____

Address: _____

City: _____ State: _____ Zip: _____

E-mail: _____ Preferred telephone: ☐ Home ☐ Work _____

State where licensed and license number: _____

CNE application fees are based upon the number of contact hours provided by the individual section. CNE fees per contact hour for ANNA members are as follows: 1.0-1.9 – $15; 2.0-2.9 – $20; 3.0-3.9 – $25; 4.0 and higher – $30. Fees for nonmembers are $10 higher.

CNE application fee for Chapter 19: ANNA member $15   Nonmember $25

ANNA Member: ☐ Yes ☐ No   ☐ Member # (if available) _____

☐ Check or money order enclosed   ☐ American Express   ☐ Visa   ☐ MasterCard

Total amount submitted: _____

Credit card number _____ Exp. Date _____

Name as it appears on the card: _____

NOTE: Your evaluation form can be processed in 1 week for an additional rush charge of $5.00.
☐ **Yes, I would like this evaluation form rush processed. I have included an additional fee of $5.00 for rush processing.**

---

1. I verify that I have read this chapter and completed this education activity. _____ Date _____
   Signature

2. What would be different in your practice if you applied what you have learned from this activity? (Please use additional paper if necessary.)
   _____
   _____
   _____
   _____

	Strongly disagree				Strongly agree
3. The activity met the stated objectives.					
a. Identify opportunities to close quality gaps through quality assessment performance improvement (QAPI) activities in the outpatient setting.	1	2	3	4	5
b. List nine QAPI indicators mandated for review by the 2008 ESRD *Conditions for Coverage*.	1	2	3	4	5
c. Identify two relevant strategies to keep QAPI on track in the outpatient setting.	1	2	3	4	5
4. The content was current and relevant.	1	2	3	4	5
5. The content was presented clearly.	1	2	3	4	5
6. The content was covered adequately.	1	2	3	4	5

7. How would you rate your ability to apply your learning to practice?   ☐ diminished ability   ☐ no change   ☐ enhanced ability

Comments _____
_____

8. Time required to read the chapter and complete this form: _____ minutes

CQI Application:
Meeting the Challenges of ESRD Networks

Deuzimar Kulawik, MSN, RN
Angeline F. Wieler, MSN, RN, CNN
Mary Fenderson, MSHSA, RN, CNN

Objectives

Study of the information presented in this chapter will enable the learner to:
1. Relate background pertaining to the ESRD Networks' work with dialysis facilities in improvement processes.
2. Discuss continuous quality improvement concepts applied to the clinical setting.
3. Describe a proposed framework for the working relationship between the ESRD Networks and dialysis providers.
4. Discuss a patient-centered approach using an established model for improvement.

Overview

This chapter exhibits a brief background pertaining to the ESRD Networks' goals, objectives, attributes, and requirements relevant to the quality improvement process. Additionally, a review of the concepts of continuous quality improvement is provided and includes how to foster its application in a standardized way that is applicable to clinicians, providers, and stakeholders. A proposed framework is presented that highlights the relationship between ESRD Networks and providers using a patient-centered approach with the use of a model for improvement, the Plan-Do-Study-Act (PDSA) cycle. The reader is offered information on unifying the PDSA cycle in the work of determining the "how to" in delivering optimal quality care for patients with ESRD.

Introduction

The quality of end stage renal disease (ESRD) care has received considerable attention by providers, beneficiaries, regulators, and other stakeholders in recent years. This attention is mainly driven from sub-optimal patient outcomes, economic constraints in the healthcare system, and complexity of the healthcare delivery system. Evidence of patient outcomes, the work to improve patients outcomes, and continued opportunities can be found in results from the Clinical Performance Measures initiative. Section 4558 (b) of the Balanced Budget Act required the Centers for Medicare and Medicaid Services (CMS) to develop and implement "a method to measure and report the quality of renal dialysis services provided under the Medicare program" (CMS, 2008e). To implement this legislation, CMS funded the development of clinical performance meures based on the National Kidney Foundation's (NKF) Dialysis Outcomes Quality Initiative (DOQI) Clinical Practice Guidelines. Data for the ESRD clinical performance measures continue to be collected annually on a national sample of adult patients on hemodialysis (HD) and peritoneal dialysis (PD)

(CMS, 2008e). In order to work toward solutions to improve quality to ESRD beneficiaries, implementation of continuous quality improvement (CQI) methods could be considered as a way to help providers meet the challenges of the ESRD Networks and implement organizational change.

Applying CQI to Improve Patient Outcomes For ESRD

In general, CQI aims to facilitate ongoing improvement by using objective data to analyze and improve processes. Emphasis is placed on efficient and effective functioning of organizational systems. CQI involves an ongoing cycle of gathering data regarding how well organizational systems are functioning, developing, and implementing improvements (Agich, 2007). An essential starting point is the systematic and objective assessment of performance and the system's ability to support good performance. Good quality information is needed so goals can be set and strategies developed for improving key areas. CQI is characterized by cyclical activities involving examination of existing processes, change, monitoring the apparent effects of the change, and further change (Beecroft, Duffy, & Moran, 2003).

Proponents of CQI believe that while the language may change, the tools and vision of CQI will persist because they are adaptive (Shortell, Bennett, & Byck, 1998). It is this positive view of the promise of CQI that calls for implementation of CQI processes in the dialysis facility's environment. CQI combines a scientific methodology with a management philosophy of improving processes continuously. The scientific methodology is known as the use of statistical data to analyze processes, and consequently, decrease existent variation (Shortell et al., 1998). The management philosophy component can be viewed as the quality management method that utilizes the Plan-Do-Study-Act (PDSA) cycle. CQI application provides the theory and methods to allow the transformation from the current convention of assuming quality to one of actually measuring and improving quality (Nelson, Batalden, & Godfrey, 2007).

Figure 20-1
End Stage Renal Disease Networks

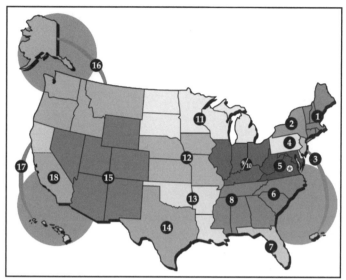

Source: National Forum of ESRD Networks, n.d., a.

Understanding the Role of the ESRD Networks

According to NKF (2008), 26 million Americans have chronic kidney disease (CKD), and 20 million more are at increased risk. Over 400,000 Americans suffer from ESRD and require either dialysis or transplantation (NKF, 2008). ESRD is the only disease-specific program that entitles people of all ages to Medicare coverage on the basis of their ESRD diagnosis. The following background information pertaining to the history of the ESRD Networks was retrieved from the CMS (2008a, 2008b) documents, "End Stage Renal Disease (ESRD) Quality Initiative Overview" and "The End Stage Renal Disease Networks Program Overview."

Goals/Objectives of the ESRD Networks

Goals and objectives of the ESRD Networks include (CMS, n.d.):
- Improve the quality and safety of dialysis-related services provided for individuals with ESRD.
- Improve independence, quality of life, and rehabilitation of patients with ESRD to the extent possible through transplantation, self-care modalities (such as PD, home hemodialysis), and in-center self-care as medically appropriate through the end of life.
- Improve patient perception and experience of care, and resolve patient's complaints and grievances.
- Improve collaboration with providers to ensure achievement of the goals through the most efficient and effective means possible.
- Improve the collection, reliability, timeliness, and use of data to measure processes of care and outcomes, maintain the patient registry, and support the ESRD Network program and quality improvement initiatives.

In 1972, the Medicare ESRD Program was established as a national health insurance program for people with ESRD. The term "ESRD" was coined to include all patients with end stage disease, regardless of the etiology of the disease. Initially, 32 ESRD Network areas were established. The program was designed to encourage self-care dialysis and kidney transplantation, and provide clarification pertaining to reimbursement procedures in order to achieve more effective cost control of the ESRD program. The Omnibus Budget Reconciliation Act of 1986 resulted in revisions of the Network Organizations' responsibilities and merging of the 32 Network areas into 18 Network areas. The number and concentration of ESRD beneficiaries in each area geographically define the 18 Network Organizations (CMS, 2006). Some Networks represent a single state, while others encompass multiple states. The responsibilities of the Network Organizations include the quality oversight of the care of ESRD beneficiaries, data collection to administer the national Medicare ESRD program, and the provision of technical assistance to ESRD providers and patients (see Figure 20-1).

The ESRD Networks are non-profit contract organizations with governing boards responsible for their business and contractual obligations. Each Network maintains medical review boards with responsibility for quality improvement and oversight initiatives in their geographic region. All ESRD Networks are members of the Forum of ESRD Networks. The Forum is a not-for-profit organization and advocates for organizations that monitor the quality of CKD, dialysis, and kidney transplant care in the United States, its territories, and the District of Columbia. The Forum facilitates the information flow and the national quality agenda with CMS and other renal organizations. The mission of the Forum is to support the ESRD Networks in promoting and improving the quality of care to patients with renal disease through education and the collection, analysis, and dissemination of data and information (National Forum of ESRD Networks, n.d., a).

Providers are required by regulation to participate in Network activities. Under the direction of CMS, the Network Organization works with consumers, ESRD facilities, and other providers of ESRD services. The vision of Network organizations is to enhance patient care delivery systems to ensure ESRD beneficiaries obtain the right care at the right time. The ESRD Networks assist providers of ESRD services with improving the quality of patient care by:
- Conducting quality improvement projects.
- Providing technical assistance to facilities.
- Investigating and resolving patient complaints.
- Validating facility and patient data.
- Sponsoring outreach and educational activities for patients and providers.
- Providing technical and educational materials to patients and providers (CMS, 2005).

The Networks' responsibilities as delineated by CMS include:
- Quality oversight of the care patients with ESRD receive.
- Collection of data to administer the national Medicare ESRD program.

- Provide technical assistance to ESRD providers and patients.

  Examples of other responsibilities of the Networks include:
- Encouraging the use of treatment settings most compatible with the successful rehabilitation of patients.
- Encouraging participation of patients, providers of services, and ESRD facilities in vocational rehabilitation programs.
- Developing criteria and standards related to the quality and appropriateness of care.
- Implementing procedures for the evaluation and resolution of patient grievances.
- Collecting, validating, and analyzing data for reporting and maintaining a national ESRD registry.
- Identifying facilities not meeting Network goals and assisting them in the development of appropriate quality improvement plans.
- Reporting facilities and providers that are not providing appropriate medical care to CMS.
- Providing technical assistance to ESRD beneficiaries and dialysis and transplant providers (National Forum of ESRD Networks, n.d., b).

To attain the vision of the ESRD Network Organizations, the Network Program assists providers in the transformation of quality to make health care safe, effective, timely, efficient, and equitable. By establishing and supporting partnerships and collaboration among the ESRD Networks, Quality Improvement Organizations, Medicare Advantage Organizations, State Survey Agencies, professional groups, patient organizations, and ESRD facilities/providers, this program improves the quality of care and life for patients with ESRD and improves data reporting, reliability, and validity.

Quality health care for Medicare beneficiaries is a high priority for CMS. In 2001, The Department of Health and Human Services (DHHS) announced the Quality Initiative to assure quality health care for all Americans via accountability and public disclosure. The intent of the initiative is to empower consumers with quality care information to be able to make informed decisions about their health care and also to encourage improvement of the quality of health care provided.

In 2004, the Quality Initiative was expanded to include kidney dialysis facilities (ESRD Quality Initiative). The aim of the initiative was to standardize dialysis care measures, ESRD data definitions, and data transmission to support the needs of Medicare's ESRD program. Examples of quality initiatives include:
- Dialysis Facility Compare.
- Fistula First Breakthrough Initiative.
- ESRD *Conditions for Coverage.*
- ESRD *Clinical Performance Measures.*
- The electronic data submission system for ESRD information system.

In addition to national initiatives, each Network conducts quality improvement projects locally, working with providers and facilities to specifically address regional and local issues (CMS, 2008a). A brief description of the quality initiatives of ESRD programs follows.

Dialysis Facility Compare

Dialysis Facility Compare is a Web site containing quality information on all Medicare-approved dialysis facilities, and provides various information and resources about CKD and dialysis for patients and family members. The site includes information pertaining to dialysis facility services. These include facility contact information, the facility's initial date of Medicare certification, modalities and types of dialysis offered, availability of evening shifts, number of treatment stations, and facility ownership and corporate name (CMS, 2005). Quality measures provide information about the care that a dialysis facility provides to its patients. This is one way to compare dialysis facilities. Quality measures include information pertaining to outcomes using the following as clinical indicators:
- Anemia management using hemoglobin less than 10.0 g/dL and the percentage of patients at a facility with a hemoglobin greater than 12.0 g/dL.
- HD adequacy using urea reduction ratio (URR) of 65% or greater.
- A facility's expected patient survival rate as compared with the actual survival rate (CMS, 2005).

There are links to dialysis-related topics on CKD, HD, PD, and kidney transplant; Web sites for children and parents, as well as caregiver and family support; and other Medicare sites. Dialysis facility publications and a *Kidney Disease Dictionary* containing definitions of commonly used dialysis and kidney disease terms, and frequently asked questions and answers are also available.

Fistula First Breakthrough Initiative

Fistula First Breakthrough Initiative is a CMS breakthrough strategy to improve the arterial venous fistula (AVF) utilization to 66% by 2009 (CMS, 2008c). The Breakthrough Initiative has convened a broad renal coalition that consists of the CMS, ESRD Networks, dialysis providers, primary care physicians, nephrologists, vascular access surgeons, interventional radiologists/nephrologists, professional societies, quality improvement organizations, and patient advocacy groups. They are working together to increase the likelihood that every suitable patient on HD will receive the optimal vascular access. In most cases, the optimal access is a native AVF and reduces the use of catheters and vascular access complications. A dedicated Web page has been developed to support the coalition's efforts (CMS, 2008c). The project also provides support to the ESRD Networks to enhance their own quality improvement capabilities by providing useful improvement tools and materials that have generated significant national progress (Peters, Clemons, & Augustine, 2005).

ESRD Conditions for Coverage

Conditions for Coverage are the federal regulations that must be met by all facilities participating in Medicare. The ESRD *Conditions for Coverage* are the minimum health and safety rules that all Medicare and Medicaid participating dialysis facilities must meet. Updates to the ESRD *Conditions for Coverage Final Rule* were published on April 15, 2008. The revised regulations are patient-centered and reflect improvements in clinical standards of care and advanced technology.

They provide a framework to incorporate performance measures viewed by the scientific and medical community to be related to the quality of care provided to dialysis patients (CMS, 2008d). The *Conditions for Coverage* require that an interdisciplinary team consisting of the nephrologist, nephrology nurse, patient care technician, dietitian, and social worker monitors aggregate data about the facility's performance. The CQI process is to be implemented by the quality assessment performance improvement (QAPI) committee (CMS, 2008d).

Clinical Performance Measures

As discussed in the introduction section of the chapter, CMS sponsored a project to measure and report the quality of renal dialysis service provided under the Medicare program (CMS, 2008e). In 1998, CMS developed ESRD clinical performance measures based on the NKF DOQI *Clinical Practice Guidelines* (CMS, 2008e; NKF, 2001). Sixteen clinical performance measures were developed for reporting of the quality of dialysis services provided in the areas of adequacy, anemia, and vascular access management. Annual data collection for a standard set of measures is used to identify opportunities for improvement. One of the roles of the ESRD Networks is to assist dialysis providers with quality improvement activities directed toward these identified opportunities.

Examples of opportunities to improve care for patients undergoing in-center HD and PD can be identified from the *2007 Annual Report ESRD Clinical Performance Measures Project* (CMS, 2007). The goal for all adult patients on in-center HD is a (sp)Kt/V equal to or greater than 1.2. In 2005, 91% of patients achieved this goal, and it was virtually unchanged when in 2006, 90% of patients were at goal (CMS, 2007). A mean Hgb greater than 11 g/dL is a goal for adult patients on PD. Eighty-three percent (83%) of these patients were at this target over a 6-month period ending in March 2007. For vascular access type, all adult patients on in-center HD, in the last HD session during the study period, revealed an increase of the percentage of patients with AVFs. However, in the category of patients with chronic catheter, data revealed the following outcomes. In 1996, fewer than 20% of adult patients on in-center HD had catheters. This number had increased to greater than 20% of patients with catheters by 2006 (CMS, 2007), showing a directional trend contrary to the goal. CPM data continue to provide the ESRD Networks comparison reporting of Network and national results, which are utilized to identify specific quality measures for improvement (CMS, 2008e). Twenty-six new clinical practice measures were implemented to further monitor the quality of care being delivered to patients with ESRD (CMS, 2008e).

Electronic Data Submission

The electronic data submission requirement is a regulation included in the updated *Conditions for Coverage* published in April 2008 (CMS, 2008d). The final rule requires the submission and maintenance of electronic patient and provider records for all dialysis facilities. Consolidated Renal Operations in a Web-Enabled Network (CROWNWeb) is a Web-based software application designed by CMS to meet this new requirement for the collection of patient records, clinical performance measures, and facility data. CROWNWeb includes a listing of all ESRD facilities within each Network, as well as employees and patients within each facility. The application contains a facility staff module to track personnel and their roles within the dialysis facility. Patients are assigned to a primary dialysis facility responsible for their treatment and can be transferred to other facilities as required. The system provides an electronic venue to track the status of patients on dialysis as they are admitted to and/or discharged from their primary facility. The system generates the CMS-mandated forms, 2728 and 2746, to be submitted electronically to the appropriate ESRD Network. Printing these documents as well as various other facility reports are additional options available to the user. CROWNWeb uses an encryption technology that assures privacy, confidentiality, and security for electronic communications consistent with applicable Health Insurance Portability and Accountability Act (HIPAA) statutes and related regulations.

ESRD Networks and CQI Application

Network – CQI Attributes

Attributes are those characteristics that appear repeatedly throughout the literature and function similarly to criteria for making a differential diagnosis, such as in medicine (Walker & Avant, 2004). CQI is a process that has received increased focus and attention over the past decade. In order to appropriately and accurately perform CQI, one needs to understand the foundational concepts. Through mastery achievement of CQI structure, the facility culture, CQI technical dimensions, and identifying the desired outcomes, one can implement a successful CQI program.

The CQI structure includes personnel qualifications, educational or training support, and various technological resources available. The structure must be based on reliable technology with key facility personnel who are competently able to understand and operationalize the technology to ensure efficiency and effectiveness of the process. Having the technology to perform CQI is inadequate if personnel are not able to utilize it to achieve positive patient outcomes that meet or exceed industry standards. Although both technology and qualified staff are essential, educational or ongoing training support is vital. That support provides the infrastructure necessary for continued growth and competence for effectively working with fast-paced changes and improvements in today's technology-rich environment (Byers & Rosati, 2005).

The culture of a facility is the key ingredient that provides the cohesive vision, which becomes the foundation for clinical practice. To ensure achievement of successful CQI, the following must happen:
- The facility's management takes on a leadership role.
- Quality training has been provided for everyone in the facility.
- CQI has become the focus of the facility.
- All levels of personnel are involved in the achievement of a positive quality culture.

The Japanese proved this strategy to be effective after World War II, when they began their journey to become quality-oriented and major suppliers to world markets (Byers & Rosati, 2005).

The technical dimensions of CQI include attitude, aptitude, motivation, and adequate resources. Although never the intent, quality efforts at addressing issues may cause harm if they are identified as "underuse, overuse, or misuse" (Byers & Rosati, 2005, p. 14), and should be considered with every decision:

- *"Underuse* happens when patients do not receive beneficial health services" (Byers & Rosati, 2005, p. 14).
- *"Overuse* occurs when patients undergo treatment or procedures from which they do not benefit" (Byers & Rosati, 2005, p. 14).
- *"Misuse* transpires when patients receive appropriate medical services that are provided poorly, exposing them to added risk of preventable complications" (Byers & Rosati, 2005, p. 14).

A positive attitude, personal aptitude, and motivation for providing quality and access to pertinent resources can prevent these types of harm. Knowledge of professional guidelines for clinical practice can provide the basis to strengthen quality care. An awareness of and access to these resources support each individual staff member's efforts in his or her pursuit of quality and the advancement of care. The National Association of Healthcare Quality (NAHQ) has defined healthcare quality professionals' *Code for Conduct and Standards of Practice,* in which they promote maintaining membership in professional organizations to promote quality and professional growth as one of the essential features (NAHQ, 2007).

Every CQI project must have a defined outcome that becomes the goal for which it strives. The 21st century brings with it a new way of looking at quality and innovative strategies in achieving goals. At the very minimum, healthcare quality must be "safe, effective, patient-centered, timely, efficient, and equitable," as defined by the Institute of Medicine (IOM) Committee on Quality in Healthcare of America (Byers & Rosati, 2005, pp. 14-15). Health care is quickly approaching the era of pay for performance, where reimbursement will be linked to quality indicators and actual outcomes. Pay for performance in ESRD "aims to track provider and facility achievement of key evidence-based clinical performance measures, including optimization of dialysis dose, achievement of phosphate control, effective anemia management, correction of serum albumin levels, and use of fewer intravascular catheters" (Desai et al., 2008, p. 1). CQI is no longer a facility choice. Rather, it is a mandatory initiative that must be undertaken with vigor and dedication to achieve optimum, patient-centered care.

The Networks use the following IOM definition in evaluating the quality of care delivered. "Quality of care is the degree to which health services for individuals and populations increase the likelihood of desired outcomes and are consistent with current professional knowledge" (IOM, 2006). In the context of a dialysis facility, this definition means several things:

- *Health services* describe all treatments, services, and interactions that are provided in the day-to-day care for a patient with ESRD.
- *Individual* means one patient in the facility.
- *Population* means the whole population of patients.

Thus, when evaluating quality of care in a facility, outcomes for both the *individual* and the *entire group of patients* must be reviewed. A good way to differentiate the two approaches is:

- Plan of care is the evaluation of care to the *individual patient.*
- The QAPI Committee evaluates care to the *population of patients.*

The QAPI team looks at the aggregate clinical outcome data, facility processes, and water and dialysate quality. Safety and risk management are reviewed, and the care to the population of patients is evaluated. Facility mortality rate is reviewed in the QAPI meeting to consider if changes in care delivery need to be made to protect other patients from adverse or preventable events.

Determining the degree to which dialysis health services increase the likelihood of desired outcomes requires the measuring and comparing of those outcomes. The QAPI team may ask themselves, "What are the desired outcomes that are consistent with current professional knowledge?" These outcomes are described in practice guidelines, national standards and recommendations, professional organizations' standards of practice, and in current literature. The *Network Quality Management Program Criteria and Standards* included in this section contains references for obtaining standards, guidelines, and recommendations. The Networks use the term *quality management* to encompass the many aspects of the work done with and by dialysis facilities regarding delivery of quality care. Quality management consists of quality planning, quality control and quality improvement (ESRD Network of Texas, Inc., n.d.).

Quality control is the job of the QAPI Committee. The interdisciplinary QAPI Committee is composed of at least the medical director, nurse manager, chief technician, facility administrator, social worker, and dietitian (CMS, 2008d). The QAPI committee should meet monthly at a minimum, and review all quality indicator data on key aspects of care. These are described in the *Network Criteria and Standards for Dialysis Facility Specific Quality Management Programs.* Quality control involves (ESRD Network of Texas, Inc., n.d.):

- Evaluating actual performance of the facility processes:
  - This step involves auditing staff practices, medical record review, and review of data.
- Comparing the actual performance with quality goals:
  - Most corporations have established goals for various clinical indicators that should be used in this step.
  - The Networks have resources available that can be used in this step to compare actual facility clinical outcomes to statewide averages and/or practice guidelines. Many corporations have programs that provide comparative regional or national data.
  - The Network Quality Improvement Department is available to provide assistance and/or direction on current quality goals in each state for corporate or independent facilities.
- Taking action on any difference between planned goals and actual performance:
  - This may entail retraining or educating staff, as well as developing policies, procedures, and processes.

Quality improvement is a process of continually striving to improve (ESRD Network of Texas, Inc., n.d.). Whenever the QAPI committee notes that actual performance does not meet desired outcomes, quality improvement should be initiated. Quality improvement employs the following:

- Identify specific needs for improvement:
  - This can be accomplished by comparing actual performance with desired performance, whether it is in the area of clinical outcomes or operations (such as water quality, treatment initiation time, staff retention).
  - Many sources are available to describe desired performance (including professional practice guidelines, national standards, and locally developed goals). Contact the Network Quality Management staff if assistance is needed.
  - For each specific improvement project, establish a QAPI team consisting of 3 to 5 individuals who actually work in the process that is to be improved.
  - Give the team a clear charge as to what they are expected to accomplish along with an expected time frame. Describe the desired change or outcome in one or two sentences.
- Provide the resources, motivation, and training needed by the teams to identify causes, plan changes, and then monitor for improvement. The Network Quality Management staff are available to work with facilities.

Network – Quality Management/Quality Improvement Requirements

Many approaches have been designed for use in quality management/quality improvement. Networks-recommended *Criteria and Standards Dialysis Facility Specific Quality Management* can be found in Appendix A (adapted from ESRD Network of Texas, Inc., n.d.).

The expectation is that facilities that identify an issue or problem with any of the areas outlined will implement appropriate actions to address and correct the area or problem. An improvement plan clearly identifies the issue and the person responsible to monitor or perform the corrective actions. The plan contains the date by which the correction or improved process must be completed and the outcome or goal that is to be achieved. After the improvement plan actions are completed, outcomes are reviewed to determine if they were achieved. Further actions may be needed to correct the issue, and those are documented. Use of the various quality improvement tools that facilitate monitoring of progress can be included in the documentation process.

Taking CQI Beyond Facility Boundaries: A Pathway Of Processes and Interventions

What generates changes in quality improvement programs? Healthcare quality improvement programs currently require a patient-centered approach. The delivery of care and processes of care are focused on patient needs, concerns, values, and priorities. Caregivers use scientific knowledge, evidence-based guidelines, and best-demonstrated practices in the care provided. Customization based on patient needs and values should be incorporated into effective care-planning processes, with the capability to respond to individual patient choices and preferences. The safety of patients receiving care in ESRD facilities has led to the design of care systems to allow staff to recognize errors, minimize adverse events, and seek process improvements.

Cultural changes have resulted in individuals with ESRD being informed, prepared, and involved in making choices through their continuum of care from ESRD to end of life. Patient education pertaining to the various choices of renal replacement therapy (RRT) prepares the individual for therapy when progressing from CKD to ESRD. This education facilitates timely vascular or peritoneal catheter access placement, transplant referral for evaluation, and discussion of all possible treatment modalities, including self-care, when appropriate.

Quality improvement programs have undergone many iterations, as have been presented in this book. Another model, Rapid Cycle Improvement, also known as a Model for Improvement, is a carefully designed program of activities (Brown, 2007). This model sets improvement goals, identifies changes that are likely to achieve improvements, and specifies how these changes can be applied in practice. It establishes methods of measuring the effectiveness of the intervention. The cycle uses standard quality tools with skilled facilitators to achieve improvements in performance within a rapid time frame.

Rapid Cycle Improvement is performed by the ESRD Networks' use of data elements, such as clinical practice measures. Information technology is used in partnership with providers to increase the efficiency, timeliness, and accuracy of data collection and reporting. ESRD Networks work collaboratively with caregivers, facilities, and other renal community representatives to assure the provision of quality care to patients with ESRD. Achieving outcome measures developed through broad consensus have a strong correlation to the patients' quality of care, quality of life, hospitalization, mortality, and perception of care. Public reporting of outcome measures to beneficiaries and open communications with providers promote informed health choices, protect individuals from poor care, and strengthen the delivery system for health care.

According to Donabedian (2002), the concept of *continuous improvement* suggests that no level of quality can be totally satisfactory, as the expectations of patients and healthcare professionals are continually shifting upward. Donabedian's (2002) framework of structure, process, and outcomes suggest that structures affect processes, which in turn, affect outcomes. Structure symbolizes the characteristics of the settings in which care occurs. These characteristics include material resources (such as facilities, equipment, and financing), human resources (number and experience of personnel) and organizational structure that pertains to medical staff, the organization itself, and peer reviews. Structure refers to characteristics that affect the system's ability to meet the needs of individual patients or a community. Structural indicators illustrate the type of resources used by the organization to deliver services and relate to material and human resources. Examples of structure would include clinical guidelines revised periodically, access to specific technology (such as vascular access monitoring), and staffing of a dialysis facility (Himmelfarb, Perreira, Wesson, Smedberg, & Henrich, 2004).

Process refers to what is actually performed in the provision of care (such as the physician's activities in making a diagnosis, recommendation or implementation of treatment, or other actions with the patient). Process indicators evaluate what was provided to the patient and how well it was executed. Process indicators measure the activities of care. Examples would include the number of patients treated according to clinical guidelines and the number of patients on HD with vascular access assessment conducted prior to treatment.

Outcome measures indicate the effects of care provided to the patient. Outcomes indicate state of health following care provided. Outcome indicators capture the effect of care processes on a patient's well being. Some examples of outcome indicators include mortality, morbidity, quality of life, and patient satisfaction (Mainz, 2003).

All three provide valuable information to measure quality; however, most literature on the quality of care focuses on measuring processes of care. How does one measure process quality? By assessing the appropriateness of care and the interventions provided. Evaluating health benefits versus health risks is a component of determining the value of the intervention. Another way of measuring process quality is to determine if the care provided meets professional standards of care by the evaluation of quality indicators (IOM, 2001).

Quality Improvement Plan Concepts

One responsibility of the ESRD Networks is to identify facilities not meeting goals. The Network quality improvement staff work with facility staff to develop quality improvement plans to improve the identified areas. Areas targeted for improvement may include poor clinical performance, noncompliance with data and forms submission, and/or multiple grievances. To be able to implement CQI to address targeted areas, facilities need to have an effective quality improvement program. The quality improvement program should align with the facility's philosophies and mission, and reflect the expectations and standards of the entity represented. Approval by the facility's governing body should be documented in the QAPI meeting minutes and a timeline should be established for annual review.

The purpose of the quality improvement program is to ensure compliance to state, federal, and regulatory guidelines. The quality improvement program facilitates processes that methodically measure, assess, and improve performance to achieve high-quality outcomes through effective and efficient use of resources. This is accomplished via the QAPI committee. The scope of the quality improvement program should extend to all employees as defined in each role description. The use of critical thinking skills relates to how people improve the quality of their thinking, enabling them to analyze and assess problems (Knapp, 2007). The use of critical thinking skills can raise vital questions to problems and collect and assess pertinent information. Applying these skills can test the data against relevant criteria and standards to determine a course of action, engaging members of the team throughout the process. In a patient-centered care environment, the patient, the patient's family/significant others, and other members of the healthcare team collaborate to ensure the plan of care supports the needs identified in the assessment process. Levels of experience and knowledge of organizational standards, policies, and procedures contribute to the planning and implementation process. Constant evaluation and re-evaluation is needed to determine the outcome.

Documentation is an essential part of the critical thinking process, as supported by the old adage, if it was not documented, it was not done. Documentation provides a means to evaluate past interventions to determine if they were successful. The scientific approach using critical thinking assists the nurse to develop evidence-based practice.

The following scenario describes how critical thinking skills can be applied.

The Network data department notified your facility that the mandatory 2728 forms were submitted past the deadline. As the facility's manager, you review the facility's process for data submission to ensure it includes the correct timeline. You then review the actual forms for completion dates and identify the ones that were submitted late. After discussion with the staff member who recently assumed this task, you discover that the employee's training did not include the required timelines for compliance with data submission. The employee was educated concerning the required timelines, and the data were subsequently completed and documented.

Collaboration is important for effective team functioning. The work of each individual on the team, however efficient that person's contribution may be, still may not serve the overall effort to meet the need being addressed. An example of this may be applied to the previous scenario of data forms being submitted late to the Network office. If the person performing the orientation was of a different discipline than the employee (the trainee), the trainer may have inadvertently excluded the submission timelines as relevant information. Both team members were diligent in completing their understood tasks, although the result produced a negative outcome (in this scenario, submission of forms after the deadline). Using the facility's workflow process for the orientation would encompass the completion of the forms as part of the training. Using these processes in parallel can foster a positive outcome.

Care Coordination

Coordinating the multiple healthcare services used by the population of patients with ESRD is a challenge facing organizations. Coordination, sometimes referred to as clinical integration, is defined as "the extent to which patient care services are coordinated across people, functions, activities, and sites over time so as to maximize the value of services delivered to patients" (IOM, 2001, p. 133). This coordination features practitioners and health information systems intent to organize health services, patient needs, and information to facilitate patient-centered care. The *Conditions for Coverage* encourage coordination of care among all parties involved in the patient's care (CMS, 2008d). Coordination of care necessitates team interactions that when not communicated effectively, may cause conflict or delay in the delivery of care. Collaboration and shared accountability promote smoother transition of care. Care coordination across clinicians and

Figure 20-2
Conceptual Framework: Enhancing the Relationship between ESRD Networks and Providers

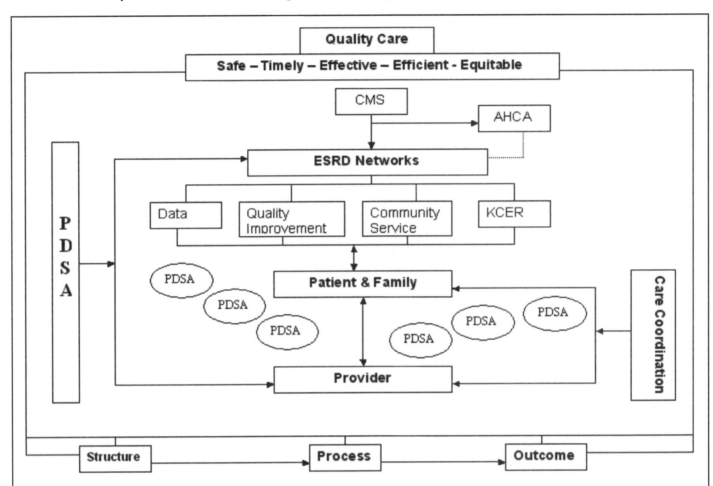

Notes: ESRD = end stage renal disease, CMS = Centers for Medicare and Medicaid Services, AHCA = Agency for Healthcare Administration, KCER = Kidney Community Emergency Response Coaltion, PDSA = Plan-Do-Study-Act.
Source: Brown, 2007; Donabedian, 2002; Himmelfarb et al., 2004; IOM, 2001.
Adapted and used with permission from Deuzimar Kulawik.

healthcare settings have been shown to result in greater efficiency and better clinical outcomes (IOM, 2001). Coordinating care for patients with several complex chronic conditions and acute episodes represents a challenge for healthcare systems and may require modification of care processes. It is important for patients and their families that the process for transferring patient-related information is accurate and available when needed.

How does one embrace this concept of care coordination? By involving patients and families/significant others in collaborating with the healthcare team to tap into all available and appropriate resources. Autonomy by some patients and their families to coordinate their care may raise opportunities for education on accessing information and technological support for conveying information to others involved in their care. A process within the healthcare delivery system is needed to ensure accurate and timely sharing of information. The monthly submission of the facility patient activity report to the

Network office is an example of coordination of care pertaining to data management. Providers' data are submitted electronically with the release of CROWN Web. CROWN Web has created a change in the data submission process by the facility, but it also provides the facility a mechanism to update patient and facility-specific data in real time. ESRD Networks play a vital role in supporting facilities with this new technology through collaboration with the facility teams.

Conceptual Framework: Enhancing the Relationship Between ESRD Networks and Providers

Using a CQI application as a framework adds an important dimension to identify boundaries of ESRD Networks and providers, establish priorities, and develop congruent interdisciplinary interventions. A framework assists the interdisciplinary team to decide what area or process needs improvement within the context of the Networks' perspective. The framework illustrates the relationship between key components, and it can be used to reinforce CQI practice. As a process, applying a framework can be a powerful tool to stimulate staff with a common set of expectations for effective program applicability (Himmelfarb et al., 2004).

The framework relies on the 10 rules for healthcare process reform suggested by the IOM (2001), which are:
- Care based on continuous healing relationship.
- Customization based on patient needs and values.
- The patient as the source of control.
- Shared knowledge.
- Evidence-based decision making.
- Safety as a system property.
- The need for transparency.
- Anticipation of needs.
- Continuous decrease in waste.
- Cooperation among clinicians (Brown, 2007).

The framework is patient-centered. Its implementation requires review of current practices in the organization and in the facility, continual rethinking of nursing practices, good understanding of care coordination, and the creation of new approaches to address patient education (see Figure 20-2).

Conclusion

The nephrology community understands that it can expect to continue to respond to changes in delivery of healthcare services to the ERSD population in the coming years. Nephrology healthcare providers may be caring for an increasingly complex patient population and providing care in a changing environment of rules and regulations as the healthcare system undergoes a transformation. Recent examples of changes having an impact on the nephrology community include CMS *Conditions for Coverage* and electronic data submission via CROWN Web (CMS, 2008d). The ESRD Networks will continue in their role of "promoting and improving the quality of care to patients with renal disease through education and the collection, analysis, and dissemination of data and information" (National Forum of ESRD Networks, n.d., a). Moving forward with a focus on the use of CQI problem-solving methodology will ensure nephrology nurses have the ability to implement changes, reach desired outcomes, and achieve excellence.

References

Agich, G. (2007). Healthcare organization responsibility for quality improvement. In B. Jennings, M.A. Baily, M. Bottrell, & J. Lynn (Eds.), *Healthcare quality improvement: Ethical and regulatory issues.* Garrison, NY: The Hastings Center.

Beecroft, D.G., Duffy, G., & Moran, J. (2003). *The executive guide to improvement and change.* Milwaukee, WI: American Society for Quality.

Brown, J.A. (2007). *The healthcare quality handbook: A professional resource and study guide* (22nd ed.). Pasadena, CA: JB Quality Solutions, Inc.

Byers, J.F., & Rosati, R.J. (2005). Foundation, techniques, and tools. In L.R. Pelletier & C.L. Beaudin (Eds.), *Q solutions: Essential resources for the healthcare quality professional* (pp. 1-76). Glenview, IL: National Association for Healthcare Quality (NAHQ).

Centers for Medicare and Medicaid Services (CMS). (n.d.). *Strategic plan ESRD network program July 06-June 09.* Retrieved December 14, 2008, from http://www.cms.hhs.gov/ESRDNetworkOrganizations/Downloads/StrategicPlanjanuary24final.pdf

Centers for Medicare and Medicaid Services (CMS). (2005). *Dialysis facility compare.* Retrieved March 4, 2009, from http://www.medicare.gov/Dialysis/Include/DataSection/Questions/SearchCriteria.asp?version=default&browser=IE|6|WinXP&language=English&defaultstatus=0&pagelist=Home

Centers for Medicare and Medicaid Services (CMS). (2006). *Summary of ESRD Network Program.* Retrieved March 4, 2009, from http://www.cms.hhs.gov/ESRDNetworkOrganizations/Downloads/ESRDNetworkProgramBackgroundpublic.pdf

Centers for Medicare and Medicaid Services (CMS). (2007). *2007 Annual Report ESRD Clinical Performance Measures Project: Opportunities to improve care for in-center hemodialysis and peritoneal dialysis patients.* Retrieved March 4, 2009, from http://www.cms.hhs.gov/CPMProject/Downloads/ESRDCPMYear2007Report.pdf

Centers for Medicare and Medicaid Services (CMS). (2008a). *End stage renal disease (ESRD) quality initiative overview.* Retrieved March 4, 2009, from http://www.cms.hhs.gov/ESRDQualityImproveInit/

Centers for Medicare and Medicaid Services (CMS). (2008b). *ESRD Network Program Goals: Strategic Plan ESRD Network Program July 06-June 09.* Retrieved March 4, 2009, from http://www.cms.hhs.gov/ESRDNetworkOrganizations/

Centers for Medicare and Medicaid Services (CMS). (2008c). *Fistula First.* Retrieved December 14, 2008, from http://www.fistulafirst.org

Centers for Medicare and Medicaid Services (CMS). (2008d). *Conditions for coverage.* Retrieved March 4, 2009, from http://www.cms.hhs.gov/CFCsAndCoPs/downloads/ESRDfinalrule0415.pdf

Centers for Medicare and Medicaid Services (CMS). (2008e). *Clinical Performance Measures Project.* Retrieved March 4, 2009, from http://www.cms.hhs.gov/cpmproject

Desai, A.A., Bolue, R., Nissenson, A., Bolus, S., Solomon, M.D., Khawar, O., et al. (2008). Identifying best practices in dialysis care: Results of cognitive interviews and a national survey of dialysis providers. *Clinical Journal of the American Society of Nephrology,* 1-11.

Donabedian, A. (2002). *An introduction to quality assurance in health care.* Oxford, United Kingdom: Oxford University Press.

End Stage Renal Disease (ESRD) Network of Texas, Inc. (n.d.). *Information for professionals.* Retrieved March 4, 2009, from http://www.esrdnetwork.org/professionals/quality-improvement/index.asp

Himmelfarb, J., Perreira, B., Wesson, D., Smedberg, P., & Henrich, W. (2004). Payment for quality in ESRD. *Journal American Society of Nephrology, 15,* 3263-3269.

Institute of Medicine (IOM). (2001). *Crossing the quality chasm: A new health system for the 21st Century.* Washington, DC: National Academies Press.

Institute of Medicine (IOM). (2006). *Crossing the quality chasm: The IOM health care quality initiative.* Retrieved March 4, 2009, from http://www.iom.edu/CMS/8089.aspx

Knapp, R. (2007). *Nursing education – The importance of critical thinking.* Retrieved March 4, 2009, from http://www.articlecity.com/articles/education/article_1327.shtml

Mainz, J. (2003). Defining and classifying clinical indicators for quality improvement. *International Journal for Quality in Health Care 15*(6), 523-530.

National Association for Healthcare Quality (NAHQ). (2007). *NAHQ code of ethics and standards of practice.* Retrieved December 23, 2008, from http://www.nahq.org/about/code.htm

National Fire Protection Association (NFPA). (2002a). *National fire alarm code.* Quincy, MA: Author.

National Fire Protection Association (NFPA). (2002b). *Standard for health care facilities.* Quincy, MA: Author.

National Fire Protection Association (NFPA). (2003). *New ambulatory health care occupancies, life safety code.* Quincy, MA: Author.

National Forum of ESRD Networks. (n.d.,a). *Welcome to the ESRD Network Forum.* Retrieved March 4, 2009, from http://www.esrdnetworks.org

National Forum of ESRD Networks. (n.d.,b). *Decreasing patient-provider conflict.* Retrieved March 4, 2009, from http://www.esrdnetworks.org/special-projects/copy_of_decreasing-patient-provider-conflict-dpc

National Kidney Foundation (NKF). (2001). *Executive summary – K/DOQI clinical practice guidelines.* Retrieved March 4, 2009, from http://www.kidney.org/professionals/kdoqi/guidelines/ doqi_upex.html

National Kidney Foundation (NKF). (2006). *Clinical practice guidelines and clinical practice recommendations: Hemodialysis adequacy: Update 2006.* Retrieved April 3, 2009, from http://www. kidney.org/Professionals/kdoqi/guideline_upHD_PD_VA/index.htm

National Kidney Foundation (NKF). (2008). *The facts about chronic kidney disease.* Retrieved March 4, 2009, from http://www.kidney. org/kidneyDisease/

Nelson, E.C., Batalden, P.B., & Godfrey, M.M. (2007). *Quality by design.* San Francisco: Jossey-Bass.

Peters, V.G., Clemons, G., & Augustine, B. (2005). "Fistula First" as a CMS breakthrough initiative: Improving vascular access through collaboration. *Nephrology Nursing Journal, 32*(6), 686-687.

Shortell, S.M., Bennett, C.L., & Byck, G.R. (1998). Assessing the impact of continuous quality improvement on clinical practice: What it will take to accelerate progress. *Milbank Quarterly, 789,* 590-634.

Walker, L.O., & Avant, K.C. (2004). *Strategies for theory construction in nursing* (4th ed.). Upper Saddle River, NJ: Prentice Hall.

Additional Readings

Bennis, W.G., & Thomas, R.J. (2002). *Geeks and geezers: How era, values, and defining moments shape leaders.* Boston: Harvard Business School Press.

Edgman-Levitan, S., Shaller, D., McInnes, K., Joyce, R., Coltin, K.L., & Cleary, P.D. (2003). *The CAHPS® improvement guide: Practical strategies for improving the patient care experience.* Cambridge, MA: Harvard Medical School.

Neufeldt, V., & Sparks, A.N. (Eds.). (2003). *Webster's new world dictionary.* New York: Simon & Schuster Inc.

Palmer, B. (2004). *Making change work: Practical tools for overcoming human resistance to change.* Milwaukee, WI: American Society for Quality.

Price, M., Fitzgerald, L., & Kisnman, L,. (2007). Quality improvement: The divergent views of managers and clinicians. *Journal of Nursing Management, 15,* 43-50.

Scott, C., (2006). How do you define process improvement? *International Journal of Newspaper Technology.* Retrieved March 4, 2009, from http://www.newsandtech.com/issues/2006/09-06/nt/09-06_cornish.htm

Stephen, C. (2008). *How to implement change effectively.* Retrieved March 4, 2009, from http://www.ehow.com/how_2181271_implement-change-effectively.html

Appendix A

Network – Quality Management/Quality Improvement Requirements

Many approaches have been designed for use in quality management/quality improvement. Network-recommended *Criteria and Standards Dialysis Facility Specific Quality Management* (ESRD Network of Texas, Inc., n.d.) include the following:

I.   Quality Management Program Structure
    A.   The facility operates a quality management program that includes:
        1.   *Quality planning*: Governing body Issues. This is the activity of developing the products and processes required to meet customer's needs.
        2.   *Quality control*: Data management and analysis. This consists of evaluating actual performance, comparing performance with goals and acting on the difference.
        3.   *Quality assessment performance improvement (QAPI)*: Identification of opportunities for and plans for improvement. This is the process of continuously striving to improve.

II. The Governing Body
    A.   Establishes the *quality mission* of the facility.
    B.   Conducts quality planning.
    C.   Allots sufficient time and resources to support an active quality management program.
    D.   Reviews the activities of the QAPI:
        1.   At a minimum quarterly.
        2.   Provides guidance.
        3.   Provides resources.
        4.   Revises goals.
        5.   Monitors improvement projects.

III. The program systematically:
    A.   Provides ongoing review of key elements of care utilizing:
        1.   Comparative data.
        2.   Trend data.
    B.   Identifies areas where performance measures or outcomes indicate an opportunity for or need for improvement.
    C.   Establishes interdisciplinary *improvement team(s)* who understand the process to:
        1.   Study and understand variation from desired outcomes.
        2.   Create and implement an improvement plan.
        3.   Evaluate success of the plan.
        4.   Conduct monitoring and improvement activities until:
            a.   Goals are achieved.
            b.   Data demonstrate that improvements have been made.
            c.   Data demonstrate that improvements are maintained.

IV. Meetings are conducted:
    A.   Monthly at a minimum by the QAPI:
        1.   Medical director.
        2.   Nurse manager.
        3.   Administrator.
        4.   Dietitian.
        5.   Social worker.
        6.   Technical services representative.
    B.   Frequently by the improvement teams.
    C.   Separately from patient care conferences.

D.   Complete and maintain minutes that reflect:
    1.   Conclusion of monitoring.
    2.   Evaluation and problem solving activities.
    3.   Include actions and dates of re-study until final resolution occurs.

V.   Quality Indicators
    A.   The facility establishes and monitors key/important aspects of care that:
        1.   Have acceptable levels of performance that are consistent with current professional knowledge.
        2.   Include, at a minimum, the ongoing monitoring of quality indicators for key aspects of patient care and facility operations.

VI. Key Aspect of Care: Hemodialysis Water Quality
    A.   Primary monitoring elements:
        1.   Maximum chloramines and maximum total chlorine.
        2.   Action and maximum bacteria for both product water and dialysate.
        3.   Action and maximum endotoxin for both product water and dialysate.
        4.   Chemical contaminants analysis and cultures.
        5.   Comprehensive water treatment logs completed accurately and appropriately.
        6.   Dialysate and acid mixing parameters, if applicable.
        7.   Other indicators of water quality specific to facility water treatment process.
    B.   Recommended reference(s) for facility standard development:
        1.   Association for the Advancement of Medical Instrumentation (AAMI) *Standards and Recommended Practices* (RD52) (CMS, 2008d).
        2.   CMS *Conditions for Coverage* (CMS, 2008d).
        3.   State-specific Department of State Health Services (DSHS) ESRD Facilities Licensing Rules.

VII. Key Aspect of Care: Dialysis and Other Medical Equipment Quality
    A.   Primary monitoring elements:
        1.   Routine preventive maintenance.
        2.   Equipment failure.
        3.   Testing equipment to include all items based upon manufacturer recommendations.
        4.   Logs complete, accurate results within acceptable limits.
    B.   Recommended reference(s) for facility standard development:
        1.   AAMI *Standards and Recommended Practices*.
        2.   State specific DSHS ESRD Facilities Licensing Rules.
        3.   CMS *Conditions for Coverage* (CMS, 2008d).
        4.   National Fire Protection Association (2002a, 2002b, 2003).
        5.   Manufacturers recommendations.
        6.   Organization policy and procedures.

VIII. Key Aspect of Care: Hemodialyzer Reuse Program
    A.   Primary monitoring elements:
        1.   Dialyzer performance measures.
        2.   Dialyzer labeling.
        3.   Sterilization.
        4.   Total cell volume on hollow fiber dialyzers.
    B.   Recommended reference(s) for facility standard development

1. AAMI *Standards and Recommended Practices.*
2. State specific DSHS ESRD Facilities Licensing Rules.
3. CMS *Conditions for Coverage* (CMS, 2008d).
4. Manufacturers recommendations.
5. NKF KDOQI Hemodialysis Adequacy (NKF, 2006).
6. Organization policy and procedures.

IX. Key Aspect of Care: Infection Control Practices
   A. Primary monitoring elements:
      1. Standard precautions for personnel and patients.
      2. Patient and employee infection control testing and monitoring:
         a. Immunizations (promotion, administration, tracking, trending).
      3. Pyrogenic reactions: Dialyzer, water, machine, and dialysate cultures.
      4. Peritonitis rate.
      5. Septic episodes.
      6. Document and investigate all episodes of infection; analyze the findings.
   B. Recommended reference(s) for facility standard development
      1. Centers for Disease Control and Prevention (CDC) *National Surveillance of Dialysis-Associated Diseases, United States Annual Report.*
      2. CDC *Recommendations for Serologic Surveillance for Hepatitis B Virus among Patients and Staff of Chronic Hemodialysis Centers.*
      3. AAMI *Standards and Recommended Practices.*
      4. State-specific DSHS ESRD Facilities Licensing Rules.
      5. CMS *Conditions for Coverage* (CMS, 2008d).
      6. Occupational Safety and Health Administration (OSHA), Occupational Exposure to Blood borne Pathogens Standard.
      7. Organizational policy and procedures.

X. Key Aspect of Care: Adverse Occurrence Reports (AORs)
   A. Primary monitoring elements:
      1. Adverse patient occurrence.
      2. Incidence rates.
      3. Ambulance transfers from facility to hospital.
   B. Recommended reference(s) for facility standard development:
      1. State specific DSHS ESRD Facilities Licensing Rules.
      2. CMS *Conditions for Coverage* (CMS, 2008d).
      3. Organizational risk management reports and statistics.

XI. Key Aspect of Care: Patient Mortality
   A. Primary monitoring elements:
      1. Each death.
      2. Facility rate.
   B. Recommended reference(s) for facility standard development
      1. CMS *Conditions for Coverage* (CMS, 2008d).
      2. *United States Renal Data Service (USRDS) Annual Report,* Reference Tables.
      3. *USRDS Standardized Mortality Ratio/Standardized Hospitalization Ratio Facility Specific Report.*
      4. Organizational risk management reports and statistics.

XII. Key Aspect of Care: Patient Hospitalization
   A. Primary monitoring elements:
      1. Each hospitalization.
      2. Facility rate.

      b. Recommended reference(s) for facility standard development.
      1. *USRDS Annual Report,* Reference Tables.
      2. *USRDS Standardized Mortality Ratio/Standardized Hospitalization Ratio Facility Specific Report.*
      3. Organizational risk management reports and statistics.

XIII. Key Aspect of Care: Complaints and Suggestions
   A. Primary monitoring elements
      1. Satisfaction evaluation:
         a. Patient and family.
         b. Staff.
         c. Report and analyze the feedback; develop action plan for improvement.
   B. Recommended reference(s) for facility standard development:
      1. CMS *Conditions for Coverage* (CMS, 2008d).
      2. Network quality improvement resource.
      3. Organizational aggregate and facility patient satisfaction survey data.

XIV. Key Aspect of Care: Staffing
   A. Primary monitoring elements:
      1. Orientation and training.
      2. Competency.
      3. Licensing and certification.
      4. Workload/ratios.
   B. Recommended reference(s) for facility standard development:
      1. State-specific DSHS ESRD Facilities Licensing Rules.
      2. CMS *Conditions for Coverage* (CMS, 2008d).

XV. Key Aspect of Care: Safety/Risk Management
   A. Primary monitoring elements:
      1. Fire/disaster preparedness.
      2. Hazardous waste disposal.
      3. Personnel protection/health monitoring.
      4. Physical plant inspection (such as floor tiles, lighting, rips or tears in chairs addressed).
   B. Recommended reference(s) for facility standard development:
      1. Network for resources.
      2. State-specific DSHS ESRD Facilities Licensing Rules.
      3. CMS *Conditions for Coverage* (CMS, 2008d).
      4. OSHA Occupational Exposure to Bloodborne Pathogens Standard; OSHA Hazard Communication Standard.

XVI. Key Aspect of Care: Medical Records
   A. Primary monitoring elements:
      1. Patient medical records.
   B. Recommended reference(s) for facility standard development:
      1. State-specific DSHS ESRD Facilities Licensing Rules.
      2. CMS *Conditions for Coverage* (CMS, 2008d).
      3. HIPAA regulations.
      4. Network resources.

XVII. Key Aspect of Care: Clinical Outcomes
   A. Primary monitoring elements:
      1. Laboratory core indicators – Adequacy, anemia, nutrition, mineral/bone metabolism, medical injuries, medical errors, health outcomes.
      2. Hospitalization rates.
      3. Vascular access types (catheters more than 90days,

arterio-venous fistulae (AVF), arterio-venous grafts (AVG).
4. Vascular access complications – Infections, patency, thrombosis events.
B. Recommended reference(s) for facility standard development:
1. CMS National Clinical Performance Measures (CPM) Reports.
2. CMS *Conditions for Coverage* (CMS, 2008d).
3. DSHS Quality of Care Indicators Report.
4. *USRDS Annual Report,* Hospitalization reference tables.
5. Organization patient outcome data and statistics.
6. NKF KDOQI *Practice Guidelines.*

XVIII. Key Aspect of Care: Patient Functional Status
A. Primary monitoring elements:
1. Vocational rehabilitation – Referrals as indicated.
2. Quality of life.
3. All patient care plans/conferences are complete and up-to-date.
   a. Follow the requirements listed in the CMS *Conditions for Coverage* (see CMS Measures Assessment Tool [MAT] [CMS, 2008d]).
4. Determine patient desire for activity:
   a. Patient education.
B. Recommended reference for facility standard development
1. CMS *Conditions for Coverage* (CMS, 2008d).
2. CMS *Conditions for Coverage* MAT.
3. *ESRD Network, Annual Statistical Data Report.*

4. *Life Options Rehabilitation Activity Report.*

XIX. Key Aspect of Care: Kidney Transplant Option Education
A. Primary monitoring elements:
1. Patient education.
2. Patient referral.
3. Transplant activity.
4. Document reason why patient is not a transplant candidate.
B. Recommended reference for facility standard development:
1. CMS *Conditions for Coverage* (CMS, 2008d).
2. *ESRD Network Annual Statistical Data Report.*
3. United Network of Organ Sharing (UNOS).
4. Organization data and statistics.

XX. Key Aspect of Care: Review Alerts/Faxes/Announcements
A. Primary monitoring elements:
1. Place a copy of the fax in QAPI minutes.
2. Implement appropriate action as described.
B. Recommended reference for facility standard development:
1. ESRD Networks.
2. State-specific DSHS.
3. CMS.
4. Federal Drug Administration (FDA).
5. CDC.
6. Manufacturers.

Appendix B

Understanding the Concept of CQI
Scenario 1 – Clinical Outcomes (Standardized Mortality Ratio)

The Network's Medical Review Board (MRB) conducted a review of the 2008 Dialysis Facility Reports to identify clinical areas for improvement. One of the clinical areas identified was a facility with a higher than expected standardized mortality ratio (SMR). The facility medical director and manager received notification from the Network that the facility was under Network focus review pertaining to the facility's high SMR. The facility was requested to complete a quality improvement plan signed off by the facility medical director to address not only the facility's mortality rate but also additional clinical indicators not meeting goals. A quality improvement plan template was provided. The facility was to submit clinical outcomes data monthly by the 15th of each month using a Network tracking tool. The letter stated that Network quality improvement staff were available to assist the facility in the development of the quality improvement plan and provide technical assistance.

Form an interdisciplinary QAPI committee and review the focus for the quality improvement plan with the medical director.

Plan
I. Prioritize and Select Opportunities
A. Identify additional quality indicators not meeting goal:
1. URR.
2. Use of central venous catheters (CVCs).
B. Brainstorm to identify root cause for each measure identified:
1. Cause and effect diagram.
2. Multi-voting to select 1 or 2 root causes for focus.
C. Develop a plan for improvement:

1. Who does what?
2. When?
3. With what tools?
4. With what training?

II. Design Monitoring
A. What baseline data?
1. 70% patients with URR greater than 65%.
2. 35% patients with CVCs.
B. Who will collect?
C. What are the goals?
1. 85% or more of patients with URR equal to or greater than 65%.
2. Decrease CVC rate to 10% or lower.
D. What are the timelines to meet the goals?
1. URR within 3 months.
2. CVC within 9 months.
E. How will we know a change has occurred?

III. Develop Quality Improvement Plan
A. Use available resources:
1. Action step: Contact Network quality improvement staff.
   a. Who: Facility manager.
   b. When: By date.
2. Action step: Review KDOQI guidelines.
   a. Who: Team.
   b. When: By date.
3. Action step: Conduct review of previous laboratory results, infections, and hospitalizations for all deaths.
   a. Who: Clinical coordinator.

      b. When: For each reported death.
      c. Where: Review in quality improvement meetings monthly.
  B. URR below target:
    1. Action step: Identify reasons patients sign off early.
      a. Who: Social worker.
      b. When: By date.
    2. Action step: Evaluate treatment times for patients with CVCs with physician.
      a. Who: Clinical coordinator.
      b. When: By date.
    3. Action step: Evaluate patients with CVC for permanent vascular access.
      a. Who: Vascular access manager.
      b. When: By date.
  C. CVC only:
    1. Action step: Identify reason for patient refusals.
      a. Who: Social worker.
      b. When: By date.
    2. Action step: Delay in referral time – Meet with surgeon(s) to develop protocol for vascular access referrals.
      a. Who: Facility manager and vascular access manager.
      b. When: By date.

Do
I. Implement the actions:
  A. SMR:
    1. Develop a tool to review clinical data on deceased patients.
  B. URR:
    1. Social worker to work with patients' issues for signing off early (for example, transportation, treatment time, and document in medical record).
    2. Clinical coordinator to obtain orders from physicians regarding treatment times and dialyzers, inform patient and staff of changes.
    3. Clinical coordinator and vascular access manager to review access referrals and adequacy results monthly using data tracking tool.
  C. CVC only:
    1. Social worker to report patient issues for patients refusing permanent access to clinical coordinator and medical director and document in medical record. Patient education will be provided for patients regarding issues and documented in medical record.
    2. Facility manager and vascular access manager will develop a procedure/algorithm based on surgeon and medical director input, and obtain governing body approval; conduct staff education.
    3. Facility manager will complete the monthly clinical indicator tracking tool and submit to the Network by the 15th of each month and report trended data in monthly QAPI meetings.

Study
I. Are mortality reviews addressed in QAPI meetings? Were any common threads identified? If so, was an action plan developed to address the issues?

II. Medical record audits will be conducted monthly to track treatment times for early patient sign off. What are the results of the audits? Review audits in QAPI meetings.

III. Was there an improvement in the URR for patients with low blood flow rates with new orders for treatment times?

IV. Are referrals for permanent access placement more timely using new protocol?

V. How is effectiveness of patient education monitored? Was a patient survey done? What were the results?

VI. Is the monthly clinical indicator tracking information submitted to the Network timely? Is the information being reviewed in QAPI meetings?

VII. Review of the improvement plan. Are there updates to the improvement plan when improvement is not evident?

Act
I. All documentation needs to be reflected in QAPI minutes.

II. Submit documentation to the Network and continue to submit monthly indicators.

III. Identify system changes implemented that have positive results for full implementation.

IV. Adopt the solutions resulting in improvement as a facility culture (not just for the project timeline).

VI. Plan ongoing monitoring of the solutions and continue to look for incremental improvements to refine the solutions.

VI. Continue to review the improvement plan in monthly QAPI meetings.

VII. For solutions not yielding positive outcomes, cycle back to the plan phase and repeat the PDSA cycle to investigate possible alternative root causes.

VIII. Communicate with the Network quality improvement staff for ongoing technical assistance of the project.

Appendix C

Understanding the Concept of CQI
Scenario 2 – Community Services

The Network did a routine review of the complaints and grievances that were received over the last quarter and identified a facility that had a pattern of complaints (3 or more complaints in the span of 3 months). The facility was contacted and a conversation was held with the clinical manager. The complaints consisted of unprofessional conduct which included different comments and behaviors exhibited by staff toward the patients.

Plan
I. Brainstorm Ways to Improve

II. Prioritize and Select Opportunities

III. Develop a Plan for an Improvement Trial
    A. Who does what?
    B. When?
    C. With what tools?
    D. With what training?

IV. Design Monitoring
    A. What baseline data?
    B. Who will collect?
    C. How will we know a change has occurred?

V. Develop an Improvement Plan
    A. Document the issue:
        1. Multiple patient complaints regarding lack of professionalism by the clinical staff.
    B. Determine interventions or changes needed (brainstorm options to prevent future occurrences):
        1. Formal professionalism training for all clinical personnel.
        2. Decreasing Patient-Provider Conflict Training (National Forum of ESRD Networks, n.d., b).
        3. Conduct staff and patient satisfaction surveys.
        4. Review staffing ratios (are there enough staff scheduled to perform the daily tasks competently and efficiently?).
    C. Designate a responsible person(s):
        1. ESRD Network patient services coordinator schedule an on-site visit to do professionalism training.
        2. Clinical manager to schedule a mandatory staff education time for patient services coordinator visit.
        3. Social worker to complete staff and patient satisfaction survey immediately and again at the completion of Decreasing Patient-Provider Conflict training.
        4. Clinical manager to review staff schedules and shift change over routines.
        5. Social worker to begin Decreasing Patient-Provider Conflict training for all staff; schedule half-hour training sessions over a period of 3 months ensuring all staff receive the entire training.
    D. Set the deadline completion:
        1. Clinical manager to collaborate with ESRD Network patient services coordinator to determine availability for training.
        2. Social worker to complete staff and patient surveys within 1 week.
        3. Social worker to begin Decreasing Patient-Provider Conflict training immediately.
    E. Clearly state the goal:
        1. The staff and patient satisfaction surveys will show increased satisfaction with care provided.

Do
I. Implement the Actions
    A. Provide educational resources to the social worker to perform with staff and patient satisfaction surveys immediately.
    B. Provide the decreasing patient-provider conflict training materials to the social worker to begin Decreasing Patient-Provider Conflict training for the staff immediately.
    C. Clinical manager to review staff schedules and shift change over routines immediately.
    D. Clinical manager to schedule ESRD Network patient services coordinator site visit as soon as possible.
    E. Communicate the deadlines and expectations.

Study
I. After the results of the satisfaction surveys are returned, review the outcomes.

II. What are the themes identified in the surveys?

III. Will the actions identified address the issues discovered in the surveys?

IV. Did the review of the staff schedule and turn around times decrease the conflict?

V. Present the findings at the monthly CQI meeting:
    A. Review the improvement plan.
    B. Update the improvement plan (did the actions get completed as outlined on the improvement plan?).

Act
I. Full documentation needs to be filed with the QAPI minutes (copies of the staff and patient satisfaction survey results, copies of the in-service sign in sheets).

II. Submit full documentation to the ESRD Network and continue to submit all relevant documentation until all training is completed.

III. Schedule follow-up staff and patient satisfaction surveys upon completion of Decreasing Patient-Provider Conflict training.

IV. Continue to review progress of the improvement plan with monthly QAPI meetings, verifying that training is going as planned and everyone is up to date with required sections of the training.

V. Corrective action for any employee not participating as required in the training process or failing to implement the patient quality of care strategies discussed in the training plan.

Appendix D

Understanding the Concept of CQI
Scenario 3 – Data Management

A facility did not meet the deadline for submitting their monthly Patient Activity Record (PAR) to the Network. The facility manager received a notification from the Network stating that the information was late and due immediately. Meeting the goals and objectives of the Network is a mandate that CMS requires from facilities for participation in the Medicare/Medicaid program. Implementation of CQI will address and correct the problem. Investigate the problem:

- Who should have submitted this form?
- Why was the PAR form not submitted?
- Was there adequate staffing?
- Was it a lack of knowledge?
- Was the information available to the assigned person (computer access, log updated as required)?

Note: The answers to these questions then become the foundation for development of the improvement plan.

In this example, the person who normally submits this information was on vacation and no other person in the organization was aware of the PAR report or the process to submit it. Upon return from vacation, the designated staff person promptly sent in the report.

Plan

I. Develop an Improvement Plan
A. Document the issue:
   1. Failure to submit PAR report timely.
B. Determine interventions or changes needed (brainstorm options to prevent future occurrences):
   1. Perform cross-training for a minimum of 2 other staff members in the execution of the report so that future reports will not be delinquent in the absence of the person primarily responsible for submitting it.
   2. Develop a binder that contains a procedure that outlines steps and directions, samples of forms, and applicable fax numbers and contact people as a resource/reference.
C. Designate a responsible person:
   1. Use the actual name of the person(s) (Jane Doe, John Smith).

D. Set the deadline for submission monthly:
   1. 5th of each month.
E. Clearly state the goal:
   1. The next month's PAR report will be submitted by the 5th day of the month.

Do

I. Implement the Actions
A. Provide the educational resources to train the staff who have been assigned the duty of submitting.
B. Communicate the deadlines and expectations.
C. Develop the binder that will be the resource/reference manual.

Study

I. Check How the Process Went on the 5th of the Next Month
A. Was the form submitted on time?
B. Did the person responsible use the binder resources?
C. Did the back up people check to make sure the PAR was submitted?
D. Was there an awareness of the importance of the PAR form?
E. Present the findings at the monthly CQI meeting.
F. Review the improvement plan and update (did the actions get completed as outlined on the improvement plan?).

Act

I. Form Successfully Submitted by the 5th of the Month and the Back-Up Personnel Aware that Form Had Been Submitted
A. The improvement plan is considered completed successfully.
B. Full documentation needs to be filed with the QAPI minutes, and the minutes should reflect the successful improvement made.
C. This new resource and training will now be routinely part of the operations of the facility.
D. If one of the designated people should resign or be unavailable for this duty, other personnel will need to be trained. This will permit at least 2 back-up personnel who are aware and competent to submit the report per the defined timeline.

Appendix E

Understanding the Concept of CQI
Scenario 4 – Disaster

You are the manager of a dialysis facility located on the Gulf Coast. The ESRD *Conditions for Coverage* require the facility to evaluate, at least annually, the effectiveness of the facility's disaster plan. Knowing this, you contact your ESRD Network to participate in a disaster drill being conducted in the local area by the Network and surrounding dialysis facilities. An evaluation of your facility's processes for disaster preparedness after the drill revealed a deficit in several areas that offered an opportunity for improvement. You discuss the outcome of the disaster drill at the next QAPI meeting with the medical director and quality improvement team with consensus to initiate a quality improvement plan. You assemble an interdisciplinary team and solicit assistance from the Network to have the Quality Improvement Coordinator participate in your improvement plan.

Plan

I.   Prioritize and Select Opportunities

II.   Identify Areas Requiring Improvement

III. Brainstorm to Identify Root Cause for Each Area Identified
A.   Cause and effect diagram.
B.   Multi-voting.

IV.   Develop a Plan for Improvement
A.   The Network staff member participates in your project and assists in establishing the channel of communication via conferencing during meetings and email.
1.   Who does what?
2.   When?
3.   With what tools?
4.   With what training?

V.   Design Monitoring
A.   What baseline data?
B.   Who will collect?
C.   What are the goals?
D.   What are the timelines to meet the goals?
E.   How will we know a change has occurred?

VI.   Develop Quality Improvement Plan
A.   Use available resources
1.   What: Network quality improvement staff/Kidney Community Emergency Response.
2.   Who: Facility manager and ESRD network staff.
3.   When: By date.
B.   Document the issues:
1.   Staff did not execute the call down system properly:
a.   Root causes identified:
i.   45% of the staff lost their call down lists.
ii.   35% of staff contact information was incorrect.
iii. 20% of patients did not have their 3 day emergency supplies.

b.   Root causes identified:
i.   Non compliance with preparedness.
ii.   Lack of funds.
C.   Determine interventions for each measure identified:
1.   Staff call down list:
a.   Update contact information.
b.   Wallet-size call down lists.
2.   3-day emergency supplies:
a.   Re-educate patients/families.
b.   Social Services consult funds/donations.

Do

I.   Implement the Actions
A.   Administrative assistant updated personnel contact information.
B.   Developed wallet-size cards to enter contact list.
C.   Education coordinator met with each patient/family to review disaster preparedness plans for emergency supplies with documentation in medical record.
D.   Social worker set up donations for emergency supplies.
E.   Repeat the disaster drill in 1 month.

Study

I.   Is there a process for monitoring call down lists for accuracy?

II.   How was patient education evaluated for effectiveness? Audit patients for emergency preparedness needs.

III. Were enough donations received to meet demands.

IV.   What were the results of the repeat drill? Were the actions implemented correctly?

Act

I.   All documentation needs to be filed in QAPI minutes.

II.   Identify system changes with positive results for unit-wide implementation.

III. Adopt solutions resulting in improvement.

IV.   Plan ongoing monitoring of the solutions, continue to look for incremental improvements to refine the solutions.

V.   For solutions not resulting in positive outcomes, cycle back to the plan phase and repeat the PDSA cycle to investigate possible alternate root causes.

VI.   Communicate with the Network quality improvement staff for ongoing technical assistance of the project.

| Chapter 20 | CONTINUING NURSING EDUCATION EVALUATION FORM | 1.4 Contact Hours |

CQI Application: Meeting the Challenges of ESRD Networks   **ANNP0920**

Applying Continuous Quality Improvement in Clinical Practice contains 22 chapters of educational content. Individual learners may apply for continuing nursing education credit by reading a chapter and completing the Continuing Nursing Education Evaluation Form for that chapter. Learners may apply for continuing nursing education credit for any or all chapters.

Please photocopy this test page, complete, and return to ANNA.
You can also download this form from www.annanurse.org (choose Education - CNE Activities - Publications)
Receive continuing nursing education credit (CNE) immediately by completing the CNE evaluation process in ANNA's Online Library. Go to www.annanurse.org, and click on the Online Library icon for more information.

Name: _____
Address: _____
City: _____ State: _____ Zip: _____
E-mail:_____ Preferred telephone: ☐ Home ☐ Work_____
State where licensed and license number: _____

CNE application fees are based upon the number of contact hours provided by the individual section. CNE fees per contact hour for ANNA members are as follows: 1.0-1.9 – $15; 2.0-2.9 – $20; 3.0-3.9 – $25; 4.0 and higher – $30. Fees for nonmembers are $10 higher.

CNE application fee for Chapter 20: ANNA member $15   Nonmember $25
ANNA Member: ☐ Yes ☐ No   ☐ Member # (if available) _____
☐ Check or money order enclosed   ☐ American Express   ☐ Visa   ☐ MasterCard
Total amount submitted:_____
Credit card number _____ Exp. Date _____
Name as it appears on the card: _____
NOTE: Your evaluation form can be processed in 1 week for an additional rush charge of $5.00.
☐ **Yes, I would like this evaluation form rush processed. I have included an additional fee of $5.00 for rush processing.**

Instructions
1. To receive continuing nursing education credit for an individual study after reading the chapter, complete this evaluation form.
2. Detach, photocopy, or download (www.annanurse.org) the evaluation form and send along with a check or money order payable to **American Nephrology Nurses' Assocation** to: ANNA, East Holly Avenue Box 56, Pitman, NJ 08071-0056.
3. Test returns must be postmarked by **April 30, 2011**. Upon completion of the answer/evaluation form, a certificate will be sent to you.

This section was reviewed and formatted for contact hour credit by Sally S. Russell, MN, CMSRN, ANNA Director of Education Services.

CNE Application Fee for Chapter 20
ANNA member = $15
Nonmember = $25

1. I verify that I have read this chapter and completed this education activity. _____Date _____
                                                                 Signature
2. What would be different in your practice if you applied what you have learned from this activity? (Please use additional paper if necessary.)
    _____
    _____
    _____
    _____

	Strongly disagree				Strongly agree
3. The activity met the stated objectives.					
a. Relate background pertaining to the ESRD Networks' work with dialysis facilities in improvement processes.	1	2	3	4	5
b. Discuss continuous quality improvement concepts applied to the clinical setting.	1	2	3	4	5
c. Describe a proposed framework for the working relationship between the ESRD Networks and dialysis providers.	1	2	3	4	5
d. Discuss a patient-centered approach using an established model for improvement.	1	2	3	4	5
4. The content was current and relevant.	1	2	3	4	5
5. The content was presented clearly.	1	2	3	4	5
6. The content was covered adequately.	1	2	3	4	5

7. How would you rate your ability to apply your learning to practice?   ☐ diminished ability   ☐ no change   ☐ enhanced ability

Comments _____
_____

8. Time required to read the chapter and complete this form: _____ minutes

Team Collaboration
In Continuous Quality Improvement

Billie Axley, MS, RN, CNN
Raymond Hakim, MD, PhD

Objectives

Study of the information presented in this chapter will enable the learner to:
1. Identify the continuous quality improvement team as an important part of the facility's quality assessment and performance improvement program.
2. Describe a formula for successful team collaboration with a common quality agenda.

Introduction

The patient dependent upon dialysis requires complex care and therapeutic input from multiple sources. A typical patient on dialysis is 65 years old and often presents with multiple co-morbidities, such as diabetes, heart disease, and/or vasculopathy, requiring treatment input from multiple medical specialties (U.S. Renal Data System [USRDS], 2008). These patients face several additional challenges. Most patients must deal with the logistics of round-trip transportation 3 times a week when dialyzed in a center. Dialysis treatments may last 4 hours or more, and patients may experience unpleasant symptoms during therapy (such as hypotension, nausea, muscle cramps). Dialysis treatments are delivered with complex equipment that patients may not understand, and as a result, may produce anxiety. Finally, patients must follow a complex diet, and many must take multiple medications.

Two formal teams are needed to provide comprehensive care to this complex patient population receiving care in a dialysis facility. One of the facility's formal teams, defined by the Center for Medicare and Medicaid Services (CMS) *Conditions for Coverage*, is an interdisciplinary team (IDT) (CMS, 2008). Its focus is to provide an individualized and comprehensive assessment of each patient's needs. The comprehensive assessment is used to develop the patient's treatment plan of care (CMS, 2008). The IDT consists of the patient or his or her designee and members of the healthcare team treating those with end stage renal disease (ESRD). The *most* important care team member is the patient, whose perspective and capabilities are needed to guide the recommendations of the IDT.

The other formal facility team is the quality assessment and performance improvement (QAPI) team. Its focus is the process of continuous quality improvement (CQI) for the quality of care provided to all patients in a facility (CMS, 2008). Professional members of the facility's IDT should participate in QAPI activities, and they are led by the facility's medical director (CMS, 2008).

The roles of each of these formal teams is defined and differentiated within the 2008 *Conditions for Coverage* (CMS, 2008). The focus of the IDT is on coordinated care for individual patients. The focus of the facility-based QAPI team is on the processes of care provided for all patients. These two formal teams are complementary in function. This chapter will focus on the facility-based, team collaboration needed in the QAPI program.

CMS Conditions for Coverage

The CMS *Conditions for Coverage* apply to patients on dialysis, and a part of these conditions require an active process for continuous quality improvement in the dialysis facility. The *Conditions for Coverage* identify the QAPI committee as the vehicle for this initiative. Each dialysis facility is expected to develop, implement, maintain, and evaluate an effective, data-driven QAPI program (CMS, 2008). The facility's IDT is also to be part of the QAPI. The team should consist of the IDT (such as the attending nephrologist), registered nurse (RN), masters-prepared social worker, and registered dietitian. Additional facility staff members can be involved in the work of the QAPI team, such as the patient care technician. In many facilities, the patient care technician, from both experience and observation in patient care, has the most face-to-face time with the patients. The patient care technician can identify processes that do not work well, as well as positively influence the culture of the clinic.

The *Interpretive Guidelines* for section V626 stipulate that the facility-based QAPI program's IDT must focus on indicators related to improved health outcomes (CMS, 2008). Data on current, professionally accepted clinical practice guidelines and standards must be used to track health outcomes. The *Interpretive Guidelines* address the requirement for prevention and reduction of medical errors, the charge for the QAPI program, and the reduction of such errors, mortality, and morbidities (CMS, 2008). CMS charges the facility's medical director to lead a CQI effort and to choose modifiable factors to measure and improve. According to Kliger (2007), it is important for the medical director to be knowledgeable about CQI and its use. Kliger (2007) also identifies resources for choosing modifiable factors to measure and improve. Patient safety initiatives include:
- National goals as defined by CMS.
- National Kidney Foundation (NKF) Kidney Disease Outcomes Quality Initiative Clinical Practice Guidelines (KDOQI™) (2009).
- Renal Physicians Association Clinical Practice Guidelines (Kliger, 2007).
- Kidney Disease Improving Global Outcomes (KDIGO) (2008).

Beyond the Minimal – Quality Assurance vs. Continuous Quality Improvement

The nephrology nurse can readily appreciate that CMS' expectation is for an effective QAPI program that is data-driven and focuses on improved health outcomes, as well as preventing and reducing medical errors (CMS, 2008). To achieve these expectations, the IDT needs to use the CQI process, and it must encompass perspectives from all members. In so doing, the team sets its own expectation that all team members are involved in the problem-solving processes.

Although processes are common to both, it is important to distinguish between a quality assurance program and a continuous quality improvement process. Quality assurance helps focus attention on important aspects of care by using retrospective audits and reviews to ensure that minimal standards are met. Quality assurance does not incorporate a prospective, "looking forward" process that focuses on a course of action that may lead to improvement in the quality of care. The quality assurance approach results in a crisis-oriented process of improvement. Wick (1993) indicated that while quality assurance increased awareness of issues/problems through data collection, it did little to produce consistent practice and process changes needed for lasting improvement. This is why the emphasis by the CMS *Conditions for Coverage* incorporates process improvement in the QAPI process.

When forming a QAPI team, the members should have intimate knowledge of the problem(s) to be addressed as well as steps needed to achieve quality outcomes. The team should be involved in defining the processes that need improvement. Teams must be interdisciplinary, and the members must have an interest in the outcome or results of the team's improvement project. Team members must work collaboratively, with regular communication about the evolving action plan for improvement. Deming's principles indicate that training and education about quality improvement concepts should be provided to all employees to enable them to work as effective and efficient teams (Deming, 2000).

Ongoing QAPI: The "Dream" Team

When CMS released the *Conditions for Coverage* in 2008, they included, for the first time, the condition of coverage specific to QAPI. This new condition speaks to the use of an IDT for CQI activities in every facility. This facility-based QAPI team is led by the medical director. The ideal QAPI team capitalizes on all talents and ideas of team members. This is based upon a central tenant of CQI that everyone is a valued team member, recognizing each one has different abilities and capabilities. Adoption of the philosophy of cooperation creates a win-win situation, fostering a sense of ownership of the improvement process by the team (Stratton, 1994). The effective QAPI team requires ongoing open dialogue and sharing of ideas, and optimizes talents of the team members. Thus, the CQI problem-solving method in QAPI is based upon teamwork and developing leadership to improve patient-specific and facility-wide outcomes, as well as using root cause analysis to define process(es) in need of improvement. (Editor's Note: Please see Chapter 3: "Root Cause Analysis for Lasting Quality Improvement," addressing the use of root cause analysis.)

For QAPI to become a reality in the dialysis facility, there is an important partnership that often correlates with the success of the program. The pivotal partnership is between the facility's medical director and the nephrology nurse functioning

as clinical manager. The facility medical director has operational responsibility for a facility's QAPI program and the delivery of patient care and outcomes in the facility (CMS, 2008). Working together, the medical director and the clinical manager are in a position to define system failures, process errors, and performance gaps. It is important for these two facility leaders, in conjunction with the facility QAPI-IDT, to prioritize facility improvement activities (CMS, 2008). (Note: One resource for addressing considerations in prioritizing improvement activities is provided by the *Conditions for Coverage* Tag V639 [CMS, 2008].) The QAPI team can use these guidelines by looking at the prevalence of a problem, the severity of a problem, the impact on clinical outcomes, and the impact on patient safety to prioritize improvement activities.

Working collaboratively, the facility medical director and clinical manager are able to set the expectations, assist in building the team, and support the culture of CQI and its activities. Examples of spreading the CQI culture include making CQI a part of every staff meeting and communicating CQI progress and ideas on a bulletin board. For example, if a team is working on a CQI process, it can post the idea on an easily accessible board in a common area. This provides an opportunity for facility staff to participate in the process by documenting their ideas on sticky notes and posting them. It is important to acknowledge staff members' involvement in the CQI process in their performance evaluations. The QAPI team also needs to interact and communicate with other nephrologists who care for patients in the facility. Although these attending physicians are not officially part of the QAPI team as mandated by CMS, they must be aware of the QAPI's activities. The role of the medical director is to share QAPI goals and performance improvement initiatives, and engage the attending physicians in the CQI process (CMS, 2008).

A Formula for a Successful CQI Project: Team Collaboration and Participatory Leadership

Deming (2000) emphasized the concept that effective leadership is required to support the "culture improvement of processes" (p. 168), and that the aim of leadership is "...to improve performance, to improve quality, to bring pride of workmanship" to the team and to "...remove causes of failure" (p. 248). Moss (1996) explains that the words "team" or "teamwork" are often used loosely, that a group is not automatically a team, and becoming a team requires leadership. Leadership must be involved in setting the expectation of not being content with how well things are going and always asking, "Can we do better?" Deming (2000) advocated for team members to rotate serving as the "leader," resulting in participatory leadership. What are the important attributes needed when leading a QAPI team? A leader exhibits a "team attitude," values every member, and leads by example. The leader works with the team to establish goals or the team's common mission. It is a common mission or goal that binds the team together and sets the stage for active staff participation through the change process (Moss, 1996). The leader is the team member responsible for establishing a communication system within the team. The leader must share knowledge, ideas, and goals in such a way as to inspire positive and effective action (Wick, 2006)

An established communication system decreases opportunities for confusion and keeps all team members informed of the status of the activities of each team member. Successful communication strategies are critical in overcoming barriers to implementation of improvement and carry an emphasis on frequent bi-directional exchange (Sharek et al., 2007). Communication strategies can consist of formal and informal methods, which may include:

- Group dialogue.
- An exchange of ideas.
- Brainstorming sources of problems.
- Discussion of action steps to address problems.

Formal methods may include:

- A staff meeting.
- The QAPI meeting.
- An action plan.
- A formal presentation of each team member's efforts and results.
- Email communication to team members.
- Written memos posted in the break room.
- Newsletters to keep all facility team members informed of the QAPI team's activities.

In addition to a communication system, the team leadership puts a team problem-solving mechanism in place. Conflict and disagreement are normal in human relationships. Team members can be in conflict for a variety of reasons. Team members may differ on the appropriate focus or critical steps to help improve an outcome, or they may differ because they do not share the same life experiences or values (Wick, 2006). Disagreement can be healthy because it can initially get all members on the team involved and help them articulate their differences. Disagreement can also provide an opportunity to learn about and recognize differences of opinion; good leadership results in the generation of new ideas. It is essential to resolve disagreements. If left unmanaged with suppressed emotions or conditions that are not expressed, conflict will become a factor that interrupts the learning and work of the team (Gerzon, 2006). A mutually acceptable solution can often be found with effective communication – talking out differences in an honest, considerate, and respectful manner (Wick, 2006). The leader must guide the team in dealing with conflict to avoid paralyzing its efforts with over-analysis of the conflict. According to Wick (2006), effective problem solving takes two rights – the right attitude and the right action plan.

The leader launches a team mechanism for evaluation and feedback, and establishes the expectation of peer-to-peer feedback. Honest and constructive feedback is critical to team members in improving their skills and ensuring their work is successful (Wick, 2006). The leader makes a plan for providing feedback on a continuous basis. One method is to provide visible measurements of success. This can include posting the achieved results on a chart in a "quality corner" of a bulletin board in a commonly accessible location. Weekly updates of progress made in the performance improvement project keeps staff members informed and engaged in the process. When team members achieve success, it is important to celebrate small improvements along the way. The price of celebrating the team's success becomes "priceless," providing positive feedback that helps the entire team feel appreciated and energized! When asked, staff members will reveal that they are especially appreciative when the physician, medical director, and/or clinical manager acknowledge the success of the team. A few examples of moderate celebrations include:

- An ice cream social.
- Pizza lunch.
- Certificate of Acknowledgment for CQI project team members after successful outcomes.
- An area-wide celebration event at the end of the year, including public acknowledgment of teams' CQI projects completed over the past year.

Inviting patients, their families, and significant others to participate in many of these activities clearly engages and reassures them in the process of improvement and celebrating its success.

A CQI Experience Driven by a Multi-Facility Action Plan

What are the characteristics of a quality improvement activity? According to Johansen (2007), a quality improvement activity should target an important clinical problem for which performance is below goal. Once the problem is identified, a QAPI team can be convened and the PDCA cycle initiated.

Selecting the Process or Problem to Improve

Example: A geographic area encompassing multiple facilities is selected for a CQI project to address reducing missed treatments.

- During a review of monthly data, an improvement opportunity was identified and was chosen to focus on decreasing the number of patients not presenting for their scheduled hemodialysis treatments. Data showed a worsening trend in "no shows"/patient/year, moving from below 1.5 up to 2.6 "no shows"/patient/year.

Team members selected for the improvement project:

- Facility assistant (unit administrative assistant)
- Social worker.
- RN.
- Patient representative.
- 2 patient care technicians.
- Renal dietitian.
- Medical director.

The performance improvement team reviewed available scientific literature to help better understand the scope of the problem. Literature analyzed included work by Unruh, Evans, Fink, Powe, and Meyer (2005), whose study utilized data from the Choices for Healthy Outcomes in Caring for End-Stage Renal Disease (CHOICE). The results of this study revealed that missed treatments equal to or greater than 3% of treatments were associated with a 69% increase in the risk for death. This estimate of risk of death from missed treatments was greater than in earlier work from the Dialysis Outcomes and Practice Patterns Study (DOPPS) study, which showed a 30% increase in the risk for death when patients missed greater than or equal to 1 treatment/month or greater than or equal to 7% of treatments (1/13) (Saran et al., 2003).

Determining the Goal

The information from the CHOICE study suggested that the dialysis team may have the potential to prevent premature death by working with targeted high-risk patients to understand their reasons for non-adherence and planning interventions with them (Unruh et al., 2003). The QAPI team developed a measurable goal to be achieved within a specific timeframe.

- Baseline data: A worsening trend over a year: 2.6 "no-shows"/patient/year at risk.
- Organizational target: Less than 1.5 "no shows"/ patient/year at risk.
- Goal: Reduce "no shows" rate to less than 1.5 "no shows"/patient/year at risk over 12 months.

Root Cause Analysis

The team met to perform a root cause analysis. The trends in data were reviewed for the past year and confirmed a worsening trend, with the last month report indicating 2.6 missed treatments/patient/year. This information triggered the need for additional analysis that included:

- Facility data analysis for patterns of missed treatments.
- Identify risk factors for patients who are missing treatments:
  - Renal dietitian to track trends of individual patients missing treatments.
  - Social worker to interview patients for reasons for missing treatments.
- Identify process related factors:
  - Treatment schedule?
  - Transportation?
  - Environmental?

Two Key Causes for Performance Improvement Focus Selected

Using the fishbone CQI tool to brainstorm for possible causes, the improvement team selected two root causes:

- Lack of team approach to problem solving of patient "no shows."
- Low level of understanding by team members of specific reasons for "no shows."

Plan (see Figure 21-1)

The medical director will provide an educational session to the performance improvement team based on the CHOICE study. This will bring all team members up to date with the same information of adverse outcomes of "no shows" for dialysis treatments. The medical director will share the quality improvement process with other attending nephrologists and encourage their active participation.

- The team will initiate a poster contest with the opportunity for staff and patients to participate. The focus is to provide education for patients on the dangers associated with missing treatments. Posters will be placed on walls in the patient waiting room.
- Renal dietitians will address the effects of missing treatments in laboratory reviews with patients.
- The social worker will focus on ensuring that transportation was not a barrier to keeping appointments.
- The patient care technician will post "No-Show Questions to Ask" next to each phone.

Figure 21-1

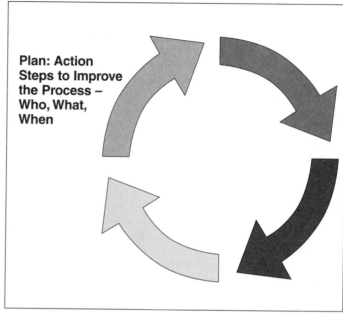

Plan: Action Steps to Improve the Process – Who, What, When

Source: Adapted from Deming, 2000.
Used with permission from Raymond Hakim and Billie Axley.

- The charge nurse or social worker will follow up with "no-show" patients at the next treatment attended.
- Staff will form "teams" of patients by shifts for team encouragement to reduce "no shows."
- The social worker will involve family members in encouraging patients to attend treatments.
- The attending physician will discuss the initiative with specific patients who are more at fault and contribute more to the "no-show" rate in a facility.

Do (see Figure 21-2)

The Poster Contest:

- Staff members and patients teamed up to make posters to ensure education of all patients on the dangers associated with missing treatments and posted it in the patient waiting room
- The teams used "Top 10 Reasons to Come and Complete Your Dialysis Treatment Every Time" for poster themes. The list included:
  - Sense of well-being.
  - More energy.
  - Improved appetite.
  - Awake refreshed and sleep better.
  - Achieve targeted weight.
  - Less itching.
  - Be mentally alert.
  - Normal breath odor.
  - Fewer hospital stays.
  - Longer life.
- Patients voted on best poster.
- Staff encouraged patients to ask questions concerning posted information.

Figure 21-2

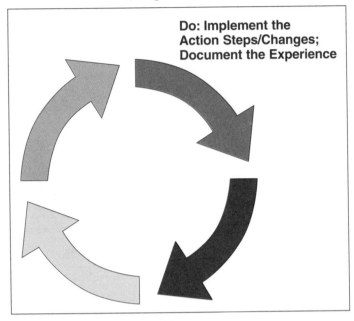

Do: Implement the Action Steps/Changes; Document the Experience

Source: Adapted from Deming, 2000.
Used with permission from Raymond Hakim and Billie Axley.

- Renal dietitians included the effect of missing treatments in laboratory reviews with patients.
- Renal dietitians put gold stars on the report cards of patients not missing any treatments in past month.

"Teams" of patients by shifts were formed for encouragement of all patients on the shift to come to treatment:
- The names of all patients who attended all treatments and completed them during the month were placed in a drawing.
- Winner received a funny "crown" made of paper and encouraged to wear it at least on drawing day.
- All patients received a happy treat (inexpensive and RD approved) on day of drawing.
- Patients were given a "certificate" to take home to family showing how many treatments the patient received in the past month.

"No-Show Questions to Ask" – Laminated and posted at each phone:
- Is there a reason you want to skip your treatment today? (If the reason is because the patient is sick, have a nurse continue through the rest of this list with the patient.)
- Do you need to go to the hospital?
- What would you like to do to make up the time you are missing? (Patient to come in later that day, re-schedule treatment, come in for at least a shorter treatment.)
- Are you worried about something that makes you feel uncomfortable to come to your treatment? Is there something we could do to help you feel more comfortable today so that you could still come to your treatment?
- Is there a specific person you would like to talk to who could help you today?

Charge Nurse or social worker follows up on "no shows:"
- Call patient's home or work.
- Call emergency contact numbers; express concern for the patient's welfare.
- If contact is unsuccessful, approach the patient at the next treatment in the facility, expressing concern for the patient's welfare.
- The patient's nephrologist is notified of "no shows" for additional patient-physician interaction and discussion; also to be addressed in the IDT plan of care.
- Sit down and offer to explore perceived barriers to attending treatment with the patient.

Check (see Figure 21-3)
Average "no-show" rate for all facilities moved from 2.6/patient/year at risk down to:
- Quarter 1 – 2.6/patient/year at risk.
- Quarter 2 – 2.5/patient/year at risk.
- Quarter 3 – 1.8/patient/year at risk.
- Quarter 4 – 1.4/patient/year at risk.

In Quarter 4, the "no show" rate was less than or equal to 1.5 no shows/patient/year at risk – Goal met!

Act (see Figure 21-4)
- Incorporate successful action steps into facility's routine/culture.
- Set new goal; 90% of "no show" patients to "make-up" missed treatment within 7 days.
- Celebrate success!
- Invite patients and their families to an informal gathering:
  - Provide renal dietitian-approved finger-foods!
  - Music!

For an algorithm depictingmissed hemodialysis treatments, see Appendix A.

Closing the Loop
The *Conditions for Coverage* (Tag V638 [b] Standard: Monitoring performance improvement) and the accompanying *Interpretive Guidelines* state that once improvement is made, the facility must have a mechanism to ensure that improvement is sustained (CMS, 2008). This mechanism could include:
- Practice audits.
- Review of laboratory data and other records.
- Repeat patient satisfaction surveys.

Closing the loop by the QAPI team can be accomplished by having them answer the following questions:
- Did outcomes improve as a result of the action steps?

If improvement did not occur:
- Did the team repeat the root cause analysis to select 1 to 2 new root causes and develop a new actions steps?

If improvement did occur:
- Were the actions resulting in improvement incorporated into the facility routine?

Figure 21-3

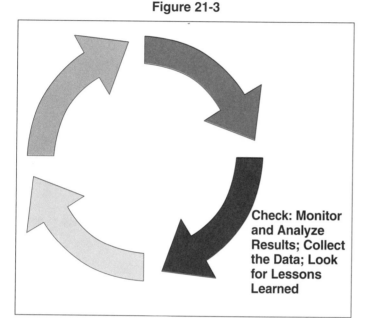

Check: Monitor and Analyze Results; Collect the Data; Look for Lessons Learned

Source: Adapted from Deming, 2000.
Used with permission from Raymond Hakim and Billie Axley.

Figure 21-4

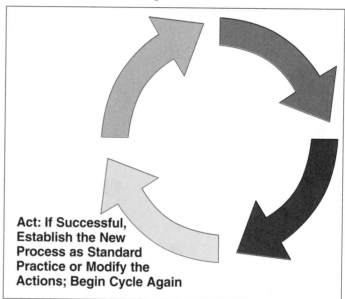

Act: If Successful, Establish the New Process as Standard Practice or Modify the Actions; Begin Cycle Again

Source: Adapted from Deming, 2000.
Used with permission from Raymond Hakim and Billie Axley.

Conclusion

The goal of the QAPI team is to improve the process leading to outcomes that are known to have an impact on patients' well being, quality of life, and survival. Nephrology nurses know that a good team will produce quality outcomes in any setting. A healthcare organization that is proud to provide quality service almost universally will have a solid team behind it. Those team members are viewed as true partners in a culture of collaboration in pursuit of improvement. Deming, in his work with quality improvement, reminds us to constantly examine our roles in improving quality and to take action (Deming, 2000). Improvement of patient outcomes is the vision, common goal, and mission. QAPI teams will always have a common goal: optimal patient care and outcomes.

References

Centers for Medicare and Medicaid Services (CMS). (2008). *ESRD facility conditions for coverage.* Retrieved February 10, 2009, from http://www.cms.hhs.gov/CFCsAndCoPs/downloads/ESRDfinalrule0415.pdf

Deming, W.E. (2000). *Out of the crisis.* Cambridge, MA: Massachusetts Institute of Technology, Center for Center for Advanced Educational Services. Retrieved February 10, 2009, from http://books.google.com/books?hl=en&lr=&id=LA15eDlOPgoC&oi=fnd&pg=PR7&dq=Deming&ots=MrdsqTkPIq&sig=corbcBkOr-TwivUXejJD8zQA5Z0#PPR15,M1

Gerzon, M. (2006). *Leading through conflict: How successful leaders transform differences into opportunities.* New York: Harvard Business School Press. Retrieved February 10, 2009, from http://books.google.com/books?id=k7sqNl6i-8sC&printsec=copyright&dq=conflict#PPP10,M1

Johansen, K.L. (2007). Value of quality improvement reporting. *Clinical Journal of American Society of Nephrology, 2,* 1104-1105.

Kidney Disease: Improving Global Outcomes (KDIGO). (2008). Homepage. Retrieved March 24, 2009, from http://www.kdigo.org

Kliger, A.S. (2007). The dialysis medical director's role in quality and safety. *Seminars in Dialysis, 20*(3), 261-264.

Moss, M.T. (1996). Self-managed work teams: The rainbow model. *Nursing Economic$, 14*(3), 185-186.

National Kidney Foundation (NKF). (2009). *The National Kidney Foundation Kidney Disease Outcomes Quality Initiative™.* Retrieved February 10, 2009, from http://www.kidney.org/professionals/ KDOQI/

Saran, R., Bragg-Gresham, J.L., Rayner, H.C., Goodkin, D.A., Keen, M.L., van Dijk, P.C., et al. (2003). Non-adherence in hemodialysis: Associations with mortality, hospitalization, and practice patterns in the DOPPS. *Kidney International, 64,* 254-262.

Sharek, P.J., Mullican, C., Lavanderos, A., Plamer, C., Snow, V., Kmetick, K., et al. (2007). Best practice Implementation: Lessons learned from 20 paratnerships. *Joint Commission Journal on Quality and Patient Safety, 33*(12), 16-26.

Stratton, B. (1994). Gone but never forgotten. *Quality progress.* Retrieved December 3, 2008, from http://deming.org/index.cfm?content=654

Unruh, M.L., Evans, I.V., Fink, N.E., Powe, N.R., & Meyer, K.B. (2005). Skipped treatments, markers of nutritional nonadherence, and survival among incident hemodialysis patients. *American Journal of Kidney Disease, 46*(6), 1107-1116.

U.S. Renal Data System (USRDS). (2008). *Annual data report – 2008: Atlas of chronic kidney disease and end-stage renal disease in the United States.* Bethesda, MD: National Institutes of Health, National Institute of Diabetes and Digestive and Kidney Diseases. Retrieved February 10, 2009, from http://www.usrds.org/adr.htm

Wick, G. (1993). Continuous quality improvement: A problem-solving approach (Part 2). *Nephrology Nursing Today, 3*(2), 1-8.

Wick, G. (2006). *Leadership: Pearls for understanding and living it.* Paper presented at the meeting of the American Nephrology Nurses' Association. April 2, 2006, Volunteer Leader Organization Workshop, Nashville, TN.

Additional Readings

Paton, S.M. (2006). *Four days with W. Edwards Deming.* Retrieved February 10, 2009, from http://deming.org/index.cfm?content=653

Plantinga, L.C., Fink, N.E., Jarr, B.G., Sadler, J.H., Levin, N., Coresh, J., et al. (2007). Attainment of clinical performance targets and improvement in clinical outcomes and resource use in hemodialysis care: A Prospective cohort study. *BMC Health Services Research.* Retrieved February 10, 2009, from http://www.biomedcentral.com/1472-6963/7/5

Appendix A

A Sample Algorithm to Address and Monitor Missed Hemodialysis Treatments: "No Shows"

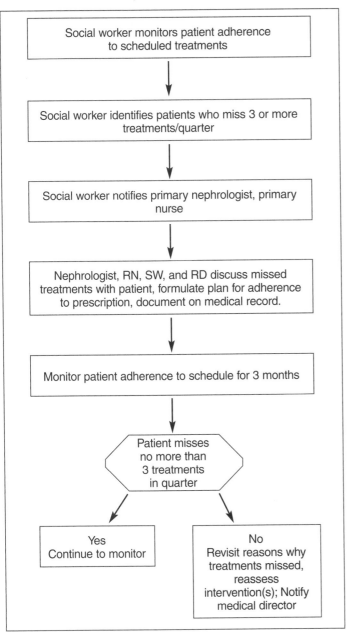

Source: Used with permission from Karen C. Robbins, 2009.

| Chapter 21 | **CONTINUING NURSING EDUCATION EVALUATION FORM** | **1.2 Contact Hours** |

Team Collaboration in Continuous Quality Improvement

ANNP0921

Applying Continuous Quality Improvement in Clinical Practice contains 22 chapters of educational content. Individual learners may apply for continuing nursing education credit by reading a chapter and completing the Continuing Nursing Education Evaluation Form for that chapter. Learners may apply for continuing nursing education credit for any or all chapters.

Please photocopy this test page, complete, and return to ANNA.
You can also download this form from www.annanurse.org (choose Education - CNE Activities - Publications)
Receive continuing nursing education credit (CNE) immediately by completing the CNE evaluation process in ANNA's Online Library. Go to www.annanurse.org, and click on the Online Library icon for more information.

Name: _____

Address: _____

City: _____ State: _____ Zip: _____

E-mail: _____ Preferred telephone: ☐ Home ☐ Work _____

State where licensed and license number: _____

CNE application fees are based upon the number of contact hours provided by the individual section. CNE fees per contact hour for ANNA members are as follows: 1.0-1.9 – $15; 2.0-2.9 – $20; 3.0-3.9 – $25; 4.0 and higher – $30. Fees for nonmembers are $10 higher.

CNE application fee for Chapter 21: ANNA member $15   Nonmember $25

ANNA Member: ☐ Yes ☐ No   ☐ Member # (if available) _____

☐ Check or money order enclosed   ☐ American Express   ☐ Visa   ☐ MasterCard

Total amount submitted: _____

Credit card number _____ Exp. Date _____

Name as it appears on the card: _____

NOTE: Your evaluation form can be processed in 1 week for an additional rush charge of $5.00.

☐ **Yes, I would like this evaluation form rush processed. I have included an additional fee of $5.00 for rush processing.**

Instructions

1. To receive continuing nursing education credit for an individual study after reading the chapter, complete this evaluation form.

2. Detach, photocopy, or download (www.annanurse.org) the evaluation form and send along with a check or money order payable to **American Nephrology Nurses' Association** to: ANNA, East Holly Avenue Box 56, Pitman, NJ 08071-0056.

3. Test returns must be postmarked by **April 30, 2011.** Upon completion of the answer/evaluation form, a certificate will be sent to you.

This section was reviewed and formatted for contact hour credit by Sally S. Russell, MN, CMSRN, ANNA Director of Education Services.

CNE Application Fee for Chapter 21
ANNA member = $15
Nonmember = $25

---

1. I verify that I have read this chapter and completed this education activity. _____ Date _____
Signature

2. What would be different in your practice if you applied what you have learned from this activity? (Please use additional paper if necessary.)

_____
_____
_____
_____

	Strongly disagree				Strongly agree
3. The activity met the stated objectives.					
a. Identify the continuous quality improvement team as an important part of the facility's quality assessment and performance improvement program.	1	2	3	4	5
b. Describe a formula for successful team collaboration with a common quality agenda.	1	2	3	4	5
4. The content was current and relevant.	1	2	3	4	5
5. The content was presented clearly.	1	2	3	4	5
6. The content was covered adequately.	1	2	3	4	5
7. How would you rate your ability to apply your learning to practice?	☐ diminished ability		☐ no change		☐ enhanced ability

Comments _____
_____

8. Time required to read the chapter and complete this form: _____ minutes

---

This educational activity is provided by the American Nephrology Nurses' Association (ANNA).
ANNA is accredited as a provider of continuing nursing education (CNE) by the American Nurses Credentialing Center's Commission on Accreditation (ANCC-COA).
ANNA is a provider approved of continuing nursing education by the California Board of Registered Nursing, provider number CEP 00910.
This CNE offering meets the Nephrology Nursing Certification Commission's (NNCC's) continuing nursing education requirements for certification and recertification.

Continuous Quality Improvement And Research in Nursing

Veronica Legg, MS, RN, FNP-BC

Objectives

Study of the information presented in this chapter will enable the learner to:
1. Define continuous quality improvement.
2. Understand basic tools of continuous quality improvement.
3. Explain the difference between continuous quality improvement and research.

Overview

This chapter highlights the history of continuous quality improvement, basic tools, and an understanding of how continuous quality improvement and research interact.

Introduction/Background

Quality assurance, quality improvement, and *continuous quality improvement* are all terms that have become integrated into the vocabulary of the healthcare system. Quality improvement awareness has its roots in the industrial sector of the 1930s, and leaders such as Walter Shewhart, J.M. Juran, Avedis Donabedian, and W. Edwards Deming introduced the concepts of measuring and enhancing quality through systematic processes and scientific inquiry.

In the healthcare industry, the road to quality began when The Joint Commission (formed in 1952 as the Joint Commission on Accreditation of Healthcare Organizations) set standards for the accreditation of hospitals. Initially, these were minimum standards, such as administrative structure, as well as physical plant and equipment (Luce, Bindman, & Lee, 1994). In 1966, Avedis Donabedian published an article describing the definition and processes of quality in health care (Donabedian, 1966). The Joint Commission broadened its standards and embraced the Donabedian model of Structure-Process-Outcomes. This model, and the many processes derived or influenced by it, is still in use throughout the healthcare industry today.

This chapter will review the definitions, models, processes, and tools used to inspect, evaluate, and improve quality and how these components relate to the research process.

Quality

In order to understand the processes and measurements used to improve quality in health care, basic concepts first need to be understood.

Quality Healthcare

The Agency for Healthcare Research and Quality (n.d.) defines quality health care as:
- Doing the right thing (getting the healthcare services you need).
- At the right time (when you need them).
- In the right way (using the appropriate test or procedure).
- To achieve the best possible results.

Further, "quality assurance can be defined as all activities that contribute to defining, designing, assessing, monitoring, and improving the quality of health care" (Quality Assurance Project, n.d.).
- Quality improvement is "an approach to the study and improvement of the processes of providing healthcare services to meet the needs of clients" (Quality Assurance Project, n.d.).
- Continuous quality improvement (CQI) builds on quality assurance and quality improvement by adding the concept of a continual process and emphasizing that it is usually the process, not the people, that are the cause of the problem (Deming, 1986).

History of Continuous Quality Improvement

Continuous quality improvement owes its conception to Dr. Walter Shewhart and Shewhart's Cycle of Plan-Do-Study-Act (PDSA) (Langley, Nolan, Nolan, Norman, & Provost, 1996). This cycle became the basis for a focused "trial and error" approach, or more aptly, a "trial and learning" method. One begins this with the plan and ends with an action which then, based on the learning gained from the previous PDSA phases of the cycle, results in the desired improvements (Benet & Slavin, n.d.). Deming built on Shewhart's Cycle of PDSA and statistical methods of quality control to build his own theory of management. He believed that improving quality would reduce expenses and increase productivity (Deming, 1986.).

It was not until the 1980s, however, that Deming's theories on management, including his "System of Profound Knowledge" (Deming, 1993) and the "14 Points for Management" (Deming, 1986) became integrated into the U.S. landscape. He believed that it is usually the processes rather than the people that are the cause of quality problems. In his 1986 book, *Out of the Crisis*, Deming emphasized:
- Having a "constancy of purpose" toward improvement.
- Making quality improvement a company-wide process.
- Looking beyond inspection to provide quality.
- Not awarding business on price alone.
- Improving constantly.
- Focusing on training and retraining employees.

Figure 22-1
Deming PDCA or the Shewhart PDSA Cycle

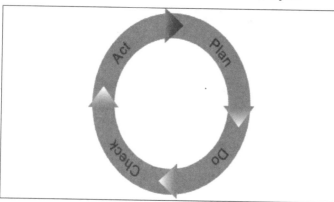

Source: Mind Tools, 2009.

Figure 22-2
Juran Management System

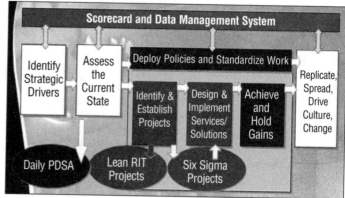

Source: Juran, n.d.

Figure 22-3
Example of a Fishbone Diagram

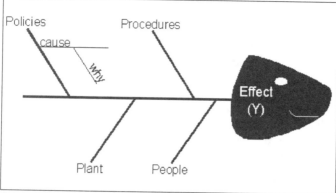

Source: Simon, K., n.d.

Figure 22-4
Variability of Hemoglobins

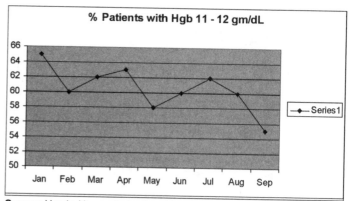

Source: Used with permission from Veronica Legg.

- Instituting and improving leadership.
- Instituting an environment where change and improvement are welcome.
- Breaking down barriers so that teamwork is developed.

Deming (1986) believed that slogans and exhortations, work quotas, and "management by objectives" are centered on individual workers rather than the system processes where quality improvement needs to focus. Instead, Deming looked at quality as everyone's job, so everyone must act to achieve that goal (see Figure 22-1) (Deming, 1986).

Donabedian (1990) pioneered quality in medical care. His *Seven Pillars of Quality* in health care state that quality is defined by 1) *efficacy* or the ability of care to improve health; 2) *effectiveness,* the degree to which these improvements are achieved; 3) *efficiency* or the best health care at the lowest cost; 4) *optimality* or the optimal balance of cost and benefit; 5) *acceptability* or achieving accessibility of health care in the patients' perceptions; 6) *legitimacy* or achieving all of the above in accordance with social norms; and 7) *equity* or fairness in the availability and benefits of health care.

Dr. Joseph M. Juran, whose work was based in Japan in the 1950s, developed the Juran Management System. The heart of his system is the "Juran trilogy of Planning, Controlling, and Improving the quality of products and services" (see Figure 22-2) (Juran, n.d.).

What Is CQI?

It has already been established that continuous quality improvement is a continuing process of looking at where we are and where we want to be. The gap between the two is the opportunity to improve. *CQI* is a team approach to solving problems, and a multitude of tools can help accomplish these goals.

With this as a background, an example of a potential CQI project could be as follows. Your dialysis unit's goal is that 70% of your patients have a hemoglobin of 11 to 12 gm/dL. Unfortunately, this month's report shows that only 55% of your patients are within that parameter. Is this an opportunity for CQI?

The unit manager appoints a team to assess anemia man-

Table 22-1
"Positive" Factors that Help Achieve the Goal and "Negative" Factors that Hinder the Goal from Being Met

Positive Forces	Negative Forces
Anemia nurse assigned to monitor labs	Labs only drawn on every 2-week cycle
MD/RN rounding	Hospitalizations
Interdisciplinary team participation at monthly Quality Assessment Performance Improvement meeting	Missed dialysis sessions/missed erythropoietic stimulating agent (ESA) doses

Source: Used with permission from Veronica Legg.

agement in the unit. First, you review the data. You use a control chart and plot the variability of the unit hemoglobins over time (see Figure 22-4). In doing so, you notice that in January, you had 65% of your patients meeting the goal. After January, your patients' hemoglobins moved up and down over the ensuing months, slowly losing ground. This variation and downward trend show that there is definitely an opportunity for improvement in this patient outcome.

By using a continuous quality improvement tool (in this case, the run chart) to look at data, it is evident that there is a great deal of variability. The question is how to decrease the variability and meet your goal (70% of our patients will have a hemoglobin of 11 to 12 gm/dL within 3 months). How do you get there?

Tools in CQI

Brainstorming

This is a creative, collaborative tool that generates a large number of ideas (Mind Tools, n.d.). In brainstorming, each person in the group is invited to present an idea that is written down in that person's own words. At the end of the session, duplicates are discarded.

Brainstorming Tool: Force Field Analysis

Kurt Lewin (iSixSigma, n.d.) developed this tool as a means of looking at the balance between the "positive" factors that help achieve the goal and the "negative" factors that hinder the goal from being met. Although Lewin rated the forces by power, simply conceptualizing these forces as either helping or hindering is a simple method of guiding brainstorming. One can then target efforts to strengthen positives and influence the negatives to achieve a goal.

A force field analysis can be used to brainstorm what needs to happen to achieve the goal for the unit. Achieving a hemoglobin of 11 to 12 gm/dL for 70% of patients within 3 months might generate identification of several forces (see Table 22-1).

The team picked two negative forces to address and developed an action plan: Improve hemoglobin after hospitalizations without waiting for the regularly scheduled laboratory draw to assess the hemoglobin status of new patients.

Brainstorming Tool: Ishikawa Fishbone Cause And Effect Diagram

This technique was pioneered by Kaoru Ishikawa to improve quality management in the Japanese shipyards (see Figure 22-3). (SkyMark Corporation, n.d). This method of discovering the root cause of a problem starts with a question: "Why do only 55% of our patient's have a hemoglobin of 11 to 12 gm/dL?"

In this diagram, the (Y) is the effect you currently have (only 55% of your patients meet the anemia management goal) (see Figure 22-4). The team would then modify the categories (as shown in Figure 22-3). They might brainstorm that the main causes or contributors to the current reality of low hemoglobins are policies, people, and miscellaneous factors. The *policies* list would include labs every 2 weeks and resume previous erythropoietic stimulating agent (ESA) orders with dose specified. *People* includes patients new to therapy, patients post-hospitalization, anemia managers, and physicians. *Miscellaneous* might include missed treatments and inflammation. Other categories are added as brainstorming continues. After brainstorming all root causes of why hemoglobins are below goal, the team would pick one or two causes to address with an action plan. After completion of the first action plan, the team would assess the outcomes of those interventions. If outcomes met the target, those changes would be implemented on a unit-wide basis to sustain the improved outcomes. If the target was not met, the team would reconvene and select other root causes to explore as part of the ongoing improvement process.

Other Brainstorming Tools

Other tools include Pareto Chart, histogram, scatter diagram, run chart, and flow chart (iSixSigma, n.d.). These tools lead the team to the Action Plan, the document that identifies what is going to be done, who is responsible, and when each step will be completed.

What Is Research?

In 1974, the United States Department of Health and Human Services (DHHS) developed regulations to ensure the protection of human subjects from research risks. These regulations, revised over the years, are referred to as "Title 45 Code of Federal Regulations Part 46, 1991 revision," or "45 CFR 46" (DHHS, 2005).

In its Code of Federal Regulations, DHHS defines research as "a systematic investigation, including research development, testing, and evaluation, designed to develop or contribute to generalizable knowledge" (DHHS, 2005). In the Belmont Report, "...the term 'research' designates an activity designed to test a hypothesis, permit conclusions to be drawn, and thereby to develop or to contribute to generalizable knowledge.... Research is usually described in a formal protocol that sets forth an objective and a set of procedures to reach that objective" (U.S. National Commission for the Protection of Human Subjects of Biomedical and Behavioral Research, 1979, p. 23193).

Research starts with a problem, a question, or development of a hypothesis. A research problem addresses a situation or condition of interest to the researcher (Polit & Hungler, 1999). Using the earlier anemia concern, the problem might be stated as, "Inadequate anemia control in patients on hemodialysis." The research question is more specific. It narrows the focus and addresses the particular query that the researcher wants to answer. Such a question might be, "Does doubling the dose of ESA at the first dialysis session following hospitalization improve anemia control in patients on hemodialysis?" If the researcher then goes on to make a prediction of the outcome, a research hypothesis is proposed and tested (Polit & Hungler, 1999}.

Research Hypothesis Example

Doubling the dose of ESA at the first dialysis session following hospitalization increases anemia control versus the standard ESA dosing in patients on hemodialysis. In this case, the standard of care might be an order to resume the previous ESA dose.

Protocol

In answering the research question or testing the hypothesis, the researcher outlines the objectives of the research, the procedures used to gather the information or test the hypothesis, and the research analysis to be done. A protocol encapsulates the research problem, the objectives, the processes, the data collection methodology, and data analysis. The United States National Library of Medicine (2008), a part of the National Institutes of Health, defines a protocol as "an action plan that describes what will be done in a study, how it will be conducted, and why each part of the plan is necessary – including details such as the criteria for patient participation, the schedule of tests, procedures, and medications, and the length of the study."

Retrospective versus Prospective

Research can be retrospective (looking back at previous events and collecting information from which to draw conclusions) or prospective (studying events as they occur). It can be observational or interventional. It includes all activities that involve a deliberate, systematic investigation designed to develop or contribute to generalizable knowledge whether or not the program is considered "research" for other purposes (DHHS, 2008).

These same regulations define a *human subject* as "a living individual about whom an investigator (whether professional or student) conducting research obtains data through intervention or interaction with the individual or obtains identifiable private information" (DHHS, 2008, p. 303).

Although there are exemptions, most research involving human subjects must be reviewed and approved by an Institutional Review Board. The duty of the Institutional Review Board is to determine that the proposed research is ethical, protects human subjects, and meets all federal, state, local, and if applicable, institutional regulations (DHHS, 2005).

CQI versus Research: When Is CQI Considered Research?

Both continuous quality improvement and research are systematic, scientific processes; both involve the collection and analysis of data; both generate knowledge (McCoy & Byers, 2006). So when does a non-research activity, such as CQI, become research, and thus, subject to the rules and regulations of 45 CFR 46? In trying to answer that question, the Centers for Disease Control and Prevention (1999) states that the primary intent of the activity is the key indicator of whether that activity is research or non-research. Therefore, the key word in the definition of research is "intent."

Research is designed to produce generalizable knowledge, and the design is selected to remove as much bias as possible so that conclusions will apply to any other similar population (Evanoff, 2005). Thus, in the anemia study, one would want to randomize (like the flip of a coin) patients into one of two groups: standard of care or double-dose of ESA on return. This randomization takes the bias out of selecting the patients into the groups so that each group is as equivalent as possible. The "gold standard" of a generalizable study is a randomized, placebo-controlled (one group receives an inactive substance), double blind study (neither the patient nor the study personnel know whether the patient is receiving a placebo or the active drug/procedure) (Kaptchuk, 2001). While not all studies can be done in this manner, the less bias there is in a study leads to more generalizable conclusions.

With this in mind, if the intent or primary purpose is to gather knowledge designed to draw conclusions, inform policy, or generalize findings (which can be applied to other populations outside of the population being studied), it is considered research (Nerenz, Stoltz, & Jordan, 2003). If the research involves human subjects and does not qualify for an exemption, then it requires Institutional Review Board approval and may require informed consent of from those participants whose personal information or participation may be needed (Office for Protection from Research Risks, 1983).

Sometimes the CQI team may find the "intent" changes as the process unfolds. Over the course of the project, one gains knowledge that is generalizable, and publishing and disseminating those findings becomes a possibility. In your anemia CQI project, you may have examined the policies and procedures used to regulate ESA dosing. As part of the process, you designed an action plan to perform early laboratory draws for new and returning patients to determine hemoglobin status prior to the regular clinic labs. Your intent is to improve your clinic outcomes, and it is a non-research activity. Let us say, however, that you then revisit your anemia CQI and add a new action item: compare the results of providing a double dose of ESA for patients returning from a missed dialysis treatment or hospitalization versus the common practice of resuming the previous ESA dose. If your intent is to see if one group of patient outcomes is better than the other, this may result in a new policy. This may have evolved into a research project that requires Institutional Review Board review, approval, and patient consent to participate.

Because the line between research and non-research can be so difficult to ascertain, the Office for Human Research

Figure 22-5
Is an Activity Research Involving Human Subjects Covered by 45 CFR part 46?

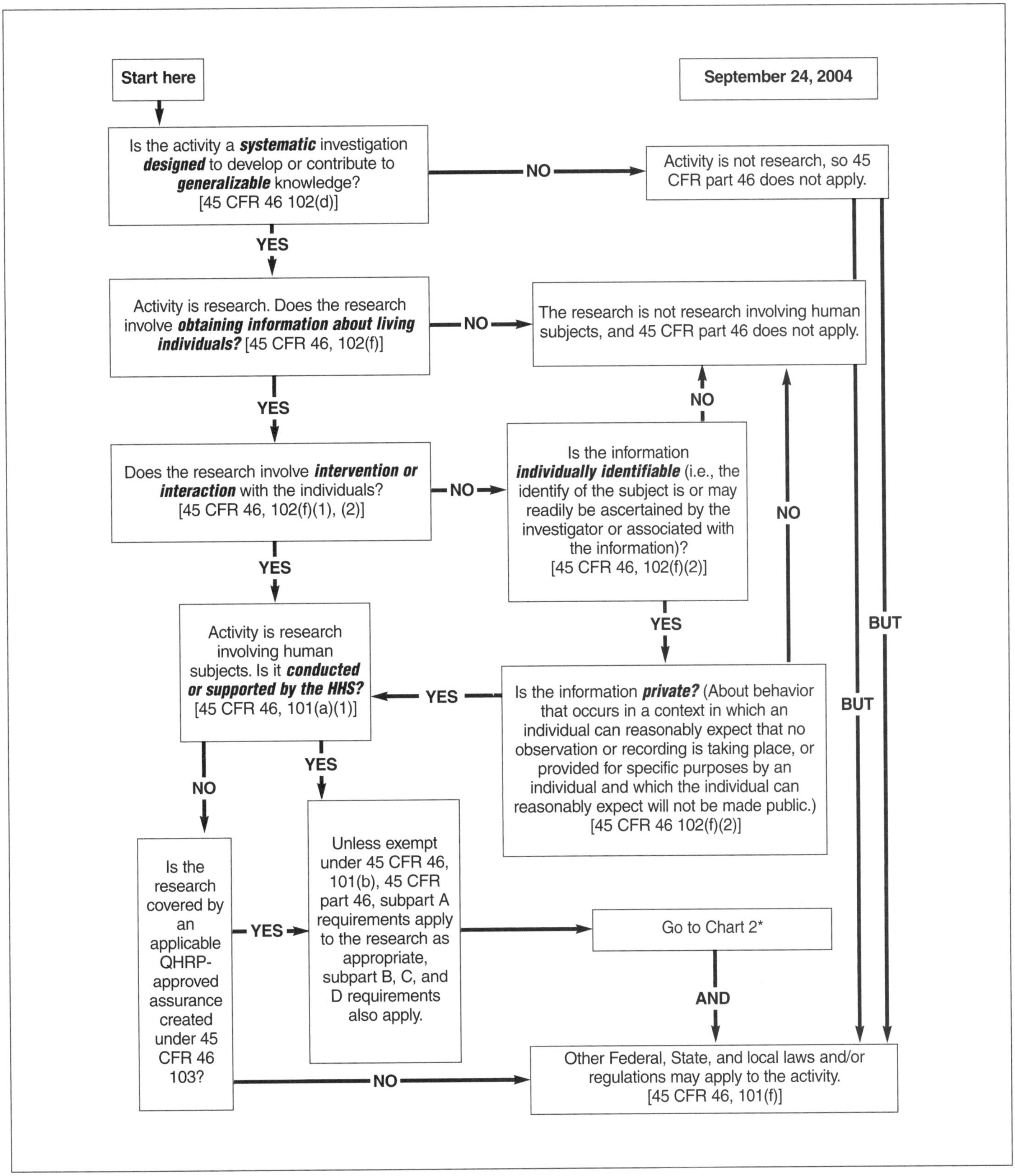

Start here

September 24, 2004

Is the activity a *systematic* investigation *designed* to develop or contribute to *generalizable* knowledge? [45 CFR 46 102(d)]

— NO → Activity is not research, so 45 CFR part 46 does not apply.

YES

Activity is research. Does the research involve *obtaining information about living individuals?* [45 CFR 46, 102(f)]

— NO → The research is not research involving human subjects, and 45 CFR part 46 does not apply.

YES

Does the research involve *intervention or interaction* with the individuals? [45 CFR 46, 102(f)(1), (2)]

— NO → Is the information *individually identifiable* (i.e., the identify of the subject is or may readily be ascertained by the investigator or associated with the information)? [45 CFR 46, 102(f)(2)]

NO

YES

Activity is research involving human subjects. Is it *conducted or supported by the HHS?* [45 CFR 46, 101(a)(1)]

← YES — Is the information *private?* (About behavior that occurs in a context in which an individual can reasonably expect that no observation or recording is taking place, or provided for specific purposes by an individual and which the individual can reasonably expect will not be made public.) [45 CFR 46 102(f)(2)]

NO

YES

BUT

BUT

NO

Is the research covered by an applicable QHRP-approved assurance created under 45 CFR 46 103?

— YES → Unless exempt under 45 CFR 46, 101(b), 45 CFR part 46, subpart A requirements apply to the research as appropriate, subpart B, C, and D requirements also apply.

→ Go to Chart 2*

AND

NO — Other Federal, State, and local laws and/or regulations may apply to the activity. [45 CFR 46, 101(f)]

Source: Office for Human Research Protections (2004).
*Chart 2 is entitled "Is the Research for Human Subjects Eligible for Exemption Under 45 CFR 46.101?" and is available on the same site.

Protections (2004) provides several decision charts. The charts address the following questions:

- Whether the activity is research and must be reviewed by an Institutional Review Board.
- Whether the review may be performed by expedited procedures.
- Whether informed consent or its documentation may be waived.

Figure 22-5 presents a chart documenting the decision-making sequence for determining the answers to the first question above.

Conclusion

Continuous quality improvement and research are important scientific processes integral to nephrology nursing and to the healthcare system. This chapter has identified some of the tools for both. Because the delineation between CQI and research is not always clear, nurses should consult their institution's review board or an independent Institutional Review Board when further clarification or guidance is needed.

References

Agency for Healthcare Research and Quality. (n.d.). *Your guide to choosing quality healthcare: A quick look at quality.* Retrieved January 27, 2009, from http://www.ahrq.gov/consumer/guidetoq/guidetoq4.htm

Bennet, L. & Slavin L. (n.d.). *Continuous quality improvement: What every health care manager needs to know.* Retrieved January 27, 2009, from http://www.cwru.edu/med/epidbio/mphp439/CQI.htm?nw_view=1233077461&

Centers for Disease Control and Prevention. (1999). *Guidelines for defining public health research and public health non-research.* Retrieved January 27, 2009, from http://www.cdc.gov/od/science/regs/hrpp/researchdefinition.htm

Deming, W. E. (1986). *Out of the crisis.* Cambridge, MA: Massachusetts Institute of Technology, Center for Advanced Engineering Study.

Deming. W.E. (1993) *The new economics for industry, government education.* Cambridge, MA: Massachusetts Institute of Technology Center for Advanced Engineering Study.

Donebedian, A. (1966). Evaluating the quality of medical care. *Milbank Memorial Fund Quarterly, 44*(3), 166-203.

Donebedian, A. (1990). The seven pillars of quality. *Archives Pathology Lab Medicine, 114*(11), 1115-1118.

Evanoff, B. (2005). Reducing bias. In D.P. Schuster & W.J. Powers (Eds.), *Translational and experimental clinical research* (pp. 67-72). Philadelphia: Lippincott, Williams & Wilkins.

iSixSigma. (n.d.). Retrieved October 10, 2008, from http://www.isixsigma.com

Juran. (n.d.). *Juran management system.* Retrieved January 27, 2009, from http://www.juran.com/HomeLeftNav/juran_mgt_system.aspx

Kaptchuk, T.J. (2001). The double-blind, randomized, placebo controlled trail: Gold standard or golden calf. *Journal of Clinical Epidemiology, 54*(6), 541-549.

Langley, G.J., Nolan, K.M., Nolan, T.W., Norman, C.L., & Provost, L.P. (1996). *The improvement guide.* San Francisco: Jossey-Bass.

Luce, J.M., Bindman, A.B., & Lee, P.R. (1994). A brief history of health care quality assessment and improvement in the United States. *Western Journal of Medicine, 160,* 263-268.

McCoy, J.M. & Byers, J.F. (2006). JHQ 1878: Using evidence-based performance improvement in the community, *Journal for Healthcare Quality, 286,* 13-17.

Mind Tools. (n.d.). *Brainstorming.* Retrieved January 27, 2009, from http://www.mindtools.com/brainstm.html

Mind Tools. (2009). *Plan-do-check-act (PDCA): Implementing new ideas in a controlled way. Also known as the PDCA Cycle, or Deming Cycle.* Retrieved January 4, 2009, from http://www.mindtools.com/amember/cecopen/TourSB3.htm

Nerenz, D.R., Stoltz, P.K., & Jordan, J. (2003). Quality improvement and the need for IRB review. *Quality Management in Health Care, 12*(3), 159-179.

Office for Human Research Protections. (2004). *Human subject regulations decision charts.* Retrieved January 27, 2009, from http://www.hhs.gov/ohrp/humansubjects/guidance/decision-charts.htm#c3

Office for Protection From Research Risks. (1983). *Protection of human subjects. Code of federal regulations 45 CFR 46.* Retrieved January 27, 2009, from http://www.hhs.gov/ohrp/humansubjects/guidance/45cfr46.htm#46.101

Polit, D.F., & Hungler, B.P. (1999). *Nursing research: Principles and methods.* Philadelphia: Lippincott.

Quality Assurance Project. (n.d.). *U.S. agency for international development: Methods and tools: QA in healthcare.* Retrieved September 11, 2008, from http://www.qaproject.org/methods/resqa.html

Simon, K. (n.d.). *The cause and effect diagram (a.k.a. fishbone).* Retrieved January 27, 2009, from http://www.isixsigma.com/library/content/t000821.asp

SkyMark Corporation. (n.d.). *Kaoru Ishikawa: One step further.* Retrieved January 27, 2009, from http://www.skymark.com/resources/leaders/ishikawa.asp

U.S. National Commission for the Protection of Human Subjects of Biomedical and Behavioral Research. (1979). The Belmont report: Ethical principles and guidelines for the protection of human subjects and research. *Federal Register 44,* 23192-23197.

U.S. Department of Health and Human Services (DHHS). (2005). *Code of federal regulations: Title 45: Public welfare. Part 46: Protection of human subjects.* Retrieved January 27, 2009, from http://www.hhs.gov/ohrp/humansubjects/guidance/45cfr46.htm#46.102

U.S. Department of Health and Human Services (DHHS). (2008). *Code of federal regulations: Title 34: Education. Part 97: Protection of human subjects.* Retrieved December 29, 2008, from http://frwebgate.access.gpo.gov/cgi-bin/get-cfr.cgi?TITLE=34&PART=97&SECTION=102&YEAR=2000&TYPE=PDF

U.S. National Library of Medicine. (2008). *FAQ: Clinicaltrials.gov – What is a protocol?* Retrieved March 24, 2009, from http://www.nlm.nih.gov/services/ctprotocol.html

Additional Readings

Donabedian, A. (1999). Evaluating the quality of medical care. *Milbank Memorial Fund Quarterly, 44,* 166-206.

North Carolina Department of Enviornment and Natural Resources. (2002). *Fishbone diagram; A problem-analysis tool.* Retrieved January 27, 2009, from http://www.isixsigma.com/offsite.asp?A=Fr&Url=http://quality.enr.state.nc.us/tools/fishbone.htm

U.S. Department of Education. (2005). *Code of federal regulations: Title 34. Part 97: Protection of human subjects, 102.* Retrieved January 27, 2009, from http://www.ed.gov/policy/fund/reg/humansub/part97-2.html#97.102

USAID Health. (2007). *Guide for interpreting the federal policy for the protection of human subjects.* Retrieved January 27, 2009, from http://www.usaid.gov/our_work/ global_health/home/TechAreas/commrule.html

U.S. Government Printing Office. (n.d.). *GPO access: Electronic code of federal regulations: eCRF, Title 21: Food and drugs. Part 56: Institutional review boards.* Retrieved January 27, 2009, from http://ecfr.gpoaccess.gov/ cgi/t/text/textidx?c=ecfr&rgn=div6&view= text&node=21:1.0.1.1.21.1&idno= 21

Value-Based Management. (2008). *Force field analysis – Lewin, Kurt.* Retrieved January 27, 2009, from http://www.valuebasedmanagement.net/methods_lewin_force_field_analysis.html

| Chapter 22 | CONTINUING NURSING EDUCATION EVALUATION FORM | 1.2 Contact Hours |

Continuous Quality Improvement and Research in Nursing

ANNP0922

Applying Continuous Quality Improvement in Clinical Practice contains 22 chapters of educational content. Individual learners may apply for continuing nursing education credit by reading a chapter and completing the Continuing Nursing Education Evaluation Form for that chapter. Learners may apply for continuing nursing education credit for any or all chapters.

Please photocopy this test page, complete, and return to ANNA.
You can also download this form from www.annanurse.org (choose Education - CNE Activities - Publications)
Receive continuing nursing education credit (CNE) immediately by completing the CNE evaluation process in ANNA's Online Library. Go to www.annanurse.org, and click on the Online Library icon for more information.
Name: _____
Address: _____
City: _____ State: _____ Zip: _____
E-mail:_____ Preferred telephone: ☐ Home ☐ Work _____
State where licensed and license number: _____

CNE application fees are based upon the number of contact hours provided by the individual section. CNE fees per contact hour for ANNA members are as follows: 1.0-1.9 – $15; 2.0-2.9 – $20; 3.0-3.9 – $25; 4.0 and higher – $30. Fees for nonmembers are $10 higher.
CNE application fee for Chapter 22: ANNA member $15   Nonmember $25
ANNA Member: ☐ Yes ☐ No   ☐ Member # (if available) _____
☐ Check or money order enclosed   ☐ American Express   ☐ Visa   ☐ MasterCard
Total amount submitted:_____
Credit card number _____ Exp. Date _____
Name as it appears on the card: _____
NOTE: Your evaluation form can be processed in 1 week for an additional rush charge of $5.00.
☐   **Yes, I would like this evaluation form rush processed. I have included an additional fee of $5.00 for rush processing.**

Instructions

1. To receive continuing nursing education credit for an individual study after reading the chapter, complete this evaluation form.

2. Detach, photocopy, or download (www.annanurse.org) the evaluation form and send along with a check or money order payable to **American Nephrology Nurses' Assocation** to: ANNA, East Holly Avenue Box 56, Pitman, NJ 08071-0056.

3. Test returns must be postmarked by **April 30, 2011**. Upon completion of the answer/evaluation form, a certificate will be sent to you.

   This section was reviewed and formatted for contact hour credit by Sally S. Russell, MN, CMSRN, ANNA Director of Education Services.

CNE Application Fee for Chapter 22
ANNA member = $15
Nonmember = $25

1. I verify that I have read this chapter and completed this education activity. _____ Date _____
                                                                        Signature

2. What would be different in your practice if you applied what you have learned from this activity? (Please use additional paper if necessary.)
_____
_____
_____
_____

	Strongly disagree				Strongly agree
3. The activity met the stated objectives.					
a. Define continuous quality improvement.	1	2	3	4	5
b. Understand basic tools of continuous quality improvement.	1	2	3	4	5
c. Explain the difference between continuous quality improvement and research.	1	2	3	4	5
4. The content was current and relevant.	1	2	3	4	5
5. The content was presented clearly.	1	2	3	4	5
6. The content was covered adequately.	1	2	3	4	5

7. How would you rate your ability to apply your learning to practice?   ☐ diminished ability   ☐ no change   ☐ enhanced ability

Comments _____
_____

8. Time required to read the chapter and complete this form: _____ minutes